RESEARCH IN ORGANIC FARMING

Edited by **Raumjit Nokkoul**

Research in Organic Farming
Edited by Raumjit Nokkoul

Published by InTech
Janeza Trdine 9, 51000 Rijeka, Croatia

Publishing Process Manager Ivona Lovric

Technical Editor Teodora Smiljanic

Cover Designer InTech Design Team

Image Copyright Christopher Meder - Photography, 2011. Used under license from Shutterstock.com

Additional hard copies can be obtained from orders@intechopen.com

Research in Organic Farming, Edited by Raumjit Nokkoul
p. cm.
ISBN 978-953-307-381-1

For EU product safety concerns:
IN TECH d.o.o., Prolaz Marije Krucifikse Kozulić 3, 51000 Rijeka, Croatia,
info@intechopen.com or visit our website at intechopen.com.

Meet the editor

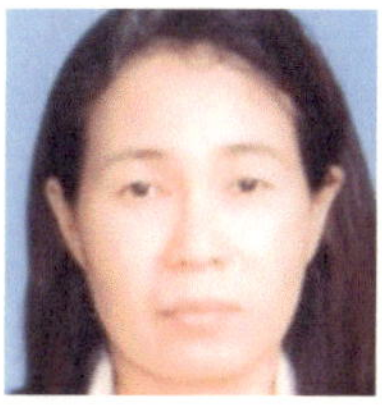

Dr. Raumjit Nokkoul, born in Chumphon, Thailand, 1967, is a lecturer at the Department of Agricultural Technology, King Mongkut's Institute of Technology Ladkrabang, Chumphon Campus, Chumphon Province, Thailand. She received her PhD in Seed Technology from the Prince of Songkla University, Thailand, and has received honors and an award for upland rice research in 2009. Dr. Nokkoul has been involved in collaboration research with many researchers since 1995, and has published on plant breeding and organic see committee of the Upper South Higher Education Network, Sub-network C—Research and Innovations Network for Dissemination of Technology to the Grassroots, CHE, Upper South.

Contents

Preface

Organic farming is based on minimizing the use of external inputs, avoiding the use of synthetic fertilizers. Pesticides system has the potential to provide benefits in terms of environmental protection, and certain methods are used to minimize pollution of air, soil and water. Organic food handlers, processors and retailers adhere to the standards set to maintain the integrity of organic agriculture products. The primary goal of organic agriculture is to optimize the health and productivity of interdependent communities of soil life, plants, animals and people.

The management system of an organic farm is crucial, as its location and product-specific issues need to be addressed to ensure sustainability. Successful cultivation depends on environmentally friendly practices in nitrogen fixation, pest control, positive hosting, sheltering etc. Various incentives can bolster transfer to organic agriculture, either consumer-driven by demand, service-driven by ecological necessity or farmer-driven by economical viability and government support. Despite its advantages, the cost and quality of produce from organic agriculture are continually under discussion. Since organic agriculture can potentially increase yield only in traditional systems and actually decrease it when compared to highly industrialized farming, it is continuously debated if the conversion of existing world farm areas would suffice for the rapidly increasing human population.

The book contains 10 chapters written by acknowledged experts, providing comprehensive information on all aspects of Organic Agriculture and Organic Food, from cultivation practices and environmental aspects, to produce certification and distribution with a clear perspective, with a balance in presentations of basic and applied research. Researchers, students, and teachers in the agricultural field in particular will find this book to be of immense use.

This book has emerged as a consequence of the difficulties we experienced in finding information when we first started researching. The goal was to produce a book where as many existing studies as possible could be presented in a single volume, making it easy for the reader to compare methods, results and conclusions. As a result, studies from countries such as Thailand, Spain, Sweden, Lithuania, Czech, Mexico, etc. have been brought together as individual chapters and references to studies from other countries have been included in the overview chapters where possible. We believe that this opportunity to compare results from different countries will open a new perspective on the subject, allowing the typical characteristics of Organic Agriculture and Organic Food to be seen more clearly. Finally, we would like to thank the contributing authors and the staff at InTech for their efforts and cooperation during the course of publication. I sincerely hope that this book will help researchers and students all over the world to reach new results in the field of Organic Agriculture and Organic Food.

Raumjit Nokkoul, PhD.
Department of Agricultural Technology
King Mongkut's Institute of Technology Ladkrabang,
Chumphon Campus, Chumphon Province,
Thailand

1

Organic Farming and Landscape: Experiences and Perceptions in Alt Empordà (Catalonia, NE Spain)

Xosé A. Armesto - López
Department of Physical Geography and Regional Analysis, University of Barcelona Spain

1. Introduction

The five sections comprising this chapter explore the word "landscape" and its meaning in the rural European Mediterranean world from the perspective of organic farmers. One of the aims of this chapter is to make the reader aware of the true nature of these landscapes, and of the need to educate inhabitants and visitors about their conservation. To this end, a case study is presented which focuses on the district of *Alt Empordà* (Catalonia, NE Spain). In the first, introductory section, some theoretical considerations concerning the concept of landscape will be discussed, and questions related to the terminology, typology and even contradictions which are encompassed in this word will be explored. The second section will consist of a brief description of the principal geographical features of the area studied, whilst the third presents the most relevant figures concerning organic farming production in Spain and Catalonia. The fourth section can be considered as representing the main body of the chapter, since it concerns the subject which has been the focus of this research: how organic farmers in the Alt Empordà district perceive the landscape. Rather than taking a rigid stance on the concept of landscape, which is after all a concept which everybody uses and is thus subject to multiple meanings and interpretations (Küster, 2004), the aim of this section is to try to describe the different perceptions that organic farmers have of this concept, and how they relate these perceptions to their activities and surroundings. Lastly, the main conclusions that were drawn from this study are summarised.
Accordingly, perhaps the best place to start this chapter is with some brief reflections on the word "landscape", and the associations and interpretations it elicits.

1.1 The concept of "landscape"

Landscape can be interpreted as a central concept within the context of the relationship which is established between humans and their surrounding environment. It is a concept which has been theorised, described and studied by numerous scientific disciplines, including Geology, Architecture, Art and Ecology. In the discipline of Geography to which the present author belongs, many authors since the 19th century have taken landscape as their central theme, exploring it from different perspectives (Schlütter, Passarge, Troll, etc.). Landscape responds to a perception, and can be defined as the appearance or aspect of a space within a specific area, thus enabling it to be distinguished from other, analogous units.

Its uniqueness renders it an unrepeatable entity. The Earth's surface, therefore, can be defined as a mosaic of unique landscapes (Ortega Valcárcel, 2000).

Landscapes are composed of both stable and dynamic elements which are determined by nature and cultural practices. Thus, landscapes where natural processes predominate and which are subject to continual change as a result of the processes of succession and evolution are habitually considered natural (Küster, H., 2004), whilst landscapes which have been shaped to a greater or lesser extent by humans are considered cultural landscapes. Agricultural landscapes are the product of human culture (Merriam, 1988) and thus form part of our common heritage (Pretty, 2001).

However, as Küster (2004) has indicated, it is becoming increasing difficult to distinguish between these two categories, and he has thus proposed the use of the word "landscape" without further distinctions.

The study of landscape is therefore an empirical exploration of a set of interconnected elements. Attempts to define the subject of study vary considerably, depending on the scientific discipline with which the researcher in question identifies. For instance, agronomists and ethnologists employ different research methodologies to study landscape, and probably, their very concept of landscape itself is different. Despite this apparent difficulty, the only perspective considered adequate at the E-conference on *Biodiversity in the Mediterranean Region* for addressing the conservation of present day biodiversity was that of the study of landscape (Hernández *et al*, 2004).

From a methodological point of view, the approach taken in the present study was not to employ exclusive criteria which could only be ascribed to one of these sciences, but rather to combine approaches from various disciplines:

a. Farms comprised the unit of analysis, as they would for an agricultural engineer.
b. The instrument used for collecting perceptions of the landscape comprised a semi-structured interview, a method halfway between the approach a sociologist and an anthropologist might take.
c. The ultimate aim was to understand not only how an area was structured but also how it was interpreted by the principal agents involved, thus pursuing a geographical objective.

The subject was addressed from a perspective which is related to agro-ecology, bearing in mind that, according to Guzmán, González & Sevilla (2000), this latter should observe the following alternative premises: a) a holistic analysis, b) a systemic focus, c) contextualisation of the subject, d) a subjective filter, and e) a pluralist conception.

According to Daniel and Vining (ob. Cit. García Asensio & Cañas Guerrero, 2002), when we employ the word "landscape", we are focusing on visual properties; however, in this study, the perceptions of landscape reported by organic farmers sometimes went beyond the merely physical.

Controversies apart, the following definition, accepted by most of the international community, can be taken as valid: "an area, as perceived by people, whose character is the result of the action and interaction of natural and/or human factors" (European Landscape Convention, 2000).

In fact, the farmers participating in this study were asked questions which transcended the basic unit of analysis, the farm, in order to avoid the bias that extrapolation to the rest of the district would cause, since according to Gliessman *et al.* (2007), agricultural production is a much wider system than the farm alone, in which many more parts are interacting, including factors which are exogenous to the farm itself.

1.2 The importance of agricultural landscapes in the rural world

Despite the fact that agricultural production has been experiencing a slow decline for more than one hundred years, and that there are now other activities which for better or worse affect a landscape, agriculture continues to play the leading role as regards determining the landscape in numerous European regions. This provides a partial context for the present study, since agriculture constitutes a set of actions of a social nature (Baldock, 2004) which have played an important role in shaping the landscape (Von Meyer, H., 1996) ever since the transformation from primitive landscape to cultural landscape began 10,000 years ago (Gastó, Vieli & Vera (2006).

In Western Europe, landscapes have evolved differently according to the region. Such evolution may be towards agricultural intensification, which generally leads to a reduction in uncultivated areas, or towards the abandonment of agricultural land, leading to an increase in uncultivated land: according to Küster (2004), it is the latter development which is mainly responsible for changes to the landscape in rural Europe. These two processes induce ecological change at a landscape level which is frequently viewed as a threat to biodiversity (Burel & Baudry, 2001; Berendse & Kleijn, 2004). Indeed, rural landscapes in Europe currently represent the outcome of a history, on the one hand, of good farming practice, and on the other, of environmental destruction (Baldock, 2004), according to the region and moment in history (Küster, 2004). The case of change in Mediterranean agricultural landscapes is a paradigmatic illustration of this trend, as their outstanding resilience has been achieved through prolonged, sensible and restrained anthropic action (Vélez Restrepo & Gómez Sal, 2008).

The magnitude of agricultural impact on the environment depends to a great extent on the structure of the landscape in which farming is practiced (Fernández Alés & Leiva Morales, 2003).

Changes to agricultural landscapes are due not only to natural factors, but are also intimately related to economic and social change. Changing forms of land ownership, fluctuations in demand for agricultural produce, changes in agricultural policies and technological progress in agriculture and livestock rearing are all decisive factors which influence the evolution of these landscapes. Thus, farmers determine the cultural landscape through their organisation and use of the land (Llausàs *et al.*, 2009), and the landscape consequently develops characteristics peculiar to each place (García Ruíz, 1988).

It should be borne in mind that the landscapes generated by farms fulfil at least four groups of functions (Rossi, Nota & Fossi, 1997): a) ecological functions related to natural features; b) economic functions related to the economy of the producers; c) social functions related to the relationships which are established between the diverse agents; d) aesthetic functions related to visual and contemplative aspects.

Considering all the above, the initial hypothesis was that organic farmers in the district of Alt Empordà would have a positive image of the landscape when considering their own farms, but would regard conventional farms as presenting poorer landscape quality. It will be interesting to see whether, as Levin (2007) claimed, the relationship between organic production and landscape composition is independent of the variables regional location, size or transformation: however, type of production, farm size and physical and geographical conditions generally exert a greater influence on landscape composition.

2. A brief geographical introduction to the study area. The district of Alt Empordà

The district of Alt Empordà is located in *Girona*'s Province, in the far north east of the Autonomous Region of Catalonia, in the north east of Spain. It covers an area of 1,357 km^2, bordering France to the north and two other Catalonian districts, Garrotxa and Pla de l'Estany, to the west. To the east, it forms the northern half of the Costa Brava tourist coastline, washed by the Mediterranean sea, whilst its neighbouring districts to the south are Baix Empordà and Gironès (Fig. 1).

From a physical point of view, three main factors should be highlighted which together help to endow this district with a distinctive personality. The first of these is the mountainous terrain to the north and the west, forming part of the foothills of the Pyrenees mountain range. To the east and south are the alluvial plains, colloquially known as the *Plana del Empordà*. And lastly, there are the areas of contact with the highest mountainous terrain in the north, which has traditionally been called the *aspres*, and the undulating hills, or *Terraprims*, in the south east. In addition, some of the most important rivers in the Catalonian Mediterranean flow through this district, the Muga and the Fluvià, historically of great importance in the plains located on their lower reaches for irrigation purposes.

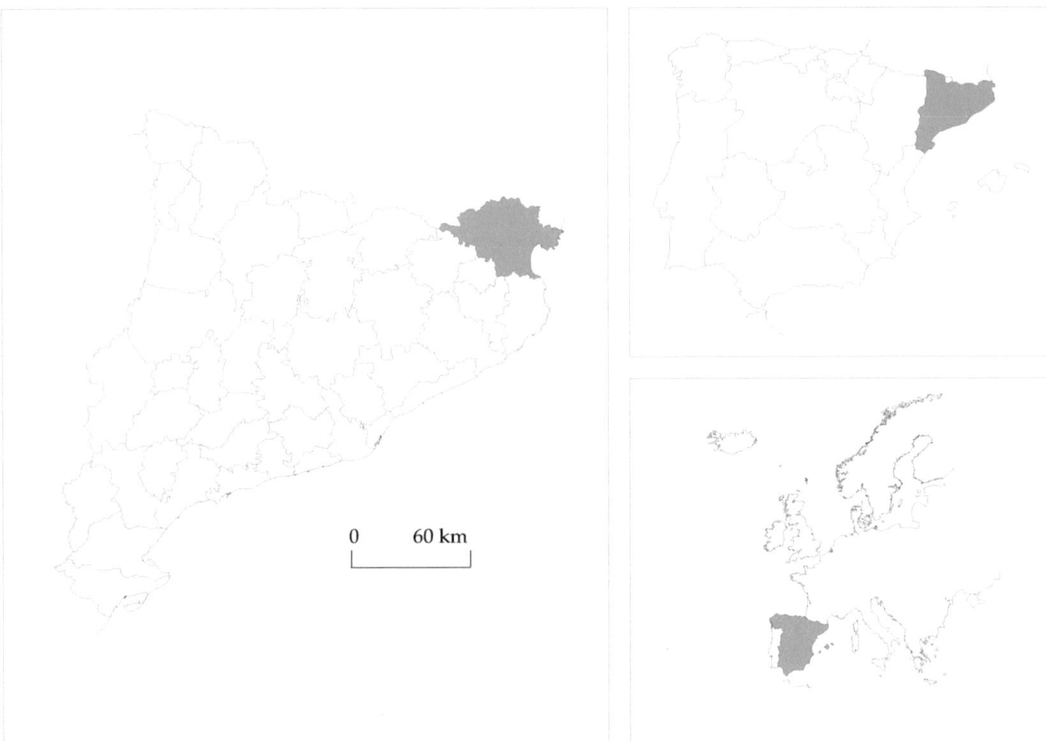

Fig. 1. Location of study area

The climate of this district is profoundly Mediterranean, although it acquires transitional sub-humid overtones in places where the relief is more pronounced. Summers are usually hot and dry, and winters are normally mild, with a mean temperature of slightly over 15 °C in the warmest areas and 12 °C in the colder zones located in the highest areas of the district. Precipitation is irregular throughout the year; however, maximum rainfall usually occurs in spring and summer (ranging from 500 mm annually in the extreme south to around 900 mm in the peaks to the north). From a climatic point of view, one of the most remarkable features of Alt Empordà, and one which exerts a strong influence on the district, is the *Tramuntana*, a strong wind from the north or north west which has traditionally conditioned farming practice. The natural vegetation occurring as a consequence of these climatic gradations presents a predominance of Mediterranean taxa together with a fair number of Euro-Siberian species in transitional climate areas.

The most noteworthy aspects of the human geography of the district can be summarised by a few figures referring to the population and the economy. Thus, in 2010, Alt Empordà had a population of 140,262 inhabitants (103 inhabitants/km^2), 40% more than in 1986, and 53% more than in 1900. The district capital, Figueres, has a population of 44,255 inhabitants (31% of the district total).

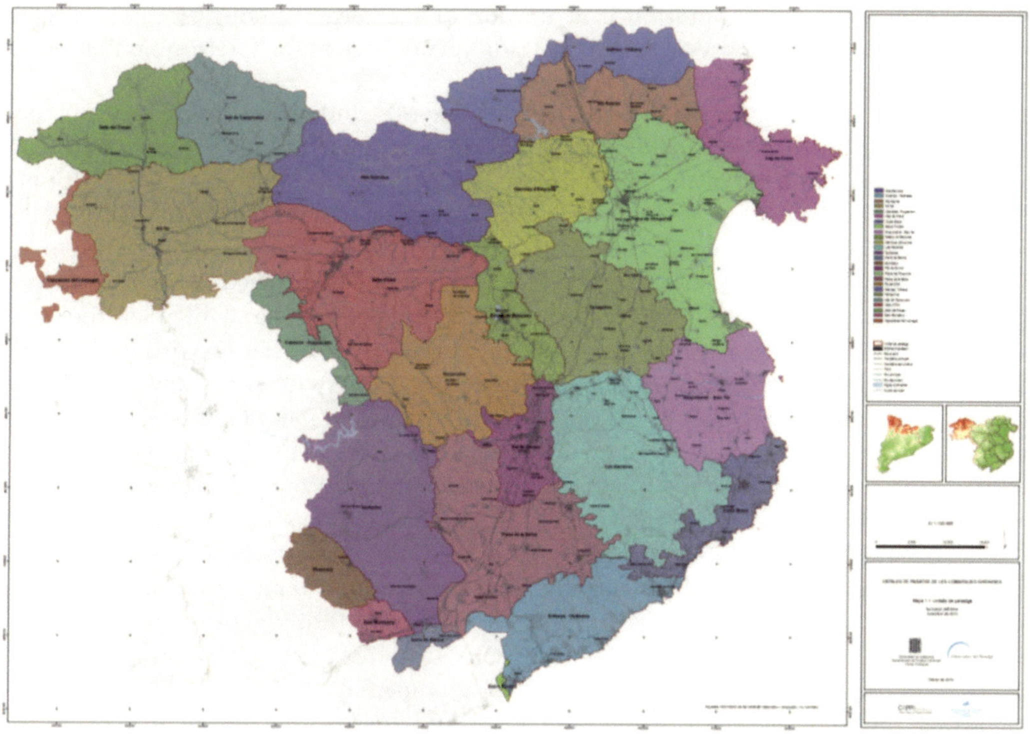

Fig. 2. Landscape units of Girona Province. Source: *Observatori del Paisatge de Catalunya* (2010)

As regards the economy, the service sector is the strongest economic sector, representing 72.5% of Gross Value Added (GVA), followed by the construction sector, representing

15.2%, industry (8.7%) and lastly, agriculture (3.6%). The proportion of the population employed in these sectors is fairly similar to the GVA figures.

Turning to the agricultural sector in the district, the main figures available indicate that there has been a slow decline in recent years in the total surface area given over to farms and farmed land. Similarly, the number of farms has reduced, although the number of livestock has increased in all categories.

A combination of physical and human factors has endowed Alt Empordà with a series of landscapes that the Catalonian Landscape Observatory (*Observatori del Paisatge de Catalunya*, 2010) has inventoried and mapped, concluding that the district presents seven different landscape categories (Fig. 2).

3. General description of organic farming in Spain, Catalonia and Alt Empordà

Organic farming in Spain is no longer a marginal and ideological sector (González de Molina, Alonso & Guzmán, 2007), due to its strong growth, rapid expansion and popularisation over the last fifteen years, aided by extensive regulatory intervention (Armesto, 2007). For the authors cited earlier, this type of production may become an alternative to conventional farming in Europe. In 2009, certified organic land in Spain accounted for 1,602,868 ha, putting it at the top of European rankings for total organic surface area, ahead of countries which have traditionally been at the forefront in this respect (Italy, Germany, France and the United Kingdom).

Spain's organic farming sector took off in the mid-90s and was consolidated in three identifiable stages: from 1997 to 1999, from 2000 to 2006, and from 2007 onwards (Fig. 3). Figures (Spanish Ministry of the Environment and Rural and Marine Affairs, 2010) also show a significant increase in the number of producers, which has now reached 25,291.

Nevertheless, it should be borne in mind that there are very marked regional differences in Spain (Table 1). More than half of the total surface area classified as organic land in Spain is unquestionably located in Andalusia, with 866,799 ha, whilst at the other extreme, there are various regions which are much smaller and where certification has not made such headway (for instance, the Basque Country, Canary Islands, Cantabria, Madrid and La Rioja all have less than 10,000 ha of certified land). Catalonia falls about midway between these two extremes of certified organic surface area, with 71,734 ha in 2009[1]. Most certified land corresponds to the category of pasture, meadows and forage crops (758,794 ha), but also includes a significant amount of woodland, cereal crops and olive groves. Organic livestock farming also presents a huge regional disparity: Andalusia once again holds more than half of the 4,547 organic livestock farms in Spain, whilst at the other extreme are those areas with less tradition of livestock farming (Murcia, the Canary Islands and Madrid all have fewer than 20 farms each). Most organic livestock farms rear cattle. It is the steady payment of agro-environmental subsidies which has been responsible for the growth of organic farming in Andalusia (González de Molina, Alonso & Guzmán, 2007).

---

[1] In contrast to whole Spain, Catalonia has already produced figures for 07/15/2011, showing that total surface area under organic production has now reached 83,506 ha (Catalan Council for Organic Agricultural Production - CCPAE - 2011).

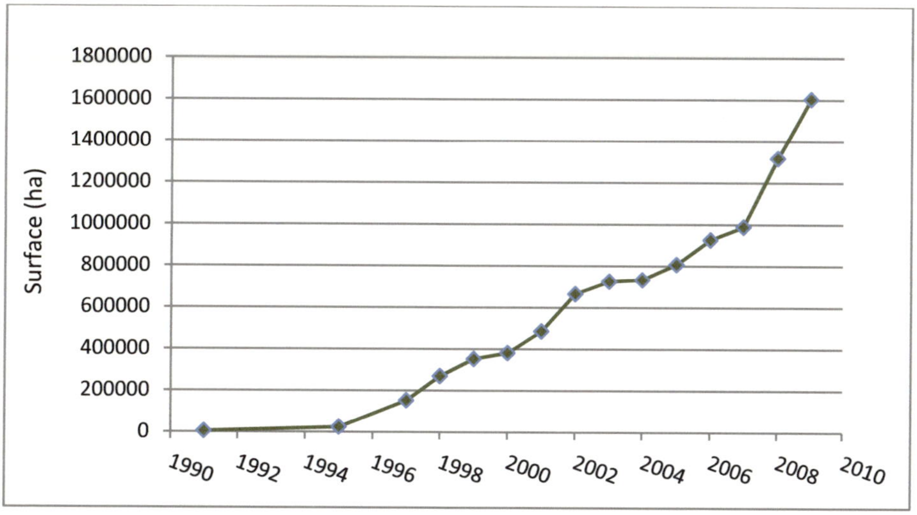

Fig. 3. Organic farming surface evolution in Spain (1991-2009) hectares. Source: MARM (2010).

	Organic Farming Surface	Number of organic farmers
Andalucía	866.799	7.794
Aragón	66.730	706
Asturias	14.019	276
Baleares	29.569	480
Canarias	4.236	665
Cantabria	5.796	128
Castilla-La Mancha	246.076	4.751
Castilla y León	22.154	334
Cataluña	71.734	899
Extremadura	115.017	3.648
Galicia	14.238	449
Madrid	6.043	199
Murcia	60.742	2.222
Navarra	30.843	556
La Rioja	8.634	205
País Vasco	1.484	170
Comunidad Valenciana	38.754	1.283
TOTAL ESPAÑA	1.670.870	24.765

Table 1. Regional surface of organic farming in Spain (2009) hectares

The case of Catalonia is almost unique within Spain, since together with Andalusia, Catalonia was one of the two regions which became a focal point for the alternative farming trends which arrived in Spain from other parts of Europe at the beginning of the 1970s. Consequently, the associated structures, regional implementation and the strength of its food industry have combined to render the region a benchmark in the context of Spain. With

397 organic livestock farms[2], Catalonia is second only in importance to Andalusia and the Balearic Isles.

Lastly, in order to contextualise the study area, Alt Empordà has a total of 3,987 ha of certified land, principally given over to pasture, meadow and forage crops and farmed by a total of 29 producers. Of these, 9 rear livestock, mainly cattle.

4. Perceptions of landscapes: Organic farmers in Alt Empordà

Following pages will show a brief methodological guide and the main discoverers due to field work.

4.1 Notes on methodology

The aim of the present study was to combine a psychological model, referring to the sensations and perception of the people who inhabited, visited or saw the landscape, with a phenomenological model focusing on subjective, individual sensations and how these were interpreted (García Asensio & Cañas Guerrero, 2002). In order to analyse some of the ecosystems, including agro-ecosystems, humans were considered as an integral part of the system under consideration (Vélez Restrepo & Gómez Sal, 2008).

As mentioned earlier, the unit of analysis for this study was the farmer, and consequently the farm, although the objective was to identify characteristic traits of perception in the agricultural district of Alt Empordà. Following Payraudeau & Van der Werf (2005), in this study an approach similar to that known as the Multi-Agent System (MAS) was employed. An in-depth, semi-structured questionnaire was administered to the farmers participating in this study. The questionnaire combined open questions with closed questions, and no time limit for completion was established.

The methodology used to construct the questionnaire was very similar to that employed by Schmitzberger et al. (2005) to analyse how agricultural styles in Austria affected biodiversity conservation in agricultural landscapes. Using the same approach as that taken by Hendriks, Stobbelaar & Van Mansvelt (1997) in their study of an organic farm in the Netherlands, the farmers were interviewed and the farm visited, but the area was examined independently of the farmers.

In addition to providing data on farmers' attitudes towards and concepts of landscape, which was the aim of the study, these interviews with the farmers also yielded information concerning how the farm was managed, together with the history of the farm and the farmer. After characterising the farm using a series of general items, the first question the farmers were asked was the same as that which Vereijken, van Gelder & Baars. (1997) asked in the introduction to their study on nature and landscape on organic farms: "what is a good landscape?". They were then asked a further five questions related to the quality of agricultural landscapes considered both at farm and district level. Next, they were asked nine questions related to diverse aspects of the landscape and its main agents. The interviewees gave a quantitative assessment on a scale of 1-7, using a variation of a psychometric scale for the first five questions, whilst the remaining four were answered on

[2] The 2010 figures for Catalonia indicate a 23.7% increase in farms over the previous year, with the number of organic farms now standing at 491 (CCPAE, 2011)

the basis of qualitative assessments with the concepts "much worse" and "much better" representing either end of the scale, respectively. The questionnaire ended with a final question to be answered on a scale of 1-7 concerning the relationship between the agricultural sector and Europe. This last qualitative item was included as part of a future plan to replicate this study in other areas of Catalonia, and although it had no statistical significance for this study, it may indicate other areas of interest.

Fieldwork was conducted in the spring of 2011. Of the 24 potential subjects identified as producers within the district studied[3], 13 participated, and these comprised the study sample. All the subjects were interviewed in situ on their farms, with the exception of one who attended the interview in a public building in the capital of the municipality where he resided. When selecting the sample, the landscape category to which the farms belonged was taken into consideration in order for all categories to be represented, as far as possible. Nevertheless, to simplify the results and guarantee interviewee anonymity, the landscape categories in Alt Empordà were reduced to three (Fig. 4): mountains, plains and hills.

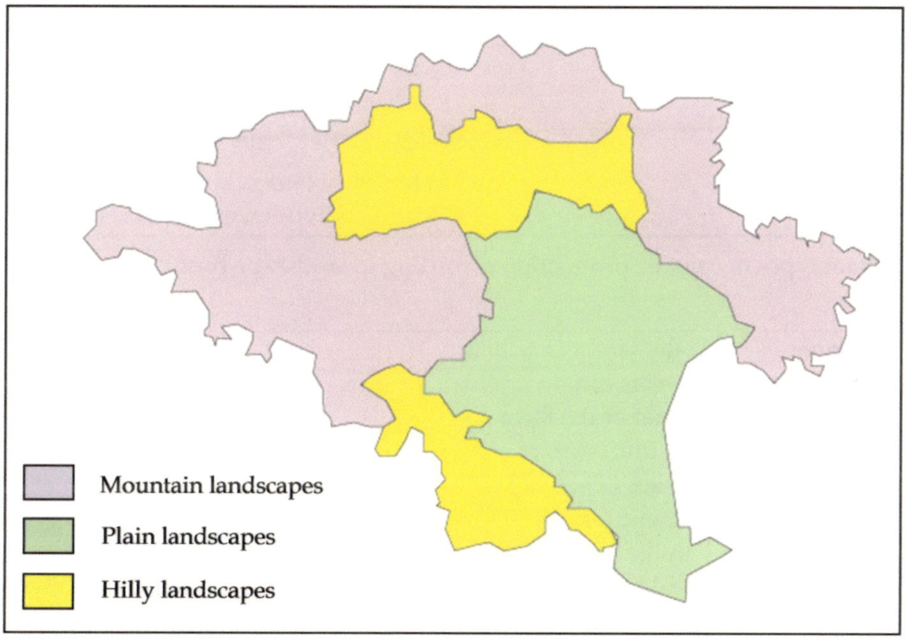

Fig. 4. Main types of Landscapes according to organic farmers

4.2 Characterisation of the farmers

All the farmers interviewed owned their farms, with the exception of one case where the interviewee was one of the sons of the owner and an active member of the family business. In total, five women and eight men were interviewed. On some occasions, the interview took place in the presence of other family members who also worked on the farm. These

[3] The official number given in figures published by the Catalan Council for Organic Agricultural Production (*Consell Català de la Producció Agrària Ecològica*) is 33, including producers, transformers and vendors. In this study, only those identified as producers or producer-transformers were interviewed.

ended up participating in the interview, and thus three more people contributed a significant number of observations which were extremely pertinent to the study. Subjects were aged between 35 and 74.

Most of the interviewees were full-time farmers, although three reported working only part-time on their farms. The majority practiced exclusively organic farming on their farms, although again, three reported maintaining some conventional production. Three of the interviewees transformed their produce on their own farms. In general, the majority of the people working on the farm were family members, although four farms also employed contracted labour on either a full- or part-time basis.

Farms varied widely in size, ranging from 7 ha to over 1,000 ha, but the most common size was between 25 and 50 ha. The farms produced a wide range of products, but in general terms the most frequent types of production are those shown in Table 2. Lastly, typical interviewee characteristics are summarised in Table 3.

Landscape type	Number of organic farms studied	Main Products
Mountain	4	Goats, cattle, forest, orchards, hens, fodder, beekeeping, fruit-trees, olive's oil
Hill	3	Fodder, barley, oats, wheat, wine, olive's oil
Plain	6	Orchards, potatoes, olive's oil, sheeps, hens, fodder, corn, pulses

Table 2. Main types of organic production according to landscape type

Organic farmer	Male 48 years old Owner of the farm Full-time worker Surface (25-50 ha) Organic farm (100%) Familiar worker aid Fodder, cereal and orchard productions with livestock. Olive's oil production oriented to self consumption

Table 3. Characteristics of intervieewed farmer

4.3 Concepts associated with landscape

In answer to the initial question "What is a good landscape?", the interviewees replied using up to a total of twenty seven different concepts. Some of these definitions coincided, and discourses related to balance or harmony, diversity and the survival of indigenous varieties as the defining elements of a quality landscape were the most frequently used concepts.

The aim of the second question was to obtain a more explicit response from the interviewees, and thus they were asked what they considered a good *agricultural* landscape.

In some cases, their reactions indicated a certain degree of surprise, since when answering the first question they had subconsciously based their response on a mental representation of the agricultural landscape about which they were now explicitly being questioned. Once the interviewer had provided the pertinent clarifications, responses differed in some respects from those made earlier. One line of reasoning in particular was employed by over half the interviewees, and thus indicated a general feeling: for there to be a good agricultural landscape, the fields must be farmed. Once again, the idea of diversity was also strongly represented. Other notable defining traits were the need for livestock and, in some cases, the presence of tree-lined riverbanks. As regards this latter point, the district studied still conserves areas where *closes* are the main landscape feature. In recent times, enclosed fields in the district have undergone drastic changes: managed by large companies, they no longer hold cattle or horses but have been turned over to poorly producing sunflower or maize crops in order to collect subsidies. In other cases, some of these fields have simply been abandoned (Llausàs *et al.*, 2009). Concepts associated with biodiversity also emerged on several occasions. The agricultural landscapes produced by smaller, less intensive farms are characterised by high biodiversity and a complex structural pattern (Küster, 2004). Conversion of conventional farms to organic farming favours an increase in biodiversity, improves the landscape and enhances the value of environment (González de Molina, Alonso & Guzmán, 2007).

In the third question, interviewees were asked what they considered to be the attractions of the Alt Empordà district, and it was this question which elicited the most extensive range of associated concepts from the organic farmers. However, to summarise the large number of features mentioned, the sea and the mountains, together with the light, were the elements that were frequently cited.

The fourth question asked the interviewees to list the dangers they felt were facing the district of Alt Empordà. After encoding their responses, it was possible to identify 25 factors which they associated with a deterioration in the district's landscape. Uncontrolled urban spread was the factor most frequently mentioned by the interviewees: it should be remembered that the study area constitutes the very essence of Costa Brava tourism, a context which has been the driving force behind economic and demographic growth in the region for the past forty years. Other issues cited by several interviewees included excessive industrial development, forest fires and the impact of projected wind farms.

In the next question, the participants in this study were asked to respond at individual farm level, in order to elicit what they identified as the attractions of the landscape for which they were directly responsible. Their responses indicated that for them, the main attractions of the land they managed were related to a subjective concept of aesthetics (Fig. 5), such as productive fields with a natural - and in some cases "wild" - appearance.

Continuing on an individual farm level, the last question in this conceptual section asked the organic farmers to explain what they felt were the dangers affecting the landscape for which they were responsible. Of all the concepts which emerged during the interviews, there were three which surfaced with the most frequency: the danger from fire (the farms of some of those interviewed either bordered wooded areas or were in part given over to woodland), and in this case an important management driver is related with wood clearance (Fig. 6), abandonment of farming (this was the second most frequently mentioned concept) and finally, what some referred to as a lack of interest on the part of the authorities in their work and methods.

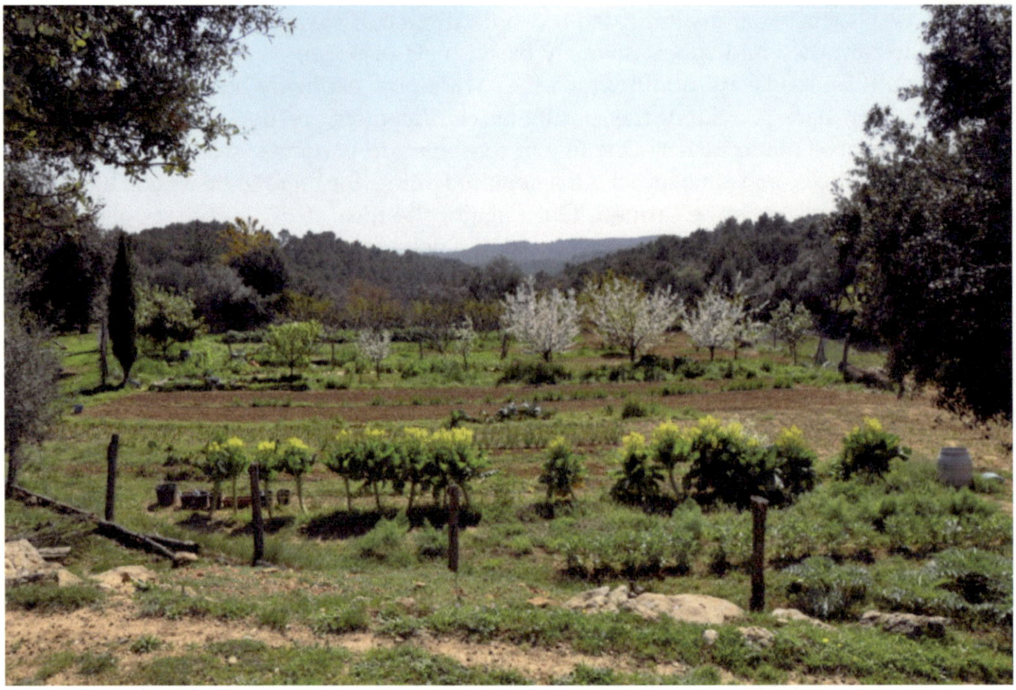

Fig. 5. Organic farm's landscape in a hilly area (Alt Empordà - April 2011)

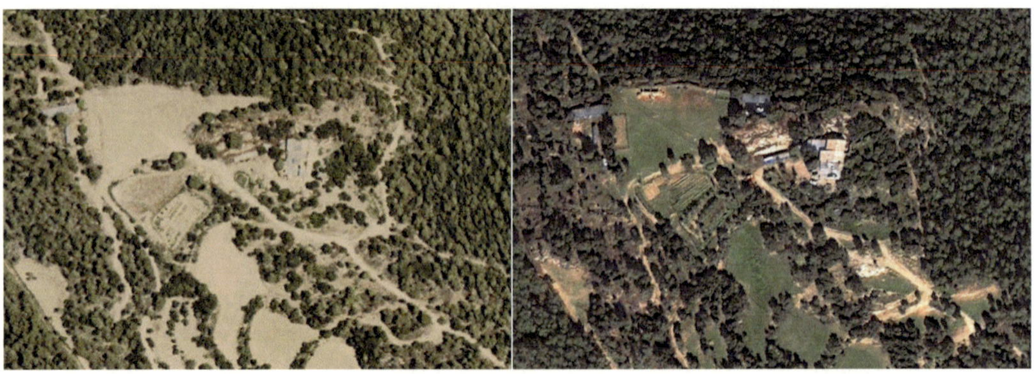

Fig. 6. Lanscape evolution in studied organic farm (2004-2010). Source: Google Earth.

4.4 Landscape assessments

The landscape assessments were obtained from six closed questions incorporating six response options, which the interviewees scored on a scale of 1-7. It goes without saying that the heterogeneity of the organic sector in Alt Empordà reflects both the variable terrain, which the farmers identified as a landscape asset, and the diversity of types of production presented by organic farmers in Catalonia. As regards this latter aspect, Armesto (2008) includes a typological essay on organic farmers in Catalonia.

The first of these questions asked farmers to rank the quality of the landscape for which they were directly responsible on a scale of 1-7, where 1 = dreadful and 7 = excellent. Of all the questions in this section, it was this one which elicited least divergence in the responses given, all of which can be considered positive.

The second question also involved ranking landscape quality, but this time, instead of assessing their own farms, participants were asked to assess neighbouring farms. Here, variability in assessments was much greater: some of the interviewees gave the lowest score possible, whilst others gave a high landscape score to their neighbouring farms.

In the third question, subjects responded to a statement which attempted to identify their perceptions of the contribution made by farmers to the physiognomy of the present day landscape in the district: in this case, 1 = zero contribution whilst 7 reflected the belief that farmers were the principal agents. Once again, divergence was enormous, in this case with various responses at either extreme. Thus, for two of the interviewees, farmers make no contribution whatsoever any more to shaping the landscape, arguing that farming is a disappearing sector without the power for autonomous management, whilst for another interviewee, farmers continue to be primarily responsible for the present day physiognomy of the landscape. In general, it could be said that the majority of respondents felt that farmers made a strong contribution to the appearance of the district's current landscape.

The fourth statement referred to the degree of involvement on the part of the authorities in maintaining the district's landscape. This question elicited the most unanimously low assessments from the respondents. Most interviewees felt that in general terms, the authorities took insufficient action.

The fifth question in this analysis concerned farmers' direct responsibility for the present day landscape in the district. Once more, the farmers interviewed gave very different responses, although in this case they generally acknowledged a certain degree of responsibility which was qualified by regulatory intervention.

The above quantitative questions specifically addressing landscape were followed by the sixth and last question, which asked the farmers to assess the effect of Spain's entry into the European Community on agricultural land twenty five years later. Inevitably, there were a range of responses accompanied by different explanations which were not ranked numerically but rather recorded during the interview. Overall, interviewees expressed moderate agreement that this had been positive.

In order to finish this presentation of the information collected regarding organic farmers' assessment of the landscape, an analysis of the four remaining questions is given below. These elicited qualitative judgements rather than a numerical score; the organic farmers participating in the study were given the choice of five possible responses: 1) much better; 2) better; 3) the same; 4) worse; and 5) much worse.

The first question referred to the farmers' perceptions of the environmental status of their farm compared to ten years previously. Answers were mainly positive. Four of the respondents had no hesitation in asserting that environmental conditions on their farms were much better, and none considered that the environmental condition of their farms was in any degree worse. In order to fully appreciate these responses, it should be borne in mind that, independently of whether their previous methods were more or less respectful to the environment, nine of those interviewed had registered their farms with the Regulatory Council of Organic Farming in Catalonia in the last ten years.

The second question continued in the same vein, although on a different level, asking how the environmental status of the district as a whole had evolved over the last ten years. In this instance, there was a clear prevalence of negative perspectives: only three respondents

considered that environmental conditions in the district had improved over the past ten years.
The third and fourth questions were similar to the previous two. Whilst well aware that some of the interviewees could not possibly have such a long historical perspective, they were nevertheless asked how the environmental conditions on their farms, and in the district as a whole, respectively, had evolved over the past fifty years. In order to correct any age-related bias, respondents under fifty were asked to think of their childhood memories or of comments and experiences recounted by family members who had been alive then. At farm level, the most frequent response was that it was not possible to say whether there had been a positive or negative evolution. However, when the perspective was broadened to include the district as a whole, responses were categorically negative: only one interviewee felt that such evolution had been positive, whilst another felt that the situation in 1960 and today was similar.

5. Conclusions

Landscape can be studied from many different perspectives, since it is a polysemic concept which has been completely assimilated into everyday language. It is the combination of natural and cultural landscapes in the rural environment that has engendered the need to interpret these landscapes, which both condition and are dependent on agricultural activity.
Organic farming is essentially a productive method which is more respectful to the environment; consequently, it is assumed to be better than conventional farming in terms of maintaining quality landscapes. In keeping with this premise, the present study, conducted with a sample of organic farmers in the Alt Empordà district (Catalonia), has demonstrated their high level of interest in the subject of the study.
Most of the organic farmers interviewed defined a good landscape as one containing balanced, diverse lands which conserved traditional structures, and in the specific case of agricultural landscapes, these needed to be spaces full of life, spaces where agricultural activity which respected the surroundings prevailed. At the same time, they identified numerous potentially attractive landscape features on their own farms and in the district as a whole, whilst also identifying possible threats on both levels.
To conclude, the aim of this study was to contribute to the geographical knowledge of an area which, due to those responsible for land use planning is under great pressure, by giving a voice to a group which, although small numerically, has an important role to play in the management of the area and the landscape.

6. Acknowledgements

This research forms part of project CSO2008-01346/GEOG funded by the Spanish Ministry of Science and Innovation.

7. References

Armesto-López, X. A. (2007). El concepto de agricultura ecológica y su idoneidad para fomentar el desarrollo rural sostenible. Boletín de la Asociación de Geógrafos Españoles, No. 43, (July 2007), pp. 155-172, ISSN 0212-9426

Armesto-López, X. A. (2008). Organic farming in Spain - Two case studies. Journal of Sustainable Agriculture, Vol. 31, No. 4, (November 2008), pp. 29-55, ISSN 1540-7578

Baldock, D. (2004). Agricultural policies sustaining the European countryside. In: *Cultural landscapes and land use,* M. Dieterich & J. Van der Straaten (Eds.), pp. 147-161, Kluwer Academic Publ., ISBN 1-4020-2104-6, Dordrecht, The Netherlands

Berendse, F. & Kleijn, D. (2004). The effectiveness of agri-environment schemes as a tool to restore biodiversity in Dutch agricultural landscapes. . In: *Cultural landscapes and land use,* M. Dieterich & J. Van der Straaten (Eds.), pp. 183-192, Kluwer Academic Publ., ISBN 1-4020-2104-6, Dordrecht, The Netherlands

Burel, F. & Baudry, J. (2001). *Ecología del Paisaje. Conceptos, métodos y aplicaciones.* Mundiprensa, ISBN 84-8476-014-6, Madrid, Spain.

Consejo de Europa (2000). Convenio Europeo del Paisaje, (07/13/2011), Available from <http://www.coe.int/t/dg4/cultureheritage/heritage/landscapeVersionsConventions/S>

Fernández-Alés, R. & Leiva-Morales, Mª J. (2003). Ecología para la agricultura. Mundiprensa, ISBN 84-8476-085-5, Madrid, Spain

García-Asensio, J. M. & Cañas-Guerrero, I. (2002). La valoración del paisaje, In: *Gestión de paisajes rurales: Técnicas e ingeniería,* Ayuga-Téllez, F., (Ed.), pp. 33-51, Fundación Alfonso Martín Escudero, ISBN 84-7114-985-0, Madrid, Spain

García-Ruiz, J. M. (1988). La evolución de la agricultura de montaña y sus efectos sobre la dinámica del paisaje. *Revista de Estudios Agrosoci*ales, No. 146, (October-December 1988), pp. 7-37, ISSN 0034-8155

Gastó, J.; Vieli, L. & Vera, L. (2006). De la silva al ager. Paisaje cultural. *Agronomía y Forestal,* No.28, pp. 29-33

Gliessman, F. J.; Rosado-May, F. J.; Guadarrama-Zugasti, J.; Jedlicka, J.; Cohn, A.; Méndez, V.E.; Cohen, R.; Trujillo, L. Bacon, C. & Jaffe, R. (2007). *Agroecología: promoviendo una transición hacia la sostenibilidad.* Ecosistemas, Vol.16, No.1 (January 2007), pp. 13-23, ISSN 1697-2473

González de Molina, M.; Alonso, A. M. & Guzmán, G. (2007). La agricultura ecológica en España desde una perspectiva agroecológica. *Revista Española de estudios agrosociales y pesqueros,* No. 214 (May-August 2007), pp. 47-73, ISSN 1575-1198

Guzmán-Casado, G.; González de Molina, M. & Sevilla-Guzmán, E. (2000). *Introducción a la agroecología como desarrollo rural sostenible,* Mundiprensa, 84-7114-870-6, Madrid, Spain

Hendriks, K.; Stobelaar, D. J. & Van Mansvelt, J. D. (1997). Some criteria for landscape quality applied on an organic goat farm in Gelderland, the Netherlands. *Agriculture, Ecosystems & Environment,* Vol. 63, No. 2-3 (June 1997), pp. 185-200, ISSN 0167-8809

Hernández-Laguna, E.; López-Bermúdez, F.; Alonso-Sarría, F.; Conesa-García, C. & Álvarez-Rogel, Y. (2004). La huella ecológica del cultivo del olivo en España y su aplicabilidad como indicador de agricultura sostenible. *Papeles de Geografía,* Vol.39 (June 2004), pp. 141-155, ISSN 0213-1781

Küster, H. (2004). Cultural lanscapes: An Introduction. In: *Cultural landscapes and land use,* M. Dieterich & J. Van der Straaten (Eds.), pp. 1-11, Kluwer Academic Publ., ISBN 1-4020-2104-6, Dordrecht, The Netherlands

Levin, G. (2007). Relationship between Danish organic farming and landscape composition. *Agriculture, Ecosystems & Environment*, Vol. 120, No. 2-4 (May 2007), pp. 330-344, ISSN 0167-8809

Llausàs, A.; Ribas, A.; Varga, D. & Vila, J. (2009). The evolution of agrarian practices and its effects on the structure of enclosure landscapes in the Alt Empordà (Catalonia, Spain), 1957-2001. *Agriculture, Ecosystems and Environment*, Vol. 129, No. 1-3, (January 2009), pp. 73-82, ISSN 0167-8809

MARM (2010). Estadísticas 2009. Agricultura Ecológica. España, In: *La agricultura ecológica en España Documentos de interés*, 2011-07-18, Available from <http://www.marm.es/es/alimentacion/temas/la-agricultura-ecologica/INFORME_NACIONAL_2009_V_14_tcm7-8092.pdf>

Merriam, G. (1988). Landscape dynamics in farmland. *Trends in ecology and evolution*, Vol.3, No.1 (January 1988), pp. 16-20, ISSN 0169-5347

Observatori del Paisatge de Catalunya (2010). Catàleg del paisatge de les comarques gironines, In: *Catàlegs del Paisatge*, 2011-07-18, Available from <http://www.catpaisatge.net/cat/cataleg_presentats_cg.php>

Ortega-Valcárcel, J. (2000). *Los horizontes de la Geografía*, Ariel, ISBN 84-344-3464-4, Barcelona, Spain

Payraudeau, S. & Van der Werf, H. M. G. (2005). Environmental impact assessment for a farming region: a review of methods. *Agriculture, Ecosystems & Environment*, Vol. 107, No. 1 (May 2005), pp.1-19, ISSN 0167-8809

Pretty, J. (2001). *Agri-Culture: reconnecting people, land an nature*, Earthscan, ISBN 85-383-925-6, London

Rossi, R.; Nota, D. & Fossi, F. (1997). Landscape and nature production capacity of organic types of Agriculture: examples of organic farms in two Tuscan landscapes. *Agriculture, Ecosystems & Environment*, Vol. 63, No. 2-3 (June 1997), pp. 159-171, ISSN 0167-8809

Schmitzberger, I.; Wrbka, Th.; Steurer, B.; Aschenbrenner, G.; Peterseil, J. & Zechmeister, H. G. (2005). How farming styles influence biodiversity maintenance in Austrian agricultural landscapes. *Agriculture, Ecosystems & Environment*, Vol. 108, No. 3 (June 2005), pp. 274-290, ISSN 0167-8809

Vélez-Restrepo, L. A. & Gómez-Sal, A. (2008). Un marco conceptual y analítico para estimar la integridad ecológica a escala de paisaje. *Arbor. Ciencia, Pensamiento y Cultura*, Vol. 184, No. 729, (January-February 2008), pp.31-44, ISSN 0210-1963

Vereijken, J. F. H. M.; Van Gelder, T. & Baars, T. (1997). Nature and landscape development on organic farms. *Agriculture, Ecosystems & Environment*, Vol. 63, No. 2-3 (June 1997), pp. 201-220, ISSN 0167-8809

Von Meyer, H. (1996). Agricultura, medio ambiente y PAC. Problemas y perspectivas, In: *Revista española de economía agraria*, Vol.176-177, pp. 193-214, ISSN 1135-6138

2

The Effect of Sustainable and Organic Farming Systems on the Balance of Biogenic Elements and Changes of Agrochemical Properties in Gleyic Cambisol

Stanislava Maikštėnienė and Laura Masilionytė
Joniškėlis Experimental Station of the Lithuanian Research Centre for Agriculture and Forestry
Lithuania

1. Introduction

In clay loam soils of glacial lacustrine origin, the abundance of clay particles results in higher sorption capacity and nutrient stability compared with light soils. However, even in these soils the level of various agrosystems' functioning is largely determined by cropping systems. When making the shift from intensive cropping system to alternative ones and replacement of fertilization systems it is important to quantify the changes in soil productivity qualitative parameters and to ascertain the effects of environmentally safe agricultural practices on crop productivity. With a higher focus on organic fertilization and reduction or complete abandonment of mineral fertilization, the content of organic carbon increases in the soil, however, this poses a problem for versatile plant nutrition (Gale & Gilmour, 1988; Deng, Motore & Tabatabai, 2000). In alternative cropping systems, when there is a shortage of specific nutrients, plants experience stress, which results in a marked reduction in crop productivity. But this will not suppress the demand for viable developmental processes and the potential collateral effects in order to avoid resource depletion. Where natural resources exist, it must be determined to what degree the environment is capable of absorbing the impact of the development. As agricultural soil is the foundation for nearly all land uses, soil quality stands as a key indicator of sustainable land use. Second, land use and its mismanagement of arable areas by farmers and grazing areas by livestock is addressed as one of the major causes of soil degradation (Zuazo et al., 2011). This discourages the development of organic agriculture, and low organic production volumes are a meagre reserve for safe food. In alternative cropping systems, plant demand for major nutrients is compensated by soil nutrient reserves and nutrients released from organic matter. With no use of mineral fertilization in alternative cropping systems, on a clay loam *Cambisol* of glacial lacustrine origin, the problem of phosphorus shortage becomes most apparent, since low phosphorus content is a genetic characteristic of this soil type.

Anthropogenic activity has a clear effect on ecosystems, because it stimulates domination of components, useful for human beings. In intensive farming, fertilization system targeted at yield increase is based on the plant nutrition needs, but little attention is paid to the maintenance of ecosystem productivity (Hoffmann & Johnsson, 2000; Nieder et al., 2003). Intensive use of chemical plant protection products and mineral fertilizers intended for crops productivity enhancement results in the atrophy of natural, self-regulation processes in soil. Rational soil management in combination with maintaining of ecological balance helps to increase fertility and to keep its potential productivity. In order to reduce environment pollution and to maintain safe environment, it is important to select prevention means appropriately by including nutrients, not absorbed by plants, into biological circulation (Di et al., 2002; Arlauskienė, Maikštėnienė & Šlepetienė, 2009; Arlauskienė, Maikštėnienė & Šlepetienė, 2011). Anthropogenic activity must be directed towards the increase of stability in farming system by improving the state of crops and fauna. The process of biologization in agriculture is one of the main factors, maintaining the natural productivity of soil as well as stability of ecosystem (Hoffmann & Johnston, 2000).

In order to protect ecosystems from effect of chemical means, alternative agricultural systems are being developed. However, these agricultural systems must often solve the problems of nutrients balance, because the issue of versatile plants nutrition arises. Mineral fertilizers help in forming the appropriate balance of nutrients ratio more easily than in cases when sustainable and organic farming is applied, where plant nutrition is solved by organic manure ant limited content of mineral fertilizers (Bhogal et al., 2000). Seeking to preserve nutrients, especially readily migration nitrogen, in the ploughlayer, to reduce nutrient leaching losses and to provide as long as possible protection of the soil surface from the direct adverse effect of the atmospheric phenomena, promoting soil degradation, we cultivated after crops after the main crops in the farming systems. Under Lithuania's conditions, during the warm period, the soil is covered with crops for only 3-4 months in a year, while in autumn with a prolonged rainy period, the risk of nutrient leaching during main crops' post-harvest arises. Catch crops accumulate in their biomass the nutrients that are left in soil after the main crops, and what is the most important, keep nitrogen in the topsoil layer (Stopes & Philipps, 1994; Marcinkevičienė et al., 2008).

The aim of this study was to estimate the effects of organic and sustainable farming systems on the balance of biogenic elements and changes of agrochemical properties in clay loam *Gleyic Cambisol.*

2. Experimental design and field management

Two bi-factor field experiments were conducted in Joniškėlis Experimental Station of the Lithuanian Research Centre for Agriculture and Forestry during 2006–2009 on a clay loam *Endocalcari-Endohypogleyic Cambisol* (*CMg-n-w-can*). The soil texture is clay loam (clay particle <0.002 mm in Ap horizont 0–30 cm make up 27.0 %) on silty clay with deeper lying sandy loam. Parental rock is limnoglacial clay on morenic clay loam. Research was done in the northern part of Central Lithuania's lowland (56°21'N, 24°10'E).

The crop rotation, expanded in time and space, consisted of perennial grasses - red clover (*Trifolium pretenses* L.) and meadow fescue (*Festuca pratensis* Huds.), winter wheat (*Triticum aestivum* L.), pea (*Pisum sativum* L.) and spring barley (*Hordeum vulgare* L.) with undersown perennial grasses. The investigated measures - farming systems were assessed in the grass-cereals sequence: perennial grasses (aftermath for green manure) → winter wheat + catch crops (for green manure) → pea.

The field experiment was arranged according to the following design:

Soil humus content (based on the humus content scale developed by several authors - Пестряков, 1977; Amacher, Neill & Perry, 2007) – **factor A**: 1) – low (1.90–2.01 %); 2) – moderate (2.10–2.40 %).
Farming systems – factor B: organic – I, organic – II, sustainable – I and sustainable – II, are presented in table 1.

Cropping system (Factor B)	Plants of the crop rotation sequence and fertilization		
	perennial grass	winter wheat	pea
Organic I (O I)	-	aftermath of perennial grass	straw + narrow-leaved lupine (*Lupinus angustifolius* L.) and oil radish (*Raphanus satinus* var. *Oleifera* L.)
Organic II (O II)	-	farmyard manure 40 Mg ha^{-1} + aftermath of perennial grass	straw + white mustard (*Sinapis alba* L.)
Sustainable I (S I)	-	farmyard manure 40 Mg ha^{-1}	straw + N_{30} + white mustard and buckwheat (*Fagopyrum exculentum* Moench.)
Sustainable II (S II)	$P_{60}K_{60}$	aftermath of perennial grass +$N_{30}P_{60}K_{60}$	straw + N_{30} $N_{10}P_{40}K_{60}$

Table 1. Cropping systems, plants of the crop rotation sequence and fertilization

The field experiment was arranged as a randomized single row design in four replicates.

2.1 Soil analyses

Soil sample for soil agrochemical properties were taken before experiment and of the end experiment in each plot treatment from the 0 – 20 cm layer. Soil samples for N_{min} (N-NH_4 + N-NO_3) estimation were taken from each plot at twenty positions, from the soil layer of 0 – 40 cm, taking average samples. Samples were taken in spring at the beginning of winter wheat vegetation, in autumn, before catch crop biomass incorporation and in spring before the sowing of peas.
Soil chemical analyses carried out by methods: pH_{KCl} – ionometrically (ISO 10390, 2005) method; the humus status – by Tyurin method; the mobile humic substance – by Tyurin method, modified by Ponamariova and Plotnikova (Пономарева & Плотникова, 1980) in 0,1 NaOH suspension; the available phosphorus (P_2O_5) and potassium (K_2O) – by Egner-Riehm-Domingo (A-L) method (GOST 26208-91:1993); N_{min}: the nitrate nitrogen (N-NO_3) ionometrically, the ammonia nitrogen (N-NH_4) photometrically (ISO 14256–2, 2005).

2.2 Plant analyses

Composite samples were taken at harvesting of the main crop in every field in main and secondary produce as well as the samples of over-ground biomass of catch crops. Crops yield was expressed by the content of absolutely dry matter Mg ha^{-1}. To determine the root biomass of catch crops, monoliths 0.25 x 0.25 x 0.24 m in size were dug out in the plots of each treatment replicated three times. The roots were washed and air-dry weight was determined. Samples of the aboveground and underground biomass were taken for the

determination of dry matter (dried to a constant weight at 105 °C), nitrogen, phosphorus and potassium.
In the biomass of main and secondary produce of rotation crops as well as in catch crops' biomass, nitrogen was determined by Kjeldahl method (ISO 20483: 2006), phosphorus was measured by spectrophotometric and potassium - by flame photometer methods.
Soil and plant analyses were done at the Laboratory of Chemical research at Lithuanian Research Centre for Agriculture and Forestry.

2.3 Statistical analysis

The statistical analysis of data was performed using *ANOVA* for two-factor experiment (Tarakanovas & Raudonius, 2003; Crawley, 2007; Ritz, 2009).

3. Results and discussion

3.1 Fertilization systems

3.1.1 Fertilization systems of winter wheat and analyses of biogenic elements

In a gleiyc *Cambisol* differing in humus status, seeking to determine the effects of various cropping systems, we used aftermath of perennial grass, farmyard manure and their combinations for winter wheat fertilization (Fig. 1). The data averaged over four years suggest that *Cambisol* received on average the lowest dry matter (DM) content of organic matter in organic I and sustainable II cropping systems, 2.1 and 2.0 Mg ha^{-1} respectively, having used only aftermath of perennial grass for winter wheat fertilization. In organic II and sustainable I cropping systems, with farmyard manure fertilization the soil received by on average 4.0 and 3.1 times higher DM contents.
It is consistent, that in organic II cropping system using farmyard manure and biomass of perennial grass aftermath for winter wheat fertilization the soil received the highest content of biogenic elements (Fig. 1). In this cropping system, in the soil with low humus status for winter wheat there was incorporated 3.5 times more nitrogen, 12.1 times more phosphorus and 6.8 times more potassium compared with organic I cropping system. In sustainable I cropping system, in which only farmyard manure was used the content of NPK incorporated into the soil was by 2.7, 11.3 and 5.9 higher compared with organic I system, in which only green manure was used. In sustainable II cropping system, having applied aftermath of perennial grass for winter wheat fertilization the soil received inappreciably lower DM content than in organic I cropping system (Fig. 1).

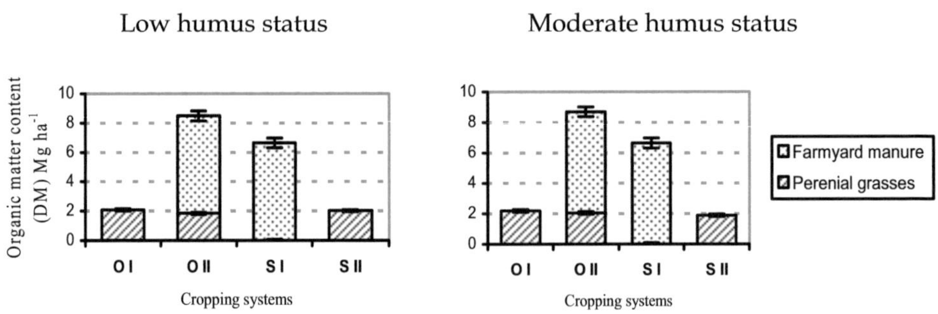

LSD$_{05}$: A-0.10, B-0.18, AB-0.27

Fig. 1. Organic matter contents (DM) incorporated into the soil with aftermath of perennial grass and farmyard manure

However, in sustainable II system, having used mineral fertilizers for additional winter wheat fertilization, the NPK content was by 1.6; 12.7 and 2.8 times higher than in organic I cropping system (Fig. 2). In the soil with moderate humus status, winter wheat received inappreciably higher contents of biogenic elements with incorporated aftermath of perennial grass compared with those in the soil with low humus status. In organic II and sustainable I cropping systems, the content of biogenic elements incorporated into the soil was markedly higher that in organic I system: of nitrogen by 3.3 and 2.4 times, of phosphorus 11.7 and 10.7 times, and potassium 6.2 and 5.2 times. In sustainable II cropping system, having used aftermath of perennial grass and additional NPK fertilization for winter wheat the content of biogenic elements incorporated into the soil was significantly higher - of nitrogen 1.4 times, of potassium and potassium by 12.0 and 2.5 times, respectively, compared with organic I system.

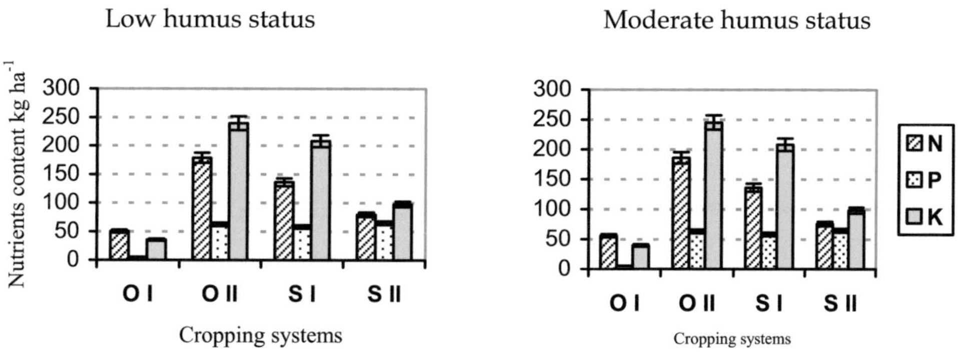

LSD05: N - A-0.53, B-0.92, AB-1.40; P - A-1.32, B-2.28, AB-3.48; K - A-2.78, B-4.81, AB-7.35

Fig. 2. Nutrient contents incorporated into the soil with aftermath of perennial grass, farmyard manure and mineral fertilizer

Nutrient content accumulated in the biomass of perennial grass, in the soil with higher humus status was not higher than that in the biomass of grass that grew in the soil with low humus status, since their development was negatively influenced by higher productivity of the cover crop and its suppressive power. In the soil of both humus levels, the trends of biogenic elements accumulation were similar. For winter wheat fertilization having used only perennial grasses' aftermath the soil received insignificant phosphorus content, per both humus levels it amounted to on average 5.3 kg ha^{-1}. These data show that in clay loam *Cambisols* whose genetic characteristic is low phosphorus level, green manure used for fertilization does not secure optimal phosphorus content in the soil for succeeding plants.

In summary, we can maintain that aftermath of perennial grasses used as green manure can meet plants' nutritional needs only for nitrogen and potassium, since only insignificant amounts of phosphorus are incorporated with their biomass.

3.1.2 Fertilization systems of pea and analyses of biogenic elements

For fertilization of pea was application biomass of catch corps and mineral fertility. Analysis of catch crops' above-ground biomass during winter wheat (pea pre-crop) post-harvest period showed that markedly higher DM content was accumulated in sustainable I cropping system when growing white mustard in mixture with buckwheat compared with organic II system when growing only white mustard, the difference in low-humus status soil made up 67.0 % in moderate-humus status soil it made up 33.3 %. Such results might have been determined not only by the biological properties of catch crops but also low nitrogen rate N_{30} applied in sustainable I cropping system for straw mineralization, which promoted catch crops' development (Fig. 3).

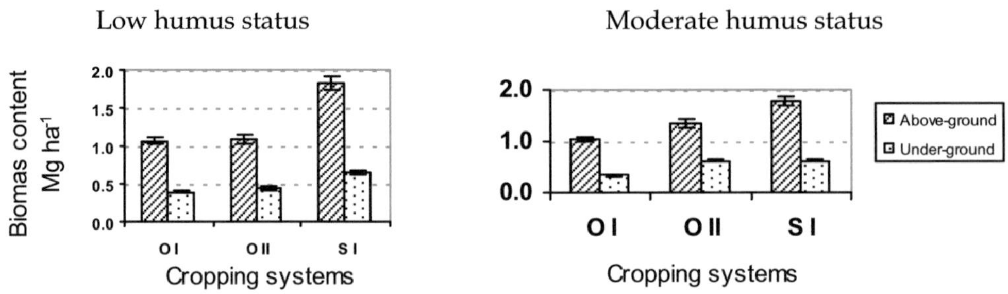

LSD05 (above-ground): A-0.22, B-0.32, AB-0.50; LSD05 (under-ground): A-0.03, B-0.04, AB-0.07

Fig. 3. Above-ground and under-ground biomass (DM) content of catch crops, Mg ha^{-1}

The lowest DM content in catch crops' above-ground biomass in the soil with low and moderate humus status was accumulated when growing narrow-leaved lupine in mixture with oil radish.

Similar results were obtained for catch crops' under-ground biomass (Fig. 3). In the soil low and moderate in humus status, DM content in the under-ground biomass of white mustard mixture with buckwheat was by 47.7 and 1.6 % higher than in organic II system, when growing only white mustard. The lowest DM content in the under-ground biomass in the soil low and moderate in humus status was accumulated when growing narrow-leaved lupine in mixture with oil radish as catch crops. Averaged over all cropping systems, the DM content in under-ground biomass of catch crops grown in the soil moderate in humus content was by 8.2 % higher than that in the soil low in humus status. It is consistent that both DM content accumulated in catch crops' biomass and biogenic elements content were markedly higher in sustainable I cropping system, in which a low nitrogen fertilizer rate N_{30} was applied for straw mineralization.

The above-ground biomass of white mustard and buckwheat mixture grown in the soil low and moderate in humus status had the highest nitrogen and potassium contents, compared with white mustard sole crop, the difference made up 36.1 and 15.7 % and 36.5 and 7.2 %, more, respectively (Fig. 4).

These data indicate that in the soil low in humus status, in worse nutrition conditions, the positive effects of catch crops' biological characteristics manifested themselves more tangibly. In sustainable I cropping system, the biomass of white mustard and buckwheat mixture contained by 40.0 % more nitrogen and by 46.4 % more potassium than in the biomass of narrow-leaved lupine and oil radish mixture in organic I cropping system. Although narrow-leaved lupine fixes nitrogen from the atmosphere and is superior to *Brassicaceae* family plants in organic agrosystems, according to its genetic origin it is a long-day plant, therefore shortening days in the autumn period have a greater negative impact.

In the soil low in humus status, when growing white mustard and buckwheat combination or white mustard as a sole crop, we established lower phosphorus content than in organic I cropping system when growing narrow-leaved lupine in combination with oil radish. However, in the soil moderate in humus status, the biomass of the latter catch crops accumulated the lowest phosphorus content. Higher soil humus status in most cases promoted more intensive biogenic elements' accumulation in the biomass of catch crops; however, the differences were not significant compared with the soil low in humus content.

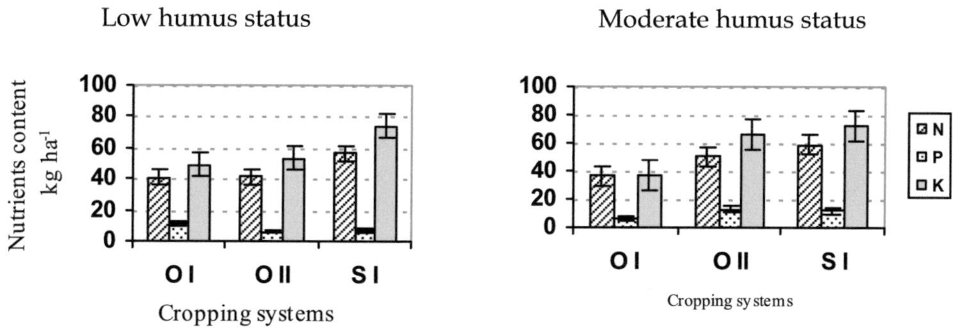

LSD05: N - A-5,68, B-8,04, AB-12,71; P - A-1,16, B-1,64, AB-2,60; K - A-9,49, B-13,43, AB-21,24

Fig. 4. Nutrients accumulated in catch crops' above-ground and under-ground biomass

The under-ground biomass of catch crops accumulated considerably less nutrients compared with the above-ground biomass (Fig. 4). In the soil low in humus status, in sustainable I cropping system, with the biomass of white mustard and buckwheat mixture the soil received the highest content of nitrogen and potassium, which was by 37.6 and 45.7 %, respectively more compared with sole white mustard grown in organic II cropping system. In the soil moderate in humus status, nitrogen and potassium accumulation in catch crops' under-ground biomass varied in a similar pattern to that in the low-humus status soil.

Averaged over all cropping systems, in the soil moderate in humus content, catch crops' under-ground biomass accumulated more nutrients compared with low-humus status soil. With catch crops' under-ground biomass the soil received insignificant contents of phosphorus.

For pea, apart from catch crops' biomass we incorporated winter wheat straw with which the soil low in humus status received NPK on average 19.3, 3.7 and 27.0 kg ha^{-1}, respectively, and the soil moderate in humus status received 22.2, 4.3 and 30.4 kg ha^{-1}, respectively.

3.2 Productivity of the crops

3.2.1 Winter wheat grain yield and biogenic elements

In organic I cropping system, when using only aftermath of perennial grass for fertilization, winter wheat yield was rather low and uncharacteristic of productive soils; in the soil low in humus it amounted to 3.0, in the soil moderate in humus to 3.3 Mg ha^{-1} DM, as a result, it accumulated rather low nutrient contents (Fig. 5).

Averaged over the four crop rotation fields, in clay loam soil, due to the slow organic matter mineralization, farmyard manure applied in organic II and sustainable I cropping systems did not give a significant increase in winter wheat grain yield compared with organic I system. The highest grain yield was produced in the more intensive - sustainable II cropping system, in which besides green manure, wheat received mineral $N_{30}P_{60}K_{60}$ fertilization. In this system, grain yield in the soil low and moderate in humus status was by 35.7 and 29.7 % respectively higher than in the organic I system. In the soil moderate in humus, in separate cropping systems we established a consistent winter wheat yield increase (on average 11.2 %) compared with that produced on the soil low in humus status.

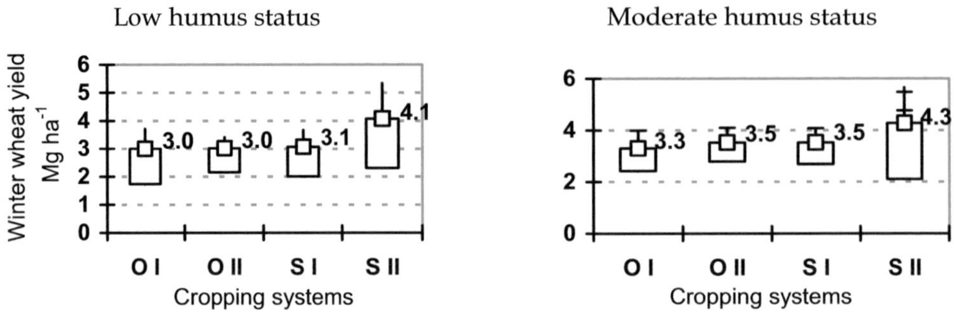

LSD05: A-0.14, B-0.25, AB-0.38

Fig. 5. The effect of fertilization on the grain yield of winter wheat

In the organic I cropping system, when using green manure, grain yield accumulated rather low contents of major biogenic elements, especially of phosphorus and potassium 11.3 and 17.8 kg ha^{-1}, respectively (Fig. 6).

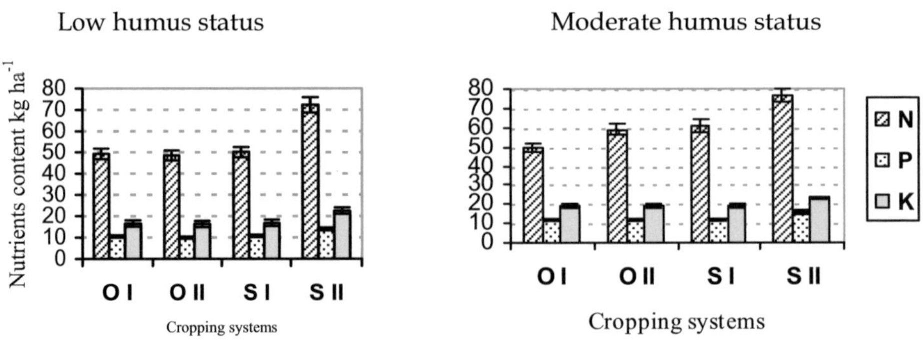

LSD05: N – A-3.20, B-5.54, AB-8.46; P – A-0.67, B-1.16, AB-1.77; K – A-0.99, B-1.71, AB-2.07

Fig. 6. Biogenic elements accumulated in winter wheat grain yield

In the soil low in humus status, the highest biogenic elements' content in winter wheat main produce was accumulated in sustainable II cropping system, with the use of moderate NPK rates in addition to green manure. In this cropping system, the contents of NPK accumulated in winter wheat yield were by 46.8, 32.1 and 36.4 % respectively higher, compared with the treatment applied with only perennial grasses' aftermath. In the soil moderate in humus status, like in that low in humus status, similar contents of biogenic elements were accumulated in winter wheat yield. Averaged over both humus levels,

significantly higher content of biogenic elements in winter wheat grain yield was in the sustainable II cropping system, where the highest grain yield was produced.
Having used minimal NPK rates in addition to aftermath of perennial grass, grain yield was found to contain more N by 43.9 %, P by 32.2 %, and K by 28.3 % compared with the treatment fertilized with only aftermath of perennial grass. When fertilizing with farmyard manure or in combination with aftermath of perennial grass, the content of biogenic elements in winter wheat grain yield was markedly lower compared with that in the treatment applied with aftermath of perennial grass and additionally NPK fertilizers.

3.2.2 Grain yield of pea and biogenic elements

Having incorporated winter wheat straw into the soil, and growing catch crops during the post-harvest period, low yields of pea were produced in the organic cropping systems (Fig. 7). This was influenced by incorporated winter wheat straw containing much lignin and therefore exhibiting slow mineralization, which utilized nitrogen present in the soil. In the soil moderate in humus status, incorporation of catch crops' biomass exerted a more marked effect on pea yield. The highest positive impact on pea yield was exerted by white mustard grown as a sole crop or in mixture with buckwheat. Incorporation of their biomass, compared with narrow-leaved lupine and oil radish mixture increased pea grain yield by 23.0 and 19.4 %, respectively. In sustainable I cropping system, having applied N_{30} for straw mineralization, pea yield significantly increased only in the soil moderate in humus status.
The highest dry matter yield of pea was produced in the sustainable II cropping system, in the soil low in humus status and in the soil moderate in humus status, the yield increase amounted to 42.9 and 46.0 %, compared with the organic I system. The higher soil humus status had a significant (33.9 %) positive effect on grain yield, compared with the soil low in humus status.

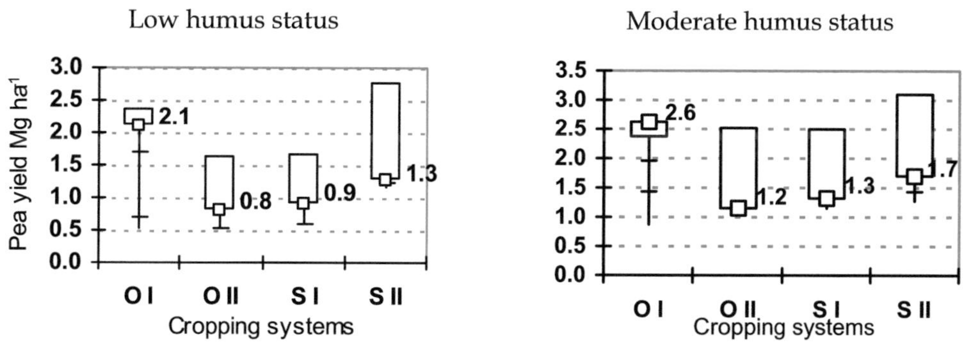

LSD05: A-0.09, B-0.16, AB-0.24

Fig. 7. The effect of fertilization on the grain yield of pea

Nitrogen accumulation in grain was positively influenced by *Fabaceae* catch crops only in the soil low in humus status, compared with *Brassicaceae* catch crops (Fig. 8). In the soil low in humus status, phosphorus and potassium contents in grain were significantly higher only in the sustainable II cropping system, where straw had been incorporated for pea fertilization and N_{30} was applied to promote straw mineralization, and minimal NPK fertilizer rates, the difference, compared with the organic I system, made up 45.9 and 32.9 %, respectively.

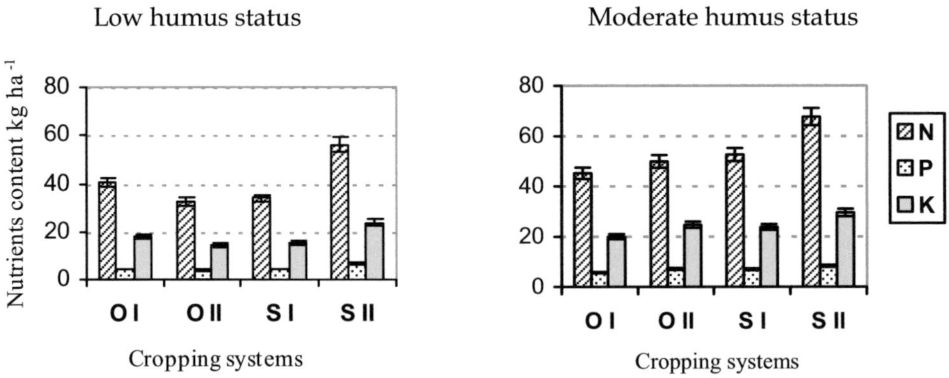

LSD05: N – A-4.04, B-6.99, AB-10.68; P – A-0.37, B-0.64, AB-0.98; K – A-1.09, B-1.89, AB-2.88

Fig. 8. Biogenic elements accumulated in pea grain yield

Different catch crops had a more marked effect on the accumulation of biogenic elements in pea grain in the soil moderate in humus status. The highest phosphorus and potassium contents were accumulated in the grain of pea crop for which biomass of sole white mustard had been incorporated, which were by 25.8 and 23.4 % respectively higher; or in combination with buckwheat by 23.4 and 19.0 % higher, compared with phosphorus and potassium contents accumulated in pea grain in the narrow-leaved lupine or oil radish treatment. In the soil moderate in humus status, the highest contents of biogenic elements were accumulated in the yield of peas grown in the sustainable II cropping system – the content of nitrogen was by 49.9 %, phosphorus by 45.6 % and potassium by 47.4 % higher compared with that in pea grain yield in the organic I system.

Averaged over all cropping systems, in the soil moderate in humus, biogenic elements' accumulation in the yield was significantly higher (of nitrogen by 32.4 %, of phosphorus 42.3 % and of potassium by 37.8 %) compared with the low humus status soil. In the soil low in humus status, incorporation of biomass of catch crops grown after winter wheat had a moderately strong effect r=0.53 $P<0.05$ on pea yield, while in the soil moderate in humus, this effect was weaker r=0.44 $P>0.05$.

3.3 Balance of nutrients incorporated into the soil and removed from the soil with the crops yield

When using organic fertilizers in the cropping systems it is rather complicated to balance the contents of nutrients incorporated into the soil and removed with the yield due to specific characteristics of loamy soils – high content of clay particles, determining slow organic matter mineralization and availability to plants. The nutrient contents accumulated in winter wheat by-produce and catch crops' biomass were returned into the soil, as a result, they were not included into the balance estimated, except for the nitrogen symbiotically fixed by narrow-leaved lupine grown as a catch crop in the organic I cropping system (Fig. 9). The balance between nitrogen introduced into the soil with organic and mineral fertilizers and that removed with the yield varied markedly between the different cropping systems. In the organic I cropping system, in both humus status levels, when using only aftermath of perennial grasses and catch crops' biomass, including nitrogen symbiotically fixed by *Fabaceae* plants, for fertilization, irrespective of the fact that removal with winter wheat and pea yield was low, N balance was negative and plant needs were compensated by 48.6 and 46.9 %, respectively. In the organic II cropping system, in which green manure and farmyard manure were incorporated into the soil low in humus status, N balance was markedly excessive, the removal with the yield of the main produce of crop rotation sequence was compensated by 152.2 %. In the soil moderate in humus status, with better plant growth conditions that determined a higher yield of plants, especially that of winter wheat main produce, N was properly balanced. In the sustainable I cropping system, nitrogen content, incorporated with farmyard manure and catch crops' biomass, in the soil low in humus status compensated N content removed with yield by 120.3 %, in the soil moderate in humus status, where the yields of the main produce were higher, N compensation rate was 86.6 %. Averaged over both soil humus levels, the nitrogen compensation rate closest to 100 % was established in the sustainable I cropping system.

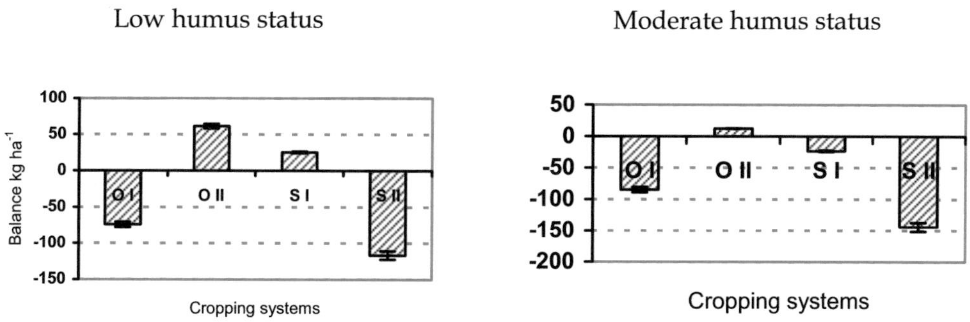

Fig. 9. N balance in the crop rotation sequence - perennial grass-winter wheat-pea

In the sustainable II cropping system, having applied mineral fertilizers for winter wheat and pea, the yield increased markedly, compared with those grown in the organic cropping systems, as is indicated when discussing yield productivity, and this resulted in higher nitrogen removal and its negative balance. In this cropping system, in the soil low and moderate in humus status, nitrogen content, incorporated with organic and mineral fertilizers, compensated the content of nitrogen removed with the yield by as little as 37.5 and 31.4 %, respectively.

Phosphorus incorporation with organic fertilizers and removal with the yield of main produce were rather low, therefore in all cropping systems, except for organic I, phosphorus balance was positive (Fig. 10). In the organic I cropping system, when only green manure was used for fertilization, phosphorus removal in the soil low in humus was compensated by 23.6 % and in the soil moderate in humus by 21.9 %. As a result, in this cropping system, in terms of phosphorus, the soil was depleted in both low and moderate humus levels; it's content in the soil over 4 years declined by 15.9 and 19.2 %, respectively. In organic II and sustainable I cropping systems, having incorporated farmyard manure for winter wheat, there was a well-marked phosphorus surplus. In these cropping systems, phosphorus removal with crop yield was compensated by phosphorus incorporation with fertilizers in the soil low in humus by 3.6 and 3.2 times; in the soil moderate in humus by 2.4 and 2.2 time, respectively.

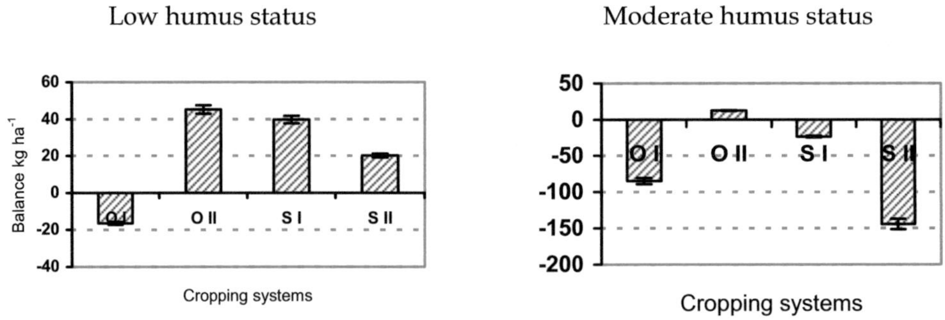

Fig. 10. P balance in the crop rotation sequence - perennial grass-winter wheat-pea

In the sustainable II cropping system, in both humus levels, organic fertilization was supplemented by mineral $N_{30}P_{60}K_{60}$ fertilization. Mineral fertilizers, due to readily plant available nutrients, gave the greatest increase in the yield of main produce and removal of nutrients. In this system, winter wheat main produce yield amounted to on average 4.2 Mg ha^{-1}; of pea to 1.9 Mg ha^{-1}. However, P content removed with the yield was sufficiently well compensated by that incorporated with fertilizers both in the soil low in humus (171.1 %) and moderate in humus (152.0 %).
Both in the soil low and moderate in humus status, K content accumulated in the main produce of crops was markedly higher than that of phosphorus (Fig. 11).

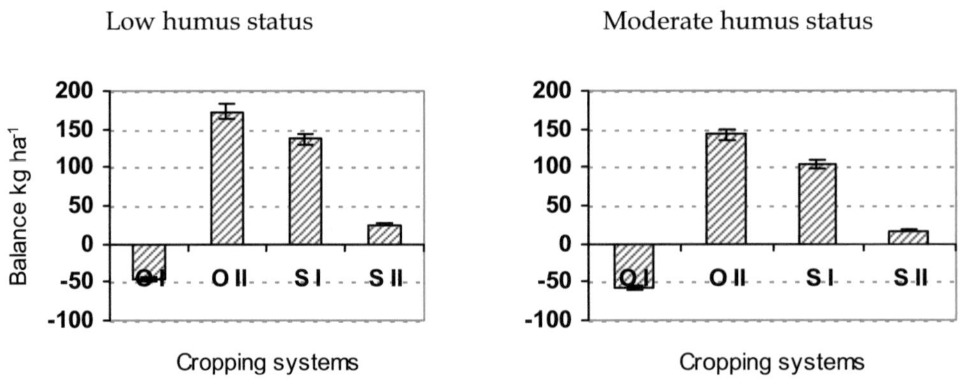

Fig. 11. K balance in the crop rotation sequence - perennial grass-winter wheat-pea

In organic I system, using only green manure for fertilization, potassium balance was strongly negative and plant needs for K in the soil low and moderate in humus were compensated by fertilizers by as little as 43.6 and 41.3 %. In this cropping system, the soil was being depleted, the content of available potassium in the soil low in humus, compared with K content at the beginning of research, declined over a 4-year period by 9.6 %, in the soil moderate in humus by 4.2 %. In the organic II and sustainable I cropping systems, in which green manure fertilization was supplemented by farmyard manure, K balance was strongly positive. In the organic II system, in the soil low and moderate in humus, K plant needs were compensated by fertilizers by 3.6 and 2.4 times, in the sustainable I system, with higher K removal with yield, by 2.9 and 2.0 times, respectively. In the sustainable II cropping system, with the use of mineral fertilizers, crop yields and nutrient removal were markedly higher, therefore potassium balance was slightly surplus, in low and moderate humus status soils it amounted to 122.7 and 114.2 %.

3.4 The effect of cropping systems on the changes of main nutrients elements in the soil

3.4.1 Available phosphorus

From the environmental protection viewpoint, seeking to explore safer systems, by biologizing agricultural production, it is important to maintain sustainability of soil productivity parameters. In the soil low in humus, which was also low in phosphorus at the beginning of research, the investigated means in the cropping systems did not secure positive changes in available phosphorus (Fig. 12).

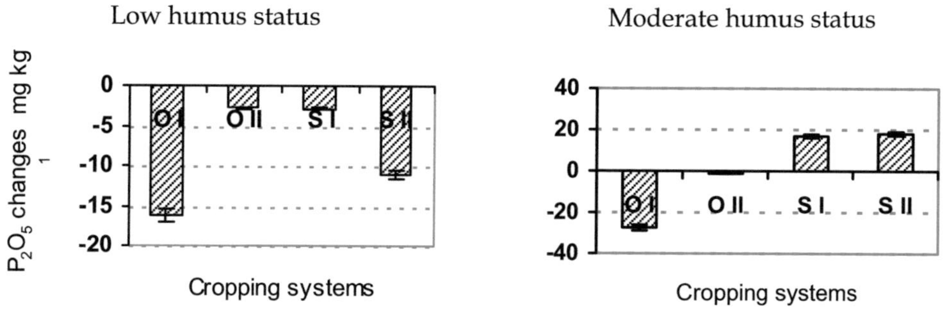

LSD05: A – 6.76, B – 11.70, AB – 17.88

Fig. 12. The effect of cropping systems on the changes in available phosphorus in the 0-20 cm soil layer, mg kg-1

Compared with the initial data, the most marked reduction in available phosphorus content in the soil occurred in the organic I and sustainable II cropping systems, in which only green manure or moderate mineral NPK rates were used for fertilization - 16.2 and 11.0 mg kg^{-1}, respectively. In the cropping systems in which phosphorus contents removed with yield were compensated by those introduced with farmyard manure, the available phosphorus level in the soil remained close to initial.

In the soil moderate in humus, the initial phosphorus level was considerably higher compared with the soil low in humus. At the end of the sequence, in the organic I cropping system, we established a significant reduction in available phosphorus content by 27.4 mg kg^{-1}, compared with the initial level. In the organic II system, it remained close to initial. In the sustainable I and II cropping systems, a marked increase in available phosphorus content in the soil was determined, which was by 16.9 and 18.1 mg kg^{-1} higher compared with that before trial establishment.

In the soil low in humus, the content of phosphorus accumulated in catch crops' biomass depended moderately on the content of available phosphorus in the soil r=0.521 ($P<0,05$). In the soil moderate in humus, the shortage of available phosphorous was less severe, therefore there was no relationship between phosphorus content accumulated in catch crops' biomass and available phosphorus content in the soil.

3.4.2 Available potassium

Heavy-textured soils are characterised by high potassium status, this shows that the soil constantly releases enough potassium compounds that are readily uptaken by plants, and the potassium content incorporated into the soil does not strongly influence plant nutrition. At the beginning of research, clay loam soil low in humus had high potassium content, and the soil moderate in humus had very high content of potassium (Fig. 13). In the soil low in humus, in organic I cropping system, using only green manure that compensated only 43.6 % of potassium removed with the yield, the changes in available potassium content were significantly negative - 21.0 mg kg^{-1}, compared with the initial level. Similar negative changes in available potassium were established in the sustainable II cropping system, in which only moderate mineral fertilizer rates were applied. In the cropping systems, farmyard manure applied once in the crop rotation determined significant positive changes in available potassium - 26.0 and 25.7 mg kg^{-1} respectively, compared with the initial status.

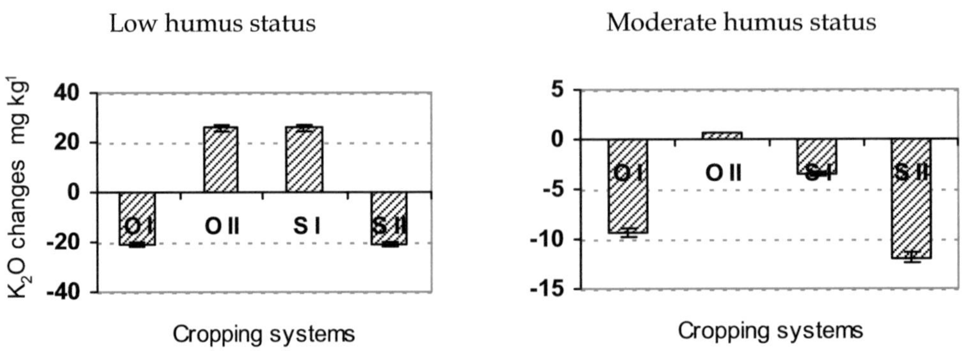

LSD05: A - 2.85, B - 4.93, AB - 7.53

Fig. 13. The effect of cropping systems on the changes in available potassium in the 0-20 cm soil layer, mg kg-1

In the soil moderate in humus, like in the soil low in humus, negative changes in available potassium were established in organic I and sustainable II cropping systems, by 55.2 and 42.6 % lower than in the soil low in humus. In organic II and sustainable I cropping systems, in which farmyard manure had been applied, the changes in available potassium were similar to initial levels. In the soil both low and moderate in humus, available potassium content weakly correlated with potassium content accumulated in catch crops' biomass.

4. Summary and conclusion

Having summarised the results of research into various alternative cropping systems, investigated over the 2006 - 2009 period in the crop rotation sequence – perennial grasses → winter wheat + catch crop → peas on a clay loam *Endocalcari-Endohypogleyic Cambisol (CMg-n-w-can)* with a different humus status, the following conclusions were made:

In the soil with low and moderate humus status, the lowest dry matters and nutrient content for winter wheat were incorporated in organic I farming system with aftermath of perennial grasses. With the application of farmyard manure 40 Mg ha^{-1} in organic II farming system and aftermath of perennial grasses with mineral fertilizers $N_{30}P_{60}K_{60}$ in sustainable II farming system, appropriate reserves of main nutrients - nitrogen, phosphorus and potassium - for optimal yields of winter wheat were incorporated.

Application of farmyard manure had not significant effect to increase the grain yield and accumulation of biogenic elements was not significantly higher than in cases, when only aftermath of perennial grasses was applied for manure. Farmyard manure due to low mineralization in clay loam *Cambisol,* it increased the yield of second rotation member (peas) more effectively, than that of the first rotation member (winter wheat yield).

Significantly higher content of accumulated biogenic elements in main production of winter wheat was observed in sustainable II farming system, when average NPK rates were applied N-43.9 %, P-28.8 % and K-28.3 % more than in cases when only aftermath of perennial grasses was applied for manure.

Catch crops', cultivated in post-harvest period as well as analysis of accumulated biogenic elements in them indicates, that the lowest content throughout averagely both humus backgrounds of accumulated dry matters and biogenic elements in their biomass was observed in mixture of narrow-leafed lupine and oil radish.

In a *Gleyic Cambisol* low and moderate humus content in the organic system with the application of organic manure - aftermath of perennial grasses for winter wheat, straw and catch crops' biomass for peas, the NPK balance was negative, despite of low removal with low crop yields.

In sustainable farming system, application of 40 Mg ha^{-1} of farmyard manure for winter wheat and N_{30} in the form of ammonium nitrate for straw mineralization, as well as catch crops' biomass for peas, NPK balance in the soil low in humus content, was positive and in the soil moderate humus status the nitrogen balance was negative, due to the better conditions for crop growth and higher removal with wheat yield. In sustainable farming system, with application of integrated system of fertilization, incorporation of aftermath of perennial grasses as well as $N_{30}P_{60}K_{60}$ for winter wheat and $N_{10}P_{40}K_{60}$ for peas, the wheat yield and accumulated content of biogenic elements in it for both humus environments were the highest; however the nitrogen balance was positive, while that of PK was insignificantly positive. Investigated farming systems demonstrates different character of available P_2O_5 and K_2O accumulation in the soil top layer during crop rotation.

5. References

Amacher M.C., O'Neill K. P. & Perry C.H. (2007) Soil vital sings: a new soil qality index (SQI) For assessing forest soil health. // *Research paper of USD of Agriculture, Forest servise.* Rocky Mountain research station. - 12 p.

Arlauskienė A., Maikštėnienė S. & Šlepetienė A. (2009) The effect of catch crops and straw on spring barley nitrogen nutrition and soil humus composition // *Zemdirbyste-Agriculture.* Vol. 96, No. 2, p. 53–70.

Arlauskienė A., Maikštėnienė S. & Šlepetienė A. (2011) Application of environmental protection measures for clay loam *Combisol* used for agricultural purposes // *Journal of Environmental Engineering and Landscape Management.* Vol. 19, Issue 1, p. 71-80.

Crawley M. J. (2007) *The R book.* - Chichester, UK, - 942 p.

Bhogal A., Rochford A.D. & Sylvester-Bradley R. (2000) Net changes in soil and crop nitrogen in relation to the performance of winter wheat given-ranging annual nitrogen applications at Ropsley, UK. // *Journal of Agricultural Science.* Vol. 135, p. 139-149

Deng S. B, Motore J. M. & Tabatabai M. A. (2000) Characterization Of Actine Nitrogen Pools in Soils Under Different Cropping Systems // *Biology and Fertility of Soils.* Vol. 32, p. 302–309.

Di H. J. & Kameron K. C. (2002) Nitrate leaching in temperate agroecosystems: sources, factors and mitigating strategies // Nutrient Cycling in Agroecosystems. Vol. 45, p. 237-256.

Gale P. M., Gilmour J. T. (1988) Net mineralization of carbon and nitrogen under aerobic and anaerobic conditions // *Soil Science Society of America Journal.* Vol. 52, p. 1006–1010.

Hoffmann M. & Johnsson H. (2000) Nitrogen leaching from agricultural land, Sweden. Model calculated effects of measures to reduce leaching loads // *Ambio.* Vol. 29, p. 67-73

Marcinkevičienė A., Pupalienė R., Bogužas V. & Balnytė S. (2008) Influence of crop rotation and catch crop for green manure on nitrogen balance in organic farming // *Žemės ūkio mokslai.* Vol. 15, No. 4, p. 16-20

Nieder R., Benbi D. K. & Isermann K. (2003) Soil organic matter dynamics // *Handbook of processes and modeling in the soil-plant system.* P. 345-409.

Ritz Ch. (2009) R for statistical analysis in toxicology. Statistics Group. *Faculty of Life Science.* - Copenhagen, Denmark, p. 13-17.

Stopes C. & Philipps L. (1994) Nitrate leaching from organic farming systems // *Soil Use and Management.* Vol. 9, p. 126-127

Zuazo V. H. D., Pleguezuelo C. R. R., Flanagan D., Tejero I. G. & Fernández J. L. M. (2011) Alternative Farming Systems, Biotechnology, Drought Stress and Ecological Fertilisation Sustainable Agriculture Reviews // *Sustainable Land Use and Agricultural Soil.* Vol. 6, p. 107-192.

Пестряков В. К. (1977) *Окультуривание почв* Северо - Запада. - Ленинград. - 343 с.

Пономарева В. В. & Плотникова Т. А. (1980), *Гумус и почвообразование* (Методы и результаты изучения). Москва. - 220 с.

Tarakanovas P. & Raudonius S. (2003) The program package „Selekcija" for processing statistical data. Akademija, Kedainiai, 56 pp.

3

Ecological Footprint and Carbon Footprint of Organic and Conventional Agrofoods Production, Processing and Services

Iuliana Vintila
Dunarea de Jos University Galati
Romania

1. Introduction

The Ecological Footprint (EF) measure the natural capital demand of human activities (Wackernagel and Rees, 1996 and 2002) and reveal the sustainability of consumption patterns on individual, local, national and global scales (WWF, 2008).
The ecological footprint measure the natural capital demand of human activities (Wackernagel and Rees, 1996) and reveal the sustainability of consumption patterns on individual, local, national and global scales (Arrow, 2002). Ecological footprint model assumes that all types of energy, material consumption and waste discharge require productive or absorptive capacity of a finite area. Six types of ecological biologically productive area (arable land, pasture, forest, sea space, built-up land and fossil energy land) are used to calculate the Ecological Footprint and ecological capacity (Wackernagel et al., 2002).
The ecological footprint estimates the ''minimum land necessary to provide the basic energy and material flows required by the economy''(Wackernagel and Rees, 1996). The consumption elements are converted into a single index: the land area to sustain the lifeliving among human consummation groups. The area of land or sea available to serve a particular use is called biological capacity (biocapacity) and represents the biosphere's ability to meet human demand for material consumption and waste disposal. The degree of unsustainability is calculated as the difference between actual available and required land. In the original ecological footprints model created by Wackernagel and Rees (1996) and reformulated by Chambers et al. (2000), the land areas included were mainly those directly required by households with autoconsumation life style. In the original ecological footprint model, land categories are weighted with equivalence and local yield factors, in order to express appropriated bioproductivity in world-average terms (Wackernagel et al., 2002). The present tendency is to emphases the potential of local food to contribute at the sustainable development, maintaining regional identities and support modern organic agricultural (Defra, 2007; Everett, 2008). Organic agro-production refers to agriculture which does not use artificial chemical fertilizers and pesticides, and respect animals lived welfare in more natural conditions, without the routine of using drugs or antibiotics, common in the intensive livestock farming. The most commonly reasons for consuming organic food are: food safety, the environment, animal welfare, and taste (Soil Association, 2003). The

principal environmental reason for localizing food supply chains is to reduce the impacts of food miles—the distance food travels between being produced and being consumed —and to reduce the energy and pollution associated with transporting food around the world. Local food is a solution to the problem of food miles (Subak, 1999).
The aim of the first part study were: (i) to compare conventional and organic agro-foods, by means of the EFE method using LCA protocol and (ii) correlate the EF values with the carbon emissions generated in the production and distribution chain.

1.1 Protocol of investigation

In the present paper research, EF was evaluated with the 3 main components (or modules):

i. EF_B, the basic or gross EF of raw materials (agriculture production surface footprint);
ii. EF_P, the EF for agro-food production and processing;
iii. EF_T, the EF of retail transport.

The EFE were conducted by grouping the raw foods under the variables of nature, type of production system and transportation facilities.
In the calculation of product-specific EF we consider all the quality-controlled life cycle information including energy, materials, transportation and wastes. To calculate EF, the inputs of different kinds are first converted to the corresponding actual area of land/water ecosystems needed to produce the resources or assimilate the emissions, converted in global hectare (gha) by means of yield and equivalence factors. The equivalence factor reflects the difference in productivity of land-use categories. The yield factor reflects the difference between local and global average productivity of the same bioproductive land type (Monfreda *et.al.*, 2004).
In LCA method, the EF of a food item is defined as the sum of direct land occupation and indirect land occupation, related to the total CO2 emissions from fossil energy associated with the transformation (industrial processing) and transportation cycle:

$$EF_i = EF_B + EF_P + EF_T \tag{1}$$

In formula (1) EF_B is the basic EF related to the land occupation 6 types identified, calculated with the formula (2):

$$EF_B = \sum_{i=1}^{n} F_i qF_i \tag{2}$$

Where: EF_B is the EF of direct land occupation (m2), F_i is the occupation of area by land use types i (m2) and qF_i is the equivalence factor of land yields based on FAO Database (FAO,2007).
The environmental impact generated by the transportation system was calculated with the original equation (3):

$$EF_T = EF_C + EF_{TS} + EF_{CO_2} \tag{3}$$

Where: EF_T is the EF value for transportation system adopted for the raw materials; EF_C is the EF value for the production of the fuel consumed in the transportation of raw foods;

EF_{TS} is the EF value for the transportation state in the refrigeration units; EF_{CO_2} is the EF value involved by the pollution generated with the emission of CO_2 in course of the transportation cycle.

1.2 Results and discussions

The CO2 Emissions and EF for farm vegetables were presented in Fig.1. The tomatoes and cucumber produced in the conventional manner shown the greatest value of CO2 emissions correlated with the EF value. The reducing of EF value by conversion to the organic agricultural procedures determined a reducing of the environmental impact with 47% in case of carrots, 29% in tomatoes case and 19% in cucumber case, respectively. The ratio of CO2 emission in conventional to organic agricultural producing methods was range from 1.05 in potatoes case to 1.896 in case of tomatoes.

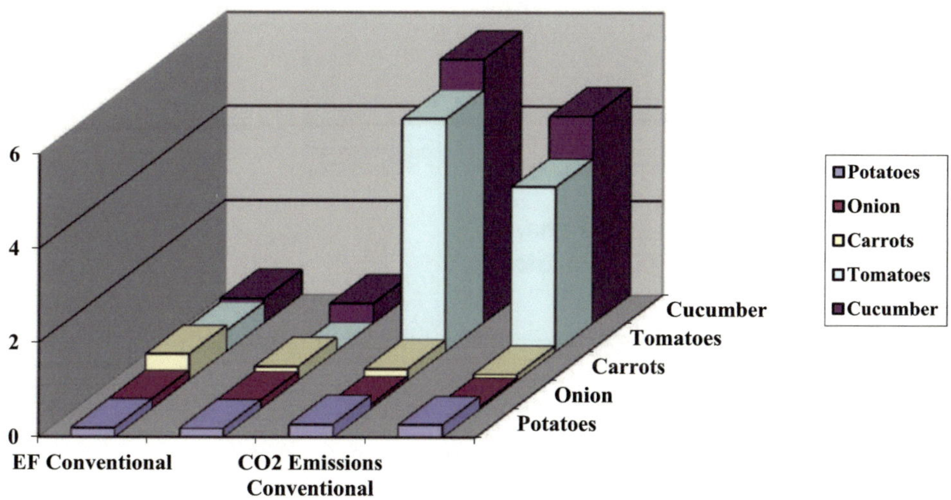

Fig. 1. CO2 Emissions (t CO_2 /t) and Ecological Footprint (gha/t) for farm vegetables

The CO2 emissions from cereals were between 0.190 and 4.60 tCO_2 /t (Tab.1).The lowest emissions were found for organic cereal production. Rice were 5 to 20 times more emissions-intense (4.55 t CO_2/t) than the regular cereals (wheat, rye).

Cereal	Carbon Emissions t CO_2/t	EF gha/t	Agro-Production System
Wheat	0.19 0.45	1.83 4.09	Organic Conventional
Rye	0.65 0.75	1.15 1.33	Organic Conventional
Rice	4.60	3.04	Conventional

Table 1.1. CO2 Emissions and EF for farm cereals

Pork meat is environmentally more favorable than chicken, which is more favorable than lamb and beef. Beef is found to be around 5 times more CO2-emissions intense than pork meat (Fig. 2), with the greatest EF value of 12, 18 gha/t in the conventional production system. The conversion to an organic production system determinate a reducing of environmental impact calculated as brut EF of 31, 03-45, 8%, depending on capacity and efficiency of the production farm. Chicken meat have the lowest impact on the total EF of ready to eat foods created with this type of meat.

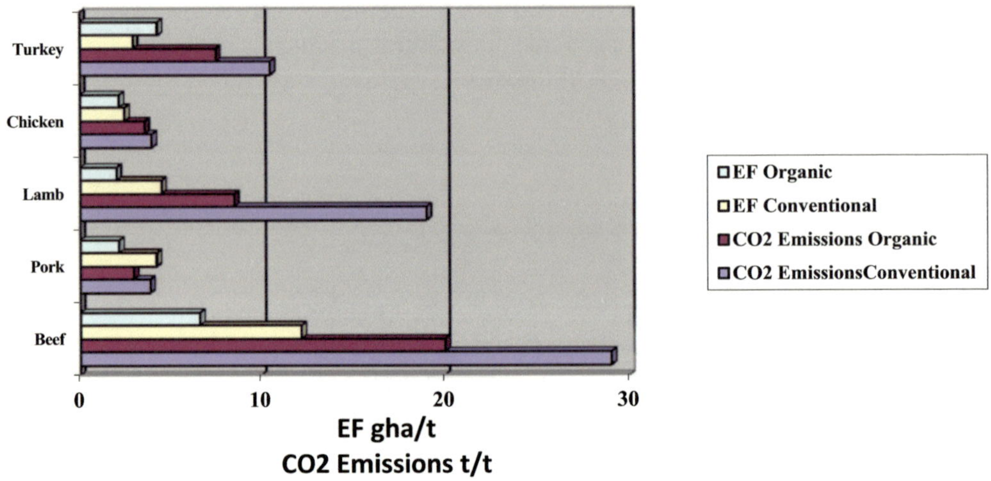

Fig. 2. CO2 Emissions (t CO_2 /t) and Ecological Footprint (gha/t) for farm meats

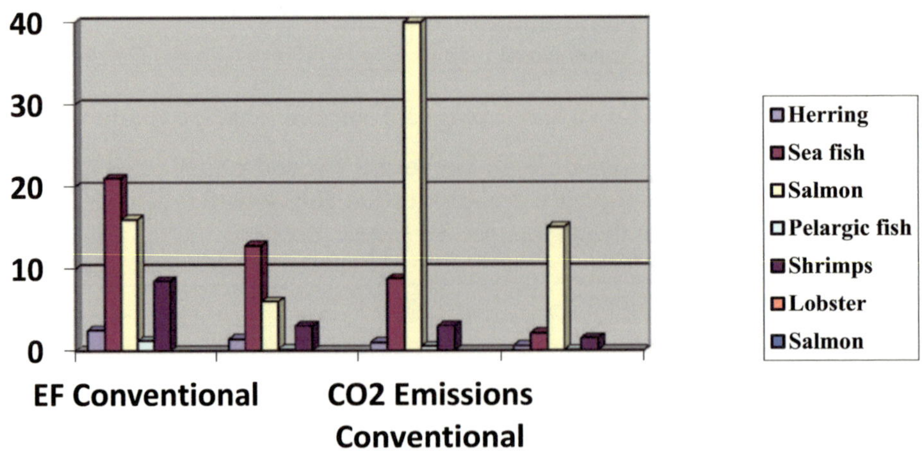

Fig. 3. CO2 Emissions (t CO_2 /t) and Ecological Footprint (gha/t) for seafoods

Pelagic fish species such as herring or mackerel have the lowest CO2 emissions in organic production case 0.08t CO2/t of fish (Fig.3). The deep-sea species and farmed carnivorous fish, such as salmon, generate the higher pressure both in term of CO2 emissions and EF impact.
Marine transport system with great capacity and efficiency generate the lowest emissions of 0.012 kg CO_2/t km in compare with an average capacity facility truck which cause emissions of 0.075 kg CO_2/ t km (Tab.2).

Transport System	Emission CO_2 kg /t km	EF gha/t
Air (EU)*	0.725	0.357
Air (transatlantic)	0.710	0.35
Rail	0.015	0.006
Trucks**	0.075	0.031
Marine	0.012	0.005

* 1 kg of diesel/kerosene corresponds to 3.15 kg CO_2
** Diesel has 85.9% carbon content by weight so the emission factor will be 0.859 × 3. 6667 = 3.15 tCO_2/t diesel (Carbon Trust, 2006).

Table 1.2. CO2 Emissions and EF for various transportation systems

The Table 3 shows that the transport of melon to Romania (Bucharest) from Brazil (Sao Paulo) by sea generate an added value of 0.033 gha/t at the brute EF of food (0. 35 gha/t), due to the greater capacity of the shipping facilities in comparison to air transport system, taking in account the potential for wastage implied by the longer travel chain. Avocado transported by air from South Africa (Cape Town) to Romania (Bucharest) imply the greatest EF correlated with the CO2 emissions 0.760 gha/t, while the transport by air generally is the most not-environment friendly type of transport. The transport by road may be 9 times more Eco-friendly than the transport by rail.

1.3 Conclusions

The conventional production system were found to have a EF value in average with 50% higher than in organic processing, mainly due to the agricultural and packing procedures. The lowest CO2 emissions were found for organic cereal production (1.15gha/t in rye case). Pork meat production is less emission intense than chicken, which is more environmentally favorable than lamb and beef. The reducing of EF in case of organic production is in the range of 1,05 (potatoes)-1,89 (tomatoes) times in vegetables case, 1.15 (rye)–2.23 (wheat) in cereals case, 1.03(chicken)-1.93(turkey) in meats case and dramatically more in case of sea foods 1.64 (shrimps)-5.9. Pelagic fish species such as herring or mackerel with low CO2 emissions register the highest reducing of EF in case of organic conversion of production and Eco-friendly distribution system.

Food, origin and transportation system	Emission in the transportation cycle kg CO_2/t	EF, gha/t	EF Transp. gha/t
Avocado, South Africa (Cape Town), aircraft	0.870	1.26	0.76
Smoked Salmon, South Africa (Cape Town), aircraft	0.870	6	0.76
Cherry , Spain (Madrid), aircraft	0.797	0.20	0.195
Melons, Brazil (Sao Paulo), marine	0.033	0.35	0.033
Tomatoes, Italy (Roma), truck	0.32	0.31	0.065
Tomatoe , Italy (Roma), train	0.030	0.31	0.006
Wine, Italy (Roma), truck	0.32	0.112	0.065
Virgin Olive oil, Italy (Roma), truck	0.32	3.17	0.065

Table 1.3. EF for Organic Agro-food transported from abroad to Romania (Bucharest)

2. Part 2

In the second stage of the research a comparative evaluation of durable development strategy for a public University UGAL (Dunarea de Jos University) using 2 assessment tools is proposed: ecological footprint(EF) versus Carbon Footprint Analysis(CF).The durable development indicators were calculated based on the evaluation of 2010 total flows for foods, energy, transport system and wastes management using Life Cycle Assessment (LCA)methodology. The general aim is to reduce the Ecological Footprint of the public institution by a rational use of natural resources and to educate the university community on the ethics of sustainability.In addition, the assesment of ecological impact of activities related with the University management due to a green strategy to addopt in the sustainability of buildings and green areas, energy and resources use.

2.1 Introduction

The actual world is moving towards a severe limitation of resources. Energy resources, essential for human well-being, are approaching to their peak point.

Human demand on ecosystem services continues to increase without a correlation with the regenerative and absorptive capacity of the biosphere. The natural capital may increasingly become a limiting factor for the future human demand. Humanity is posed in front of a major nature transformation and to face serious environmental challenges at global and local scales. The ecological attitude and sustainable behaviour has become a necessity in the recent decades (Chambers et al., 2000). In the original ecological footprint method, only emissions of CO2 from energy use were considered without the influence of greenhouse gases, land clearing, enteric fermentation in livestock, industrial processes, waste, coal seams, venting and leakage of natural gas. Since the formulation of the ecological footprint, a number of researchers have criticised the method as originally proposed (Arrow, 2002; Costanza, 2000). In nowadays, the EU caterers are concerned about the environmental and sustainability issues, including the provenance and production methods of procured food, waste management, energy and water consumption (Dawe et al., 2004). Universities are public institutions that move to become more sustainable. New ways to measure progress are being sought such as Carbon Footprint Analysis (CFA) and Ecological Footprint Analysis (EFA). Many universities have adopted broad environmental responsibility and/or sustainability policies (Van Den Bergh, 2010). All the public Universities have a particular social responsibility in encouraging best environmental practice, due to their considerable influence on societal development (Albino and Kühtz, 2002).

A number of campuses have published EFA assessment results (Burgess and Lai, 2006; Conway et al., 2008; Dawe et al., 2004; Flint, 2001; Li et al., 2008; Venetoulis, 2001; Wright, 2002) but only two studies regarding a large public university (Janis, 2007; Klein-Banai et al., 2010). A comprehensive and consistent comparative study of EFA versus CFA results for a Eastern Public University is not available in the scientific literature.

The objective of the present research is to evaluate the actual Eco-impact of UGAL activities by using the EFA and CFA methodology. In the medium term, UGAL intention is to promote a sustainable green policy with the following major objectives:

1. decreasing the material (foods, packages, utilities etc.) and energetic waves as daily activities inputs;
2. improvement of the air quality;
3. improvement of the energetic quality performance and green energy production;
4. improvement of the water management system;
5. improvement of the green facilities management.

The present part of research compare the results generated by 2 Eco-Indicators (Ecological Footprint and Carbon Footprint) as important markers in the evaluation of future greening strategy that will be adopted for the first time by a Eastern public University from Romania (UGAL).

2.2 Materials and methods

The data involved in the Eco-Indicators assessment were obtained directly from the UGAL campus and general administrative management office. The UGAL campus population in 2010 consisted of 10.000 full-time students, 8000 part-time students and 1358 employed staff. The total UGAL facilities area is in average 11gha and the building area is about 5.4 gha. The EFA methodology was based on Wackernagel and Rees procedure (1996). In the calculation of specific EF we take into account all the quality-controlled life cycle information including energy, materials, transportation and wastes. To calculate EF, the inputs of different kinds are first converted to the corresponding actual area of land/water ecosystems needed to produce the resources or assimilate the emissions. The EFA results were expressed as units of EF in global hectare with world average biological productivity, for the purposes of adding areas together and comparing results across land types. The CFA is based on the calculation of CF for materials and processes with known quantity of fuel, energy or raw material multiplied by an conversion factor, which is a rate of tons of CO2e emitted per quantity of the material consumed (DEFRA, 2009). Greenhouse gases emitted through transport and the production of food, energy, utilities (electricity, gas, coal, water) for University activities and services are expressed in terms of the amount of CO2e emitted, in tonnes units. The methodology is highly compatible with ISO 14042 requirements. Both methodologies generate the information and data necessary for the Eco-indicators assessment by analyzing and quantifying the flows of all resources (inputs) and produced waste (outputs) on the campus (canteen and student's residence) and in all UGAL facilities. The input data for the Eco-Indicators assessment were presented in Table2.1, Table 2.2.1, Table 2.2.2 and Table 2.3.

Element	*Value*
UGAL total students	18000
Full time students	10000
Part-time students	8000
UGAL total employes	1358
In-campus students	3400
Average total menus served per day	400
Active weeks per academic year	45
Total menus served per academic year	82000
Snack menus served per academic year	4100
Lunch semi-complet menus served per academic year	41000
Lunch complet menus served per academic year	4100
Dinner menus served per academic year	32800

Table 2.1. General assessment elements

Utility item	Consummation
Electricity, MWh	1423
Gas, m3	175313
Water, m3	72808.76
Coal, Gcal	5557.08
Car traffic, km	29588

Table 2.2.1. Utilities consummation in UGAL

Wastes categories	Total Quantities kg/year
Domestic waste	5291.81
Food wastes	419.26
Garden wastes	2439.76
Paper ,packages waste	636.84
Plastic waste	538.52
Glass waste	646.18
TOTAL	9972.37
TOTAL per Employee	7.34

Table 2.2.2. Wastes collected in UGAL

Commodities Item	Consummation, t/year
Beef meat	0.626
Pork meat	2.906
Poultry	5.337
Fish	0.089
Vegetables	19.568
Pulses, Flavourings	0.436
Eggs	0.602
Milk	1.362
Cream	0.423
Cheese	0.372
Pasta	0.403
Rice	0.648
Sugar	0.090
Vegetable oils	3.274
Flours	0.357
Cereals	1.468
TOTAL	35.862

Table 2.3. Commodities Consummation in UGAL canteen

2.3 Results and discussions

The results of EFA include the basic lifecycle data for food consummation, energy demand, food wastes and transportation (Table2. 4). The results of CFA include the basic lifecycle data for food consummation, energy demand, food wastes and transportation (Table2. 5).

Component	EF, gha
Energy	12301.674
Electricity	1302.045
Gas	5953.629
Coal	5046
Water	380.425
Wastes	3.025
Transport	1479.4
Traffic car	1479.4
Commodities (Foodprint)	559.565
EF UGAL 2010	14724.089
EF per student	0.818
EF per capita	0.760
Ecological Foodprint per in campus students	0.016
Ecological Foodprint per student which serve the meal in the campus area	1.39

Table 2.4. UGAL Ecological Footprint Assessment

Component	CF, tCO2Eq
Energy	1358.451
Electricity	1148.361
Gas	143.406
Coal	66.684
Water	0.80
Wastes	3.3
Transport	5177.9
Autoutilitares (175 g/km)	5177.9
Commodities	43.722
Total CF, UGAL 2010	6584.173
CF per students	0.365
CF per capita	0.340

Table 2.5. UGAL Carbon Footprint Assessment

The calculated EF value per students is 0.818 gha and per capita 0.760 gha. The Eco-Indicators values are reasonable in compare with the WWF recommendation (average of 1.9 gha per capita) and the values reported by the other universities (Table 6). Energy, transports and foods are the most important parts of the total EF value. In the food processing department, vegetables, poultry, beef and vegetable oils have the greatest ratio in the total EF due to the greatest amount in the daily canteen use. In fact, only beef induce the leading impact on the total agro-foods EF and CF, respectively. Vegetables, milk, fruits and cereals have the lower value of EF and the ratio proposed in the optimized Eco-menus must be increased in order to generate a significant reducing of the total EF. The poultry items present the lowest ecological and emissive impact, in average with 3 times less than beef items. The regular use of low-carbon fish (mackerel, herring) could reduce substantially the meal's average carbon footprint. The food commodities created by an intensive processing such refining (oils, sugar), dry substance concentration (cream, cheese, pasta, cans) or extraction (flour) multiply the EF value of the raw material with the number of concentration /extraction degree. This is a strong reason for avoid the large quantities of industrialized foods, herbs, eggs and red meats and valorise the raw, unprocessed and fresh local/traditional products as input in the canteen production. In terms of gas emissive effect, the EC per student is calculated at 0.365 tCO2Eq/ year and EC per capita is 0.340 tCO2Eq/ year. The electricity represent 84.5% from total emission generated by all forms of energy used in UGAL facilities and the transportation system cover 78.64% from total CF. Food commodities have a minor impact on the total CF (0.066%) and the undercollected wastes (7.34 kg/year, employees) represent an insignifiant part (0.005%, 3.025 EF units per year). In the food processing department the pork items are environmentally more favourable than chicken and the chicken items are more environmentally favourable than lamb and beef. Beef is found to be around four times more CO2-emissions intense than pork meat. The comparative results of the present research and prior studies conducted in other campuses and universities are presented in Table 2.6.

	University								
	Dunarea de Jos University Galati (UGAL)	University of Illinois at Chicago	University of Newcastle	Holme Lacy College, UK	Northea-stern University, China	University of Toronto at Missis-sauga	Colorado College	Kwantlen University College	Ohio State University Columbus
Year	2010	2008	1999	2001	2003	2005	2006	2006	2007
EF, gha	14724.08	97601	3592	296	24787	8744	5603	3039	650,666
Ratio EF to land area	897.81	1005	26	1.23	50	97	154	81	916
EF per capita	0.76	2.66	0.19	0.57	1.06	1.07	2.24	0.33	8.66
Energy %	83	72.66	47	19	67.97	69.40	87	28.90	23.30
Trans-port,%	10	12.60	46	23	0.08	16.10	1.40	53	72.24
Mate-rials and Waste, %	0.02	11.83	2	32	5.74	4	na	na	4.46
Paper, %	na	na	na	na	2	na	na	7.20	na
Food, %	3.8	2.60	2	25	21.80	9.20	10	9.60	na
Built-up land,%	na	0.18	2	1%	0.44	1.20	na	1.10	w/ transport
Water %	0.02	0.14%	1	w/built-up land	2	0.20	1	0.16	na
Source	Vintila, 2011	Vene-toulis, 2001	Flint, 2001	Dawe et al., 2004	Li et al., 2004	Conway et al., 2004	Wright, 2002	Burgess and Lai, 2006	Janis, 2007

Table 2.6. Comparison of EF for colleges and universities

The results are very much similar with the others presented in the previsious works, in terms of EF per capita and ratio of the principal UGAL EF elements (energy 83%, transport 10%, water 2.5%, food 3.8%, wastes 0.02%) from the total EF value. The proportion of the energy module is overload because of the traditional technologies involved in the general management and the ratio of food is underload because only 11.7% of the total UGAL in-campus students eat in the canteen facilities every day.

2.4 Conclusions

Both EF and CF represent efficient and consistent tools to measure sustainable development by comparing scolar communities consumption of natural resources and the corresponding bio-capacity. The principal conclusions of the Eco-Indicators assessment are as followings:

- the energy consummation for food processing is in average 3.967MWh/t, 10% from total energy consumed in UGAL;

- meats commodities are the greatest emissive items involved in the daily menus and the potential environmental damage is estimated at 74.56% from the total foods EF (Foodprint value);
- the primary agricultural products present the lowest EF value; in contrast, a greater industrialisation food degree due to a proportionally increasing of foodprint value (in case of refined foods as oils, sugar or food derivates such as cream, butter or cheese);
- as a general rule, the degree of the principal compound from the dry substance concentrated in the industrialisation process represent the factor of multiplying the EF value of the raw food;
- the average wastes generated in a day is 0.036t and in average the ratio food/food wastes is 3.59/1;
- the smallest impact on both gas emissive effect (CF) an EF value is generated by the wastes 0,02% from total EF, followed by water 2.5% and food 3.8%.

As a general rule, the choice of raw materials have a considerable impact on greenhouse emissions. Different food ingredients such low-carbon fish and meats can reduce substantially a meal's average foodprint.

3. Part 3

In the third stage of the research, the ecological footprint analysis (EFA) was conducted in order to analyze the environmental impact of improved catering processing system by using an increasing amount of 15-25% regional organic agro-foods and 50% less amount of meat in the daily meals created for "Dunarea de Jos" University Galati (UGAL) students in 2010. The ecological footprint (EF) was proposed as a tool to measure progress towards the future goal of increasing the "Dunarea de Jos" University (UGAL) sustainability.
In the calculation of product-specific EF were considered all the life cycle assessment (LCA) elements including energy, materials system and wastes.Comparative analysis of agro-food origin (local, regional, national, EU) were conducted for the 6 main ingredients included in the daily menus of UGAL students. The variables of EF for the transportation system were capacity and distance. Independent studies, students collected data for the calculation of UGAL canteen footprint and analysis of surveys were conducted as methodology of the present research.

3.1 Introduction

Nowadays, the EU caterers are concerned about environmental and sustainability issues, including the provenance and production methods of procured food, waste management and energy and water consumption (Lintukangas *et al.*,2007). In the last 5 years, there has been a growing interest in the phenomenon of 'alternative agro-food networks', and locally sourced organically produced food has been suggested as a model of sustainable consumption for a range of economic, social and environmental reasons (Mikkola, 2008). Today, the most commonly cited reasons for consuming organic food are: food safety, the environment, animal welfare, and taste (Soil Association, 2002). Food co-operatives, farmers' markets, community supported agriculture groups among others were formed in order to provide consumers with organic and locally grown food. They aim to revitalise local food economies and to protect the environment (Walker and Preuss, 2008). Political

recommendations encourage catering organisations to increase the use of local and organic food 10–15% annually. Caterers often perceive the procurement of local and organic food as a problem in terms of budgets, tenders and logistic efficiency (Taskinen and Tuikkanen, 2004). A professional social service include the issue for ecological sustainability in their professional daily operation (Koester et al., 2006).
The present paper research investigate the impact on menu EF of introducing more local organic foods and less meat, at the same nutritional balance imposed by the EU regulation for healthy young's nutrition in public establishments.

3.2 Model for calculating the ecological footprint for daily menus of UGAL students

The EF is a function of population and per capital material consumption. In order to evaluate the improving of student's daily menu EF by replacing 50-100 % of red meat products (beef) with fishy products in the weekly meals created for UGAL student's in 2010, the researchuse the ecological footprint evaluation (EFE).
According to the original calculation model of Wackernagel and Rees [6] a modified original calculation model for the menu EF calculation is proposed:

$$EF = \sum_{I=1}^{N} EF_i \bullet f_i \tag{3.1}$$

In the Equation (3.1), EF_i is the EF per menu ingredient i (m^2) calculated with LCA methodology; f_i are the ratio of natural ingredient i in the daily menu; N is the number of food ingredients considered from the menu structure (N=6 in the present research). The meal components (N) included in EFE were red meat, poultry, fish, vegetables (fresh fruit, garnish vegetables), milk products and bread.
The data of food origin and transportation system for EFE were obtained directly from the UGAL canteen management office. The EFE were conducted by grouping the raw foods under the following variables of origin and transportation system:

i. local-low capacity isotherms, transportation cycle under 50km;
ii. Regional-big capacity isotherms, transportation cycle under 200km;
iii. National- big capacity isotherms, transportation cycle under 1000km;
iv. UE- big capacity isotherms, transportation cycle under 10000km.

From the analysis of the students survey questionnaires, 60% of total UGAL students have 5 meals on a week in the canteen and the fish products are the main course (150g) once in a week. In average, 702 meals with fishy products are designed in a week and the total consuming value in an academically year (9 months) is about 947.7 kg. The total consummation of red meat is 300g/student, week and in an academically year the canteen process 1895.40 kg.
The UGAL student's daily meals were composed with hors d'oeuvre, main dish & garnish & salad and dessert (total meal weight 380g). Four meals, two traditional (MC1, MC2) and two Eco (EC1, EC2) were composed and subsequently analysed under EFE protocol:
MC1-Red Meat (beef) 50%; Veg-25%; Milk dessert 15%; Bread 10%.
MC2- Meat (poultry) 50%; Veg-25%; Milk dessert 15%; Bread 10%.
EC1-Red Meat (beef) 25%; Fish 25% Veg-25%; Milk dessert 15%; Bread 10%.
EC2- Fish 50%; Veg-25%; Milk dessert15%; Bread 10%.

The EC1 menu were designed for a reducing with 50% of the meat content and in EC2 red meat is completely eliminated and replaced with fishy products in the main dish recipes. The ratio Animal Origin Product/Vegetable Origin Product (AOP/VOP) was designed at 65/35%.
The increasing amount of local organic foods (fish, vegetables, milk, products, bread) in EC1 and EC2 were of 25% and 50% respectively, compared with MC1, MC2.

3.3 EFA methodology based on Life Cycle Assessment (LCA) method

In the calculation of product-specific EF we consider all the quality-controlled life cycle information including energy, materials, transportation and wastes.
In LCA method, the EF of a food item is defined as the sum of direct land occupation and indirect land occupation, related to the total CO2 emissions from fossil energy associated with the transformation (industrial processing) and transportation cycle:

$$EF_i = EF_B + EF_P + EF_T \tag{3.2}$$

In Equation (3.2) EF_B is the basic EF related to the land occupation 6 types identified, calculated with the formula (3.3):

$$EF_B = \sum_{i=1}^{n} F_i qF_i \tag{3.3}$$

Where: EF_B is the ecological footprint of direct land occupation (m2), F_i is the occupation of area by land use types i (m2) and qF_i is the equivalence factor of land use (Table 3.1). Fish yields for the RO and world yields were based on FAO evaluation (FAO, 2007).

EF Parameters	Value
Equivalence factor Forest	1.4
Equivalence factor built-up area	2.2
Equivalence factor primary cropland	2.2
Equivalence factor hydropower area	1.0
Equivalence factor pasture	0.5
Equivalence factor marine area	0.4
Fraction CO2 absorbed by the ocean	0.3
Sequestration rate of CO2	0.4
Fossil fuel emission intensity of CO2	0.07

Table 3.1. The equivalence factors and primary parameters involved in the EF calculation

In the EF methodology Yield and Equivalence factors averages is used in the area component in order to make adjustments due to bio-productivity differences of the same land type between various regions and of different land types globally. EF_P is calculated from the EF_B value with the average yield of the catering processing in the UGAL canteen.

The environmental impact generated by the transportation system was calculated with the original Equation (3.4):

$$EF_T = EF_C + EF_{TS} + EF_{CO_2} \tag{3.4}$$

Where: EF_T is the EF value for transportation system adopted for the raw materials; EF_C is the EF value for the production of the fuel consumed in the transportation of raw foods; EF_{TS} is the EF value for the transportation state in the refrigeration units; EF_{CO_2} is the EF value involved by the pollution generated with the emission of CO_2 in course of the transportation cycle.

3.4 Results and discussions

The 6 main ingredients used in the structure of the daily menus of UGAL canteen were analyzed under EFE methodology using the LCA assessment protocol. The EF depending on origin and transportation system, in terms of distance and thermal state, were presented in Figure3.1. The red meat induced the leading impact on the total menu EF, beef especially because 1 Kg of meat imposed a consummation of minimum 5-6 kg of crops. The indigen fish species show a medium environmental impact, similar with the pork and poultry meat. The main fish species with UE origin analysed in the present research were hake (Merluccius merluccius), Sardina pilchardus, and Mackerel. If we consider the red meat EF as a reference, at the local level, we can reduce with 62.87% the menu EF if we replace the equivalent quantities with poultry and with 56.06% by replacing it with fishy product. The calculation of the integral bread EF were realised for EF of wheat equal with 8.31 and we obtain a value with 4.76 times lower than our reference. Vegetables and milk from local origin have the lower value of EF and the ratio proposed in the optimised Eco-menus must be increased in order to generate a significant reducing of total menu EF.

In the menu cases, the origin and transportation systems have a secondary impact in face of item ratio in recipe formula (Figure3.2). In all origin case investigated, MC1 trial with the greatest content of red meat, show the most extended value of EF, ranged from 12.82 units to 13.76 m2/menu.

The origin of farm from canteen proximity imposed for all menu ingredients determined a reducing with 6.83% of the total EF reported at the UE origin and 3.97% reported at the national item origin. The MC2 menus trial show the lowest value of total EF due to the total replacing of beef with poultry, the category of meat with the lowest EF impact. In EC1 cases, a more balanced ratio of meat products were proposed in which half of red meat is replaced by fish and the EF were reduced with 27.45% in local origin of menu items and with 25.36% in UE origin case. EC1 is the most equilibrate menu in terms of nutritional balance, costs and environment impact. EC2 menus trial show a good total EF, slightly up to MC2 due to the impact of fish EF similar with poultry EF but with 2.27 times less than red meat (beef). The inclusion of ecologist wave strategy in the canteen future policy will due to a reducing of UGAL canteen EF with 17.27% in the food module and, also, a reducing of food costs with 20.83% only by doubling the MC2 menu in a week instead of doubling the MC1. In the actual state of UGAL canteen system, in 9 months of academically activity, EF per capita of student were evaluated at 0.9132 gha. The EF evolution trend could be improved at 0.7554 gha, by the simple replacing of analysed items with local sources and regular replace once in a week of beef with poultry or fish products.

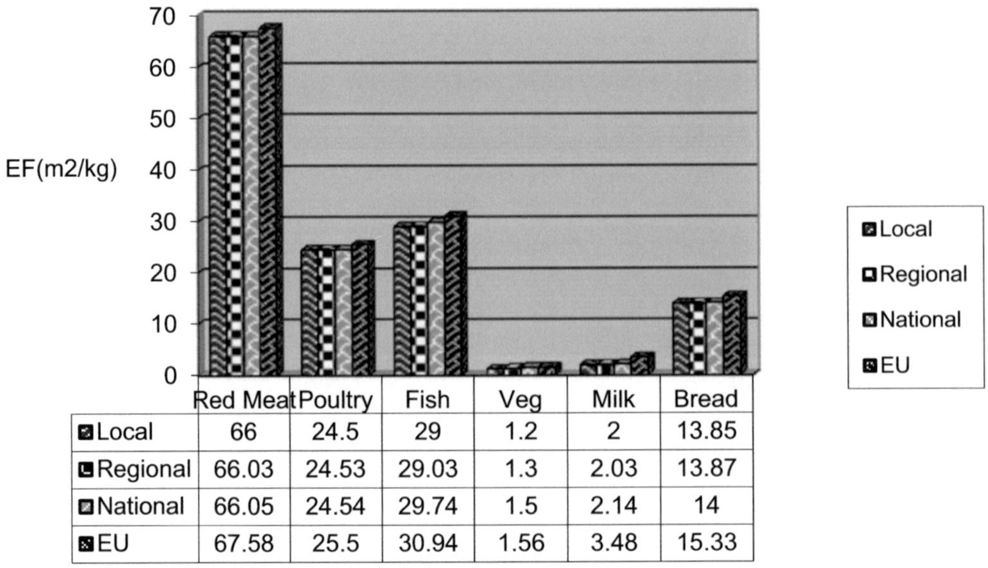

	Red Meat	Poultry	Fish	Veg	Milk	Bread
Local	66	24.5	29	1.2	2	13.85
Regional	66.03	24.53	29.03	1.3	2.03	13.87
National	66.05	24.54	29.74	1.5	2.14	14
EU	67.58	25.5	30.94	1.56	3.48	15.33

Fig. 3.1. Ecological Footprint value (m^2/menu) for menus ingredients

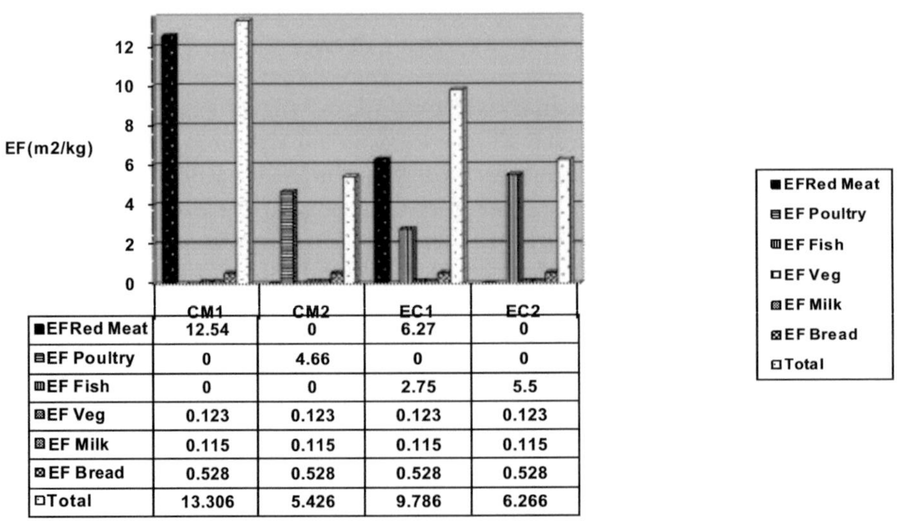

	CM1	CM2	EC1	EC2
EFRed Meat	12.54	0	6.27	0
EF Poultry	0	4.66	0	0
EF Fish	0	0	2.75	5.5
EF Veg	0.123	0.123	0.123	0.123
EF Milk	0.115	0.115	0.115	0.115
EF Bread	0.528	0.528	0.528	0.528
Total	13.306	5.426	9.786	6.266

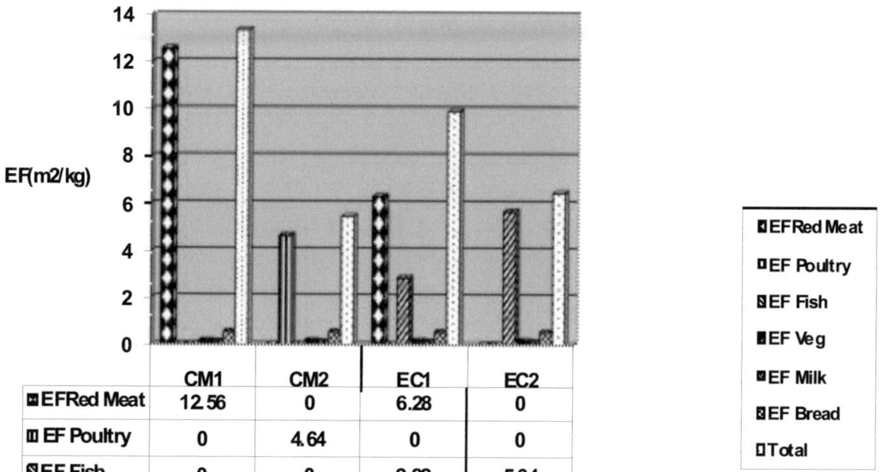

	CM1	CM2	EC1	EC2
EFRed Meat	12.56	0	6.28	0
EF Poultry	0	4.64	0	0
EF Fish	0	0	2.82	5.64
EF Veg	0.142	0.142	0.142	0.142
EF Milk	0.121	0.121	0.121	0.121
EF Bread	0.532	0.532	0.532	0.532
Total	13.355	5.437	9.895	6.435

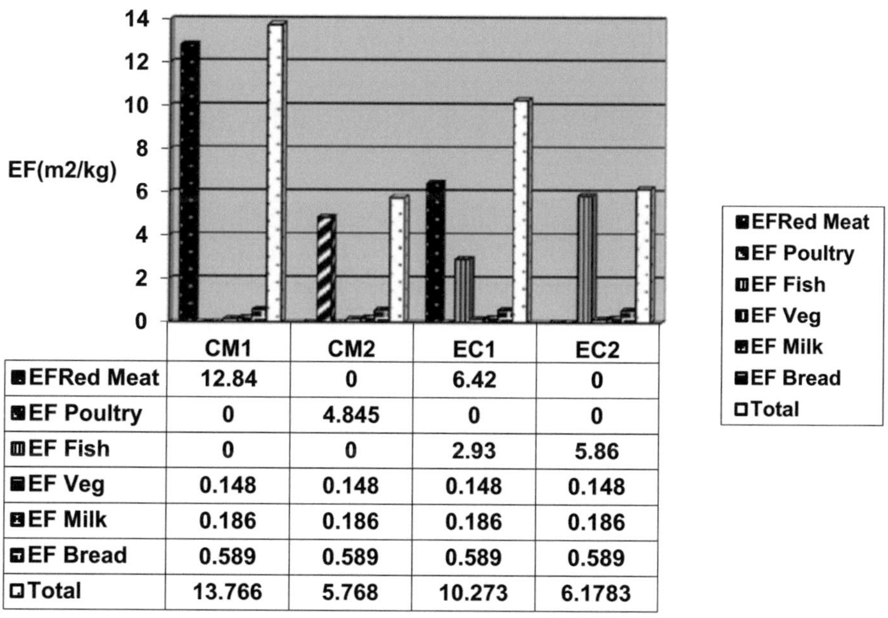

	CM1	CM2	EC1	EC2
EFRed Meat	12.84	0	6.42	0
EF Poultry	0	4.845	0	0
EF Fish	0	0	2.93	5.86
EF Veg	0.148	0.148	0.148	0.148
EF Milk	0.186	0.186	0.186	0.186
EF Bread	0.589	0.589	0.589	0.589
Total	13.766	5.768	10.273	6.1783

Fig. 3.2. Ecological Footprint value (m^2/menu) for conventional and Eco-friendly menus designed with local, regional, national and EU origin ingredients

3.5 Conclusions

The EF has become a new efficient method to measure regional sustainable development by comparing humanity's consumption of natural resources and world biocapacity. EF estimates the environmental impact due to energy use and direct land occupation expressed in global hectares.

The following results were obtained in case of Eco-strategy implementation in the UGAL canteen: (1) reducing of UGAL canteen EF with 17.27% in the food module; (2) reducing of EF per student 0.7554 gha from 0.9132 gha; (3) a reducing of food costs with 20.83%.

The choice of raw materials can have a considerable impact on emissions. Different food ingredients such low-carbon fish and meats can reduce a meal's average carbon foodprint substantially. Actual statistics discussing about the contraction of the student population with 20% in the next 10 years and in the condition of resources limitation the Eco-management became a necessity in order to respect the regional biocapacity.

4. Part 4

In the final research stage, the ecological footprints (EF) analyses were conducted in order to evaluate the environment impact of improving actual catering system by replacing 50-100% of red meat products (beef) with local/regional fishy products in the weekly meals created for "Dunarea de Jos" University (UGAL) students in 2010. Product-specific EF was calculated from consistent and quality-controlled life cycle information of food products and services, including energy, materials, transport, waste treatment and infrastructural processes. The reducing of red meat products in the student's daily menus with 50% and the reducing of long food chain at the local/regional level determined a 36.24% average decreasing of actual menu EF and the replacing of red meat with fishy products a 72.2% reducing of Eco-menus EF. At least 20.83% less amount of money could be saved in the menu creations and if we replace one day in a week 50% meat with local fishy products and the average reducing EF for menu creation in an academic year could be in average 17.27%.

4.1 Introduction

The ecological footprint (EF) was initially conceptualised by William Rees (1992) and further developed by Mathis Wackernagel (1994). The EF estimates the "minimum land necessary to provide the basic energy and material flows required by the economy" (Wackernagel & Yount 1998, 2000; Wackernagel & Silverstein 2000; Petrescu et al 2010). EF provides a measure of the extent to which human activities exceed two specific environmental limits – the availability of bioproductive land and the availability of forest areas to sequester carbon dioxide emissions. The EF integrates (i) the area required for the production of crops, forest products and animal products, (ii) the area required to sequester atmospheric CO_2 emissions dominantly caused by fossil fuel combustion, and (iii) the area required by nuclear energy demand (Monfreda et al 2004).

In 2005 the global EF was 17.5 billion global hectares (gha), or 2.7 gha per person (a global hectare is a hectare with world-average ability to produce resources and absorb wastes). The total productive area (earth biocapacity) was 13.6 billion gha, 2.1 gha per person respectively. Humanity's footprint first exceeded the Earth's total biocapacity in the 1980s. The 2005 overshoot of 30% would reach 100% in the 2030 even if recent increases in agricultural yields continue (Flint 2001). This means that biological capacity equal to two

planets would be required to keep up with humanity's resource demands and waste production (FAO, 2002).
With an average growth rate of 6.9% per year, aquaculture is the fastest growing food production sector in the world. This rapid growth faces, however, some limitations in the availability of suitable sites and in the ecological carrying capacity of actual sources. The discipline of ecological engineering addresses and quantifies the processes that are involved with management of wastes as a resource (Coll et al 2006).
Ecosystem-based management (EBM) is an integrated approach that encompasses the complexities of ecosystem dynamics, the social and economic needs of human communities, and the maintenance of diverse, functioning and healthy ecosystems (Christensen & Walters 2004).
The public universities have a particular social responsibility in being role models for encouraging best environmental practice, due to their considerable influence on societal development. Recent studies concerning ecological footprints have been focussed in University settings, given their significant social responsibility. The demand for green product rises with the number of consumers who are sensitive to environment matter and especially their degree of sensitivity (Viebahn, 2002).
The present part of research investigate the impact on menu EF of introducing more local fishy products and less red meat, at the same nutritional balance imposed by the EU regulation for healthy young's nutrition in canteens.

4.2 Method of investigation

In order to evaluate the improving of student's daily menu EF by replacing 50-100 % of red meat products (beef) with local/regional fishy products in the weekly meals created for UGAL student's in 2010, this paper use the ecological footprint evaluation (EFE). The data of food origin and transportation system for EFE were obtained directly from the canteen management office of UGAL. The EFE were conducted for fresh fishy products with the following variables of food origin and transportation system:

i. Local- low capacity isotherms, transportation cycle under 50 km;
ii. National- big capacity isotherms, transportation cycle under 1000 km;

In the calculation of product-specific EF we consider all the quality-controlled life cycle information including energy, materials, transport, waste treatment and infrastructural processes. 60% of total UGAL Students have 5 meals on a week in the canteen and the fish products are the main course (150g) once in a week. In average, 702 meals with fishy products are designed in a week and the total consuming value in an academically year (9 months) is about 947.7 kg. The total consummation of red meat is 300g/student, week and in an academically year the canteen process 1895.40 kg. The UGAL student's daily meals were composed of hors d'oeuvre, main dish with garnish and salad and dessert (total 380g). The meal components evaluated in EFE were red meat, poultry, fish, vegetables (fresh fruit, garnish vegetables), milk products and bread. Four meals, two traditional (MC1, MC2) and two Eco (EC1, EC2) were composed and subsequently analysed under EFA experimental protocol:
MC1-Red Meat (beef) 50%; Veg-25%; Milk dessert 15%; Bread 10%.
MC2- Meat (poultry) 50%; Veg-25%; Milk dessert 15%; Bread 10%.
EC1-Red Meat (beef) 25%; Fish 25% Veg-25%; Milk dessert 15%; Bread 10%.

EC2- Fish 50%; Veg-25%; Milk dessert15%; Bread 10%.
The EC1 menu were designed for a reducing with 50% of the meat content and in EC2 case meat is completely eliminated in face of fishy products included in the main dish recipes. The ratio Animal Origin Product/Vegetable Origin Product (AOP/VOP) was designed at 65/35%. The increasing amount of regional organic foods (fish, vegetables, milk, products, bread) in EC1 and EC2 were of 25% and 50% respectively, compared with MC1, MC2. In term of costs management, the calculation of costs reducing were realised with an average market acquisition value of 2.85 Euro/kg in case of red meat and 1.66 Euro/kg in fish product case.

4.3 Results and discussion

The fishy ingredients used in the UGAL canteen (Horse mackerel *Trachurus trachurus*, Blue Fish *Pomatomius saltatrix*, Sprat *Sprattus sprattus sulinus* Antipa, Bonito *Sarda sarda*) are top quality, high nutritional value and with significant health benefits. The regular integration in the institutionalised canteens of the universities generated a reducing of the environmental impact, which is 2.69 times decreased compared with the red meat of local origin (Figure 4.1).
The proximity of Danube source give a better raw EF value for fish, reduced with 2% than national origin fishy products and the overall environmental impact will be decreased with 2.48% all the time when the local produced fish will be favourites in the canteen acquisition.

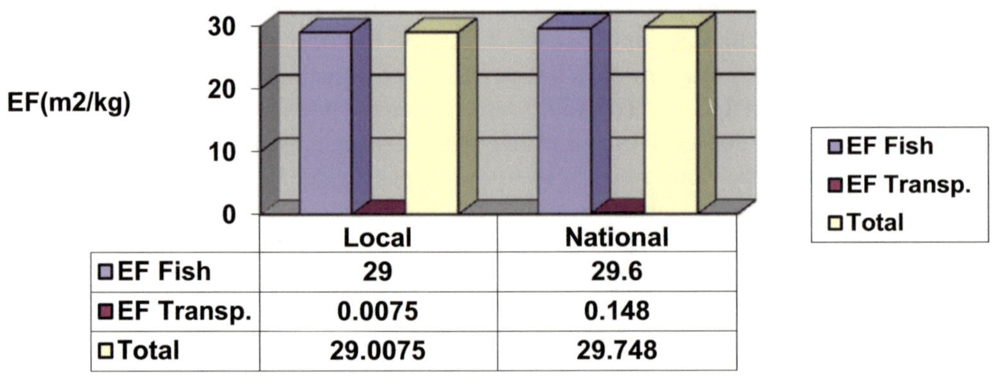

	Local	National
EF Fish	29	29.6
EF Transp.	0.0075	0.148
Total	29.0075	29.748

Fig. 4.1. Ecological Footprint value (m^2/kg) for fishy products

On the national origin basis, the results of EFE for one menu item utilised as main course in the weekly cycled menus for UGAL students show that the regular use of local instead national origin fishy products determined a reducing of the EF for transportation cycle of 94.93 % (Figure 4.2).
In all cases, the items with national origin determined an important increase of the recipe item EF despite the more productive value of the primary cycle compensated by the increasing of the resources consuming with the transportation in the refrigerated state. In the red meat case (beef), the EF value for raw brut products were reduced with 0.15% in case of national centralised farms. The high capacities of production farms due to high efficiency

in the abatorization processing system but the transportation cycle with high capacity isotherms in the refrigerated state increase the meat EF with 0.148 units instead of 0.0075 in the local origin case (Figure4.3).

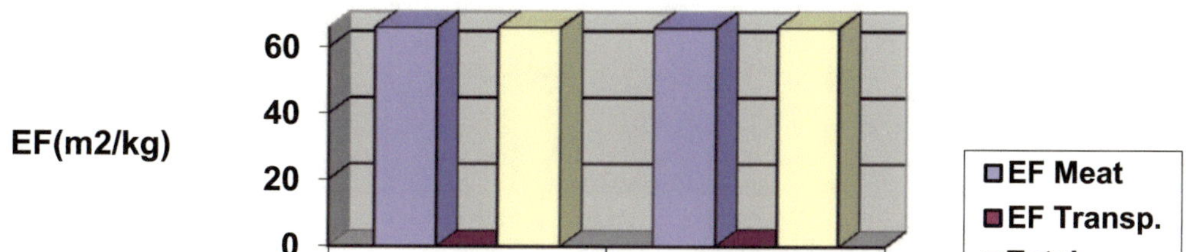

	Local	National
EF Meat	66	65.9
EF Transp.	0.0075	0.148
Total	66.0075	66.048

Fig. 4.2. Ecological Footprint value (m^2/kg) for red meat products

The EF for national common vegetables (potatoes, carrots, bean, fruits) is 1.5 units, with 20% greater than in the case of a local vegetables and with 13.33% increased in compare with the regional level (under 200km) source, respectively.
In the menu cases, the 50% replacing of red meat (beef) content in the daily menus with local fishy products in EC1 case and with 100% in EC2 case, on the conventional MC1 menu basis, generate a reducing of overall menu EF with 27.45% in EC1 case and with 54.83% in EC2 case.

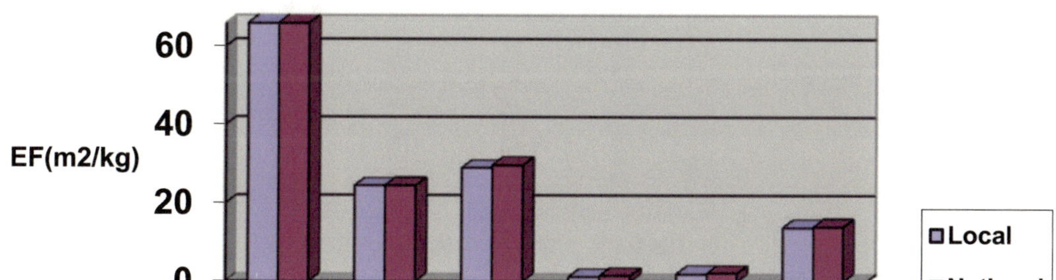

	Red Meat	Poultry	Fish	Vegetable	Milk	Bread
Local	66	24.5	29	1.2	2	13.85
National	66.05	24.54	29.74	1.5	2.13	14

Menu ingredient

Fig. 4.3. Ecological Footprint value (m^2/kg) for menus natural ingredients with local and national origin

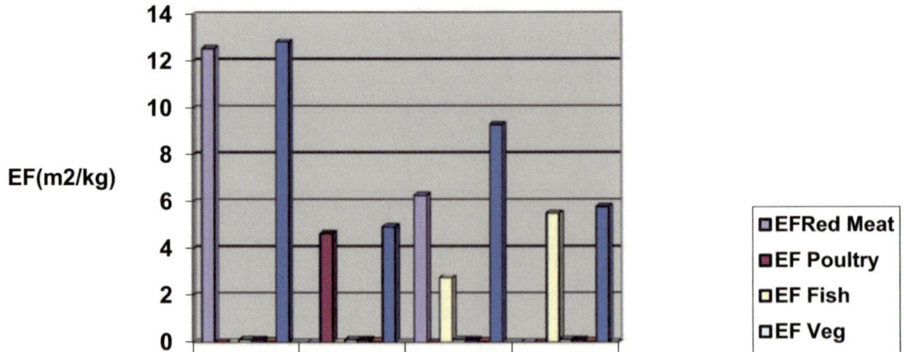

	CM1	CM2	EC1	EC2
EFRed Meat	12.54	0	6.27	0
EF Poultry	0	4.655	0	0
EF Fish	0	0	2.755	5.51
EF Veg	0.114	0.114	0.114	0.114
EF Milk	0.114	0.114	0.114	0.114
EF Bread	0.052	0.052	0.052	0.052
Total	12.82	4.935	9.305	5.79

Fig. 4.4. Ecological Footprint value (m²/menu) for Conventional and Eco-friendly menus designed with local natural ingredients

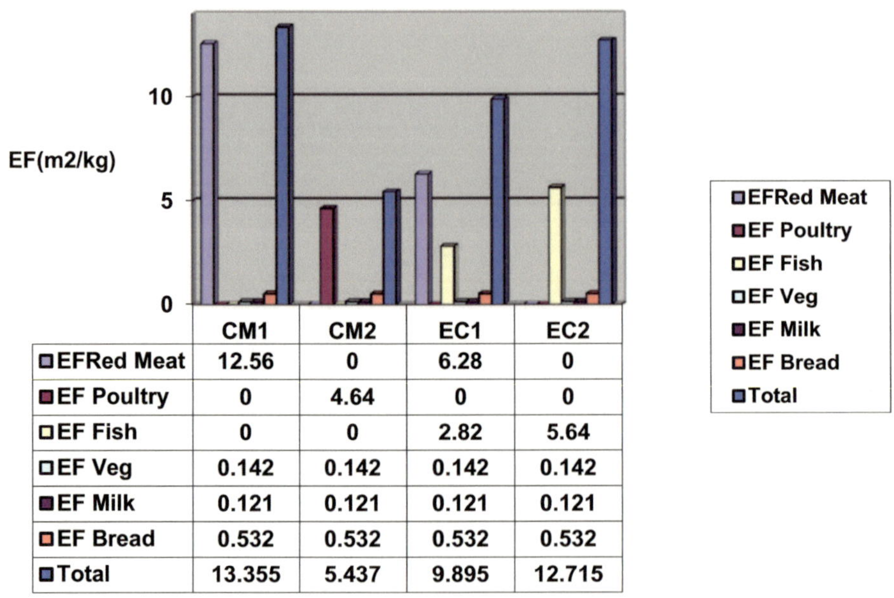

	CM1	CM2	EC1	EC2
EFRed Meat	12.56	0	6.28	0
EF Poultry	0	4.64	0	0
EF Fish	0	0	2.82	5.64
EF Veg	0.142	0.142	0.142	0.142
EF Milk	0.121	0.121	0.121	0.121
EF Bread	0.532	0.532	0.532	0.532
Total	13.355	5.437	9.895	12.715

Fig. 4.5. Ecological Footprint value (m²/menu) for conventional and Eco-friendly menus designed with national ingredients

In case of national origin ingredients, a part of menu EF increasing produced by the replacing of red meat with fish is lost in the transportation cycle. The overall menu EF decreased at 25.91% in EC1 case and with 51.79% in EC2 case at CM1 basis (Figure 4.5).
The total EF of final menu depends on the items ratio at the same origin and transportation system. Raw beef have the greatest EF amount in the all experimented menu and the vegetables the lowest value added to total EF of menu. The white meat of local origin has a reduced impact on the total menus EF because the poultry EF were with 62.87% reduced compared with red meat at the same origin and transportation system. For this reason, a replacing of red meat with poultry determined a reducing of MC2 EF with 61.54% compared with MC1. The replacing with fishy local products in EC2 case determined a reducing with almost 54.83%of the overall menu EF, because the fish EF is with 15.5% greater than poultry EF. The menu formula MC2 show the best EF values if is composed with local origin ingredients. From the environmental, nutritional and financial point of views we recommended the EC2 formula at least once in a week and MC2 formula twice in every chart pre-planification of UGAL canteen. In the situation in which the management of UGAL canteen decide to change the actual state of menu chart 2 MC1 formula +MC2+ EC1+ EC2/week with 2MC2+MC1+ EC1+ EC2/week, the canteen food EF module could be reduced with 17.27% in an academic year, with the promotion of the local acquisition circuits.
The menus designed with all ingredients of national origin showed a increasing of the overall EF of 3.8-9.2% in CM1-CM2 menus cases, 5.9-10 % in EC1-EC2 menus cases, respectively. The transportation system in the refrigerated state of fish and milk due to a increasing of resources using measured with EF value of 94.93%. On the CM1 basis, there is the possibility to reduce the menu EF with 18.6% in the EC1 case and 19% in EC2 case. On the CM2 basis, the total EF reducing value for the complete menu were of 23.07% for EC1 menu and 51.79% for EC2 menu, respectively. In the same time, the price were consistently reduced for Eco-friendly menus which replace the red meat with local origin fishy products, with about 41.66% (from 1.80 Euro in case of CM1 menu to 1.05 Euro in EC2 case) in the same nutritional equivalence of the final menu.

4.4 Conclusions

The dominating components of ecological footprint were raw material production system and energy necessary for transportation. The reducing of red meat products in the student's daily menus with 50% and the reducing of long food chain at the local/regional level give a 36.24% average decreasing of EC1 menu EF and the replacing of red meat with fishy products a 72.2% reducing of EC2 menus EF. At least 20.83% less amount of money could be saved in the menu creations if we replace one day in a week 50% meat with local fishy products and the average reducing EF for menu creation in an academic year could be 17.27%. In the same time, the catering systems create an important bridge between young's and the local products and the sustainable development of the regions will be encouraged. The local origin of agro-foods reduce the environment impact despite the fact that the total efficiency is lower than in centralized regional or national farms, in terms of productivity and primary processing yield. The red meat induced the leading impact on the total agrofoods EF. Vegetables, fruits and cereals with local origin have the lower value of EF and the ratio proposed in the optimized Eco-menus must be increased in order to generate a significant reducing of total EF. The results also indicate that using low-carbon fish (mackerel, herring) and meats (chicken, turkey) can reduce substantially a meal's average carbon footprint. *Promoting the daily menu planning including vegetable from proximity sources (short chain producers), the public catering system could have three types of advantages: nutritional, ecological and financial.* A rational and efficient network composed from a biological agriculture source of agrofoods and an environmental friendly transportation facilities generate the best result in the reducing total EF of the final ready to eat product. By reducing the quantities of meat, especially beef and sea fish and increasing the proportion of locally organic cereals, potatoes and fruits a reducing with 50% of total daily food EF is possible in case of a eco-attitude adopted in the public institution.

With the further development of international free market economy, the living standard and living quality of people will be improved constantly, which certainly will due to a constantly increasing of energy and raw material consummation.

A global eco-strategy must be constructed in the near future in order to reduce our actual EF on the individual, institutional and national scale

5. Acknowledgment

The author would like to thank the UGAL Rector Prof. Minzu Viorel, UGAL General administration Head Ms.Narcisa Condrea, UGAL Canteen Administration Head Mr.Bichescu Cezar and his collaborator Ms.Onofrei Nicoleta. Further, the author would to express a special thank you to all the collaborators from AgroBio 35 Mr.Jaffre, Conseil Regional de Bretagne Ms. Rouger, Manger Bio35 Mr.Gabillard, Association Solidarite 35 Mr.Venien and Ms.Sinequin, Scarabee BioCoop Mr.Chevalier, FRCIVAM Mr.Marechal, Inter Bio Bretagne Ms.Fassel, Les Quisines du Quotidien Mr.Mariot.

6. References

Arrow K., Bolin B., Costanza R., Dasgupta P., Folke C., Holling C.S., Jansson B.-O., Levin Bagliani M., Ferlaino F. and Procopio S. (2002). Ecological footprint and input-output methodology: the analysis of the environmental sustainability of the economic sectors of Piedmont Region (Italy), *14th International Conference on Input-Output Techniques*, Montréal

Albino V. and Kühtz S. (2002). Environmental footprint of industrial districts using input/output tables based on production processes, *14th International Conference on Input-Output Techniques*, Montréal

Burgess, B., Lai, J.(2006). Ecological Footprint Analysis and Review: Kwantlen University College

Chambers, N., Simmons, C., Wackernagel, M. (2000). Sharing Nature's Interest: Ecological Footprints as an Indicator of Sustainability. *Earthscan Publications* Ltd.,London

Chambers N. and Lewis K. (2001). Ecological footprint analysis: towards a sustainability indicator for business. Research Report No. 65, *Association of Chartered Certified Accountants, London*

Carbon Trust.(2006). Energy and Carbon Conversion. The Carbon Trust, London

Christensen V., Walters C.(2004). Ecopath with Ecosim: methods, capabilities and limitations. *Ecological Modelling* Vol.172, No.2-4,pp.109-139

Coll M., Shannon L. J., Moloney C. L., Palomera I., Tudela S.(2006). Comparing trophic flows and fishing impacts of a NW Mediterranean ecosystem with coastal upwellings

Costanza R. (2000). The dynamics of the ecological footprint concept, *Ecological Economics*, Vol.32,pp. 341-345

Conway, T.M., Dalton, C., Loo, J., Benakoun, L. (2008). Developing ecological footprint scenarios on university campuses. A case study of the University of Toronto at Mississauga. *Int. J. Sustainability High.* Ed. 9, pp.4-20

DEFRA. (2007). Environmental footprint and sustainability of horticulture (including potatoes): A comparison with other agricultural sectors, University of Warwick

DEFRA (2009). Guidelines to Defra.version 2.0. AEA for DECC and Defra.

Everett, S. & Aitchison, C.(2008). The role of food tourism in sustaining regional identity: a case study of Cornwall, South West England, *J.of Sustainable Tourism,* Vol. 16 ,No.2 ,pp. 150-167

FAO (2002). The State of World Fisheries and Aquaculture. UN Food and Agriculture Organisation, Rome.

Flint, K. (2001). Institutional ecological footprint analysis: a case study of the University of Newcastle, Australia. *Int. J. Sustainability High.* Ed. 2,pp.48-62.

Klein-Banai, C., Theis, T.L., Brecheisen, T.A., Banai, A. (2010). A greenhouse gas inventory as a measure of sustainability for an urban public research university. *Environ. Pract.,*Vol. 12, pp.35-47.

Janis, A. J. (2007). Quantifying the Ecological Footprint of the Ohio State University. Ph.D Thesis, The Ohio State University, Columbus.

Li, G.J., Wang, Q., Gu, X.W., Liu, J.X., Ding, Y., Liang, G.Y. (2008). Application of the componential methodology for ecological footprint calculation of a Chinese university campus. *Ecol. Indic.* Vol.8, pp.75-78.

Rees, W.E. (1992).Ecological footprints and appropriated carrying capacity: what urban economics leaves out. *J. Environment and Urbanisation* ,Vol.4,No.2,pp.121-130.

Rees, W.E., Wackernagal, M. (1996). Urban ecological footprints andwhycities cannot be sustainable - and why they are a key to sustainability. *Environ. Impact Assess.Rev.* 16,pp. 223-248.

Rees, W.E. (2003). Impeding sustainability? The ecological footprint of higher education. Plan. High. Ed. March-May.

Van Den Bergh, J., Grazi, F. (2010). On the Policy Relevance of Ecological Footprints Environ. *Sci. Technol.* Vol.44, pp.4843-4844.

Venetoulis, J. (2001). Assessing the ecological impact of a university: the ecological footprint for the University of Redlands. *Int. J. Sustainability High.* Ed. 2,pp. 180-196.

Wackernagel, M.(1991).Land Use: Measuring a Community's Appropriated Carrying Capacity as an Indicator for Sustainability and "Using Appropriated Carrying Capacity as an Indicator, Measuring the Sustainability of a Community.", Report I & II to the UBC Task Force on Healthy and Sustainable Communities, Vancouver.

Wackernagel, M., Rees, W. (1996). Our Ecological Footprint: Reducing Human Impact on the Earth. New Society Publishers, Gabriola Island, BC.

Wackernagel et al.(2002). Tracking the ecological overshoot of the human economy, Edward O. Wilson, Harvard University, Cambridge, MA.

Wright, E.P.(2002). The Ecological Footprint of the Colorado College: An Examination of Sustainability, Independent Study.

4

Assessment of Proximate and Phytochemical Composition for Evaluation of Nutritive Values of Some Plant Foods Obtained from Iran and India

Ali Aberoumand
Behbahan Khatemolanbia Technology University, Khuzestan Province, Iran

1. Introduction

The green Revolution and subsequent efforts through the application of science and technology for increasing food production in India have brought self-reliance in food. The impetus given by the Government, State Agricultural Universities, State departments of Agricultural and other organizations through the evolution and introduction of numerous hybrid varieties of cereals, legumes, fruits and vegetables and improved management practices have resulted increased food production. However, the nation still faces the problem of the use of improper methods for the storage of food stuffs, leading to great wastage of the food produced. Such loses in the food front aggravate the existing syndromes of under nutrition and malnutrition.

Fruits and vegetables, which are among the perishable commodities, are important ingredients in the human dietaries. Due to their high nutritive value, they make significant nutritional contribution to human well-being. The perishable fruits and vegetables are available as seasonal surpluses during certain parts of the year in different regions and are wasted in large quantities due to absence of facilities and know-low for proper handling, distribution, marketing and storage. Furthermore, massive amounts of the perishable fruits and vegetables, produced during a particular season result in a glut in the market and become scarce during other seasons. Neither can they all be consumed in fresh condition nor sold at economically viable prices.

In developing countries agriculture is the mainstay of the economy. As such, it should be no surprise that agricultural industries and related activities can account for a considerable proportion of their output. Of the various types of activities that can be termed as agriculturally based, fruits and vegetables processing are among the most important. Therefore, fruits and vegetables processing has been engaging the attention of planners and policy makers as it can contribute to the economic development of rural population. The utilization of resources both material and human is one of the ways of improving the economic status of family.All forms of preserved fruits are in the reach of only the urban elite, and the rural masses who produce more than 90% of theses fruits and vegetables are usually deprived of their usage.

India has made a fairly good progress on the Horticulture Map of the world with a total annual production of Fruits and Vegetables touching over 131 Million Tonnes during 1998-99. Today, India is the second largest producer of the Fruits (44 Million Tones) and vegetables(87.5 Million Tones) as mentioned in Indian Horticulture Database-2000 published by National Horticulture Board. Our share in the world production is about 10.1 per cent in fruits and 14.4 per cent in vegetables. The Horticulture crops cover about 8 per cent of the total area contributing about 20 per cent of the gross agricultural output in the country. India produces 41.7% of the world mangoes. 25.7% of the bananas and 13.6 per cent of the world onion. However, the productivity of fruits and vegetables grown in the country is low as compared to the developed countries. The overall productivity of fruits is 11.8 tonnes per hac. And vegetables is 14.9 tonnes per hac.

Fruits		Vegetables	
Country	Production (tones per hac)	Country	Production (tones per hac)
WORLD	434703	WORLD	606053
INDIA	44042	INDIA	87536
CHINA	53926	CHINA	237136
BRAZIL	37179	USA	34924
USA	31494	TURKEY	21743
ITALY	17676	ITALY	14501
SPAIN	13323	JAPAN	13629
MEXICO	12342	IRAN	12751
FRANCE	10863	EGYPT	12379
TURKEY	10263	RUSSIAN	12098
PHILIPPINES	10160	SPAIN	11496

Table 1. Major World Producers of Fruits and Vegetables(1998-1999)*

Through India is the second largest producer of fruits and vegetables in the world, out per capita consumption of fruits and vegetables for over one billion population is very low. More than 25 per cent of fruits and vegetables production is unfortunately wasted due to inadequate facilities for processing. Despite such a large production, their processing is yet to be developed properly. The processing includes pre-processing of fruits and vegetables before these are fit to be used for final conversation into processed foods. Delay in the use of harvested food takes away its freshness, palatability, appeal and nutritive value. Tropical fruits are luscious, juicy and pulpy. They can not be plucked early, cold-stored or subjected to controlled and long drawn out process as is possible in the case of fruits grown in temperate or cold regions. They are harvested at optimum maturity and processed or consumed promptly as they ripen because they require special attention and techniques. The Food preservation and processing industry has now become more of a necessity than being a luxury. It has an important role in the conservation and better utilization of fruits and vegetables. In order to avoid the glut and utilize the surplus during the season, it is necessary to employ modern methods to extend storage life for better distribution and also processing techniques to preserve them for utilization in the off season on both large scale and small scale.

Both established and planned fruit and vegetable processing projects aim at solving a very clearly identified development problem. This is that due to insufficient demand, weak infrastructure, poor transportation and perishable nature of the crops, the grower sustains substantial losses. During the post-harvest glut, the loss is considerable and often some of the produce has to be fed to animals or allowed to rot. Food processing, therefore, refers to the application of techniques to foods in a systematic manner for preventing losses through preservation, processing, packaging, storage and distribution, ultimately to ensure greater availability of a wide variety of foods which would help to improve the food intake and nutritional standards during the period of low availability.

2. Nutritional values of fruits and vegetables

The recommendation that the diet contain four servings fruits and vegetables does not emphasize the choices to be made within this group. Because foods in this group are so diverse in nutritional value, nutrition education programs promote the use of one serving of a citrus fruit or another fruit or vegetable high in ascorbic acid every day and a serving of dark green, yellow, or orange vegetables as a sources of vitamin A every other day. Because of the low caloric content of this group of foods, the INQ for vitamin C,A, and iron usually exceeds. In addition, valuable amounts of folacin, magnesium, and calcium will be contributed. In the vegetables and fruits, the amount of vitamin C present differs with the variety, the degree of maturity, the season, climatic conditions, the length and conditions of storage, ands the part of the plant used. The loss of nutrients in fruits and vegetables begins right after harvest and may be especially rapid in the first few hours. In addition to losses caused by oxidation, further loss can be attributed to the removal of parts of the plant during preparation to make the product moiré palatable. Since relatively few of the few of the dark green or yellow fruits and vegetables that are rich sources of carotene are popular or inexpensive items in the diet, a realistic approach to a food guide suggests the use of these every other day. this is additionally justified because of the stability of vitamin A and carotene and because foods that are rich sources usually provide more than the day's allowance in one serving. Thus a daily intake of foods high in vitamin A value, although desirable, id not absolutely necessary. The vitamin A value of typical dark green and yellow vegetables varies with the degree of pigmentation. Aside from the unique contribution of carotene and vitamin C, the fruits and vegetables group contributes about 25% of the day,s intake of iron. The amount of iron varies with the foods and parts chosen: iron content is higher in leaves than in stems, fruits, or underground portions. The absorption of iron from fruits and vegetables is less than 5%, primarily because of the high cellulose and phytic acid found in most vegetables. On the other hand, the vitamin C found in many fruits enhances iron absorption. The trace mineral content of fruits and vegetables depends on the amount present in the soil in which the plant was grown. The diverse geographical sources of fruits and vegetables and modern systems of transporting produce to market reduce the chance of a low intake. Calcium intake from fruits and vegetables is small compared to that from the milk group but will assume more importance if milk intake is low. If peas or beans are chosen , a rich source of thiamin is provided, and if dark green leafy vegetables such as spinach are used, riboflavin intake will be high.

Generally fruits and vegetables are poor sources of protein, and that present is of low biological value because of a lack of some essential amino acids. Roots and tubers contain

2% protein and 20% carbohydrates, whereas legumes such as pea and beans have 4% protein and 13% carbohydrate.

The energy contribution of the fruit and vegetable group is generally low because of the high proportion of cellulose and water and low fat content. Immature seeds, such as peas and beans, and starchy tubers, such as potatoes, contribute two to eight times as many calories per serving as do celery , carrots, spinach, and cabbage, which are high in cellulose and water but low in starch. One must remember, however, that the caloric contribution of a fruit or vegetable dish may be double or triple that of the basic food alone, depending on the way it is prepared. Another important nutritional benefit from the use of fruits and vegetables is the bulk provided by fiber. This promotes normal gastrointestinal motility and greatly facilitates the passage of food through the digestive tract, helping to prevent constipation. Recent evidence that low dietary fiber may be responsible for the increasing incidence of diverticulosis and that it may be associated with cancer of the colon is further reason to use fruits and vegetables.

Millions of people in many developing countries do not have enough food to meet their daily requirements and a further more people are deficient in one or more micronutrients (FAO 2004).Thus, in most cases rural communities depend on wild resources including wild edible plants to meet their food needs in periods of food crisis. we introduce plants selected for present investigation, from nutritive values point of view. Plant species selected were: *Alocacia indica Sch.,Asparagus officinalis DC., Chlorophytum comosum Linn., Cordia Myxa Roxb., Eulophia Ochreata Lindl., Momordica dioicia Roxb., Portulaca oleracia Linn. and Solanum indicum Linn.* It contains importance of selected food plants, their necessity of utilization and the occurrence in natural conditions in south regions of Iran and Maharashtra state such as around of Pune in India.

Selected wild edible plants were collected from various localities of Maharashtra(India) and Iran. Three wild edible plants were collected from India to names of *Alocacia indica, Momordica dioica* and *Eulophia ochreata* in September 2006. Five wild edible plants were collected from Iran to names *Asparagus officinalis, Chlorophytum comosum, Codia myxa, Portulaca oleracia* and *Solanum indicum* collected from Iran in October 2006 and April 2007. Efforts made to collect these plants in flowering and fruiting conditions for the correct botanical identification. Healthy and disease free edible plant part/s selected and dried them under shade so as to prevent the decomposition of chemical compounds present in them. All the dried material powdered in blander for further study.

3. Materials and methods

3.1 Plant material

Plant foods such as Cordia myxa R. fruit ,Alocacia indica S. Stem، Asparagus officinalis DC. Stem ، Momordica dioicia R. fruit، Eulophia ochreata L. tubers، Solanum indicum L. leaves، Portulaca oleracia L. Leaves and Stem، Chlorophytum comosum L. root tubers used as experimental material were collected from farm lands in Agricultural Research Central of Dezful , Khuzestan province, Iran and around Pune, India in October 2007. The collected plant material was placed in a polyethylene bag to prevent loss of moisture during transportation to the laboratory. Taxonomic identification of the plant was carried out at the Botany unit, Ramin Agricultural University, Ahvaz. Iran.

4. Preparation of the plant material for chemical analyses

These fruits or vegetables were washed with distilled water and dried at room temperature to remove residual moisture, then placed in paper envelope and oven-dried at 55°C for 24 hours (Abuye, Urga., Knapp, Selmar, Omwega, Imungi, & Winterhalter 2003). The dried fruit were ground into powder using pestle and mortar, and sieved through 20-mesh sieve. The edible plant powder was used for the nutrients analyses.

5. Proximate analysis

The methods recommended by the Association of Official Analytical Chemists (AOAC) were used to determine ash (#942.05), crude lipid (#920.39), crude fibre (#962.09) and nitrogen content (#984.13)(AOAC 1990).

6. Determination of crude lipid and crude fibre content

Two grams of dried fruit or vegetable were weighed in a porous thimble of a Soxhlet apparatus, with its mouthed cotton wool plugged. The thimble was placed in an extraction chamber which was suspended above a pre-weighed receiving flask containing petroleum ether (b.p. 40-60°C). The flask was heated on a heating mantle for eight hours to extract the crude lipid. After the extraction, the thimble was removed from the Soxhlet apparatus and the solvent distilled off. The flask containing the crude lipid was heated in the oven at 100°C for 30 minutes to evaporate the solvent, then cooled in a dessicator, and reweighed. The difference in weight was expressed as percentage crude lipid content.
Crude fibre was estimated by acid-base digestion with 1.25% H_2SO_4 (prepared by diluting 7.2 ml of 94% conc. acid of specific gravity 1.835g ml-1 per 1000 ml distilled water) and 1.25% NaOH (12.5 g per 1000 ml distilled water) solutions. The residue after crude lipid extraction was put into a 600 ml beaker and 200 ml of boiling 1.25% H_2SO_4 added. The contents were boiled for 30 minutes, cooled, filtered through a filter paper and the residue washed three times with 50 ml aliquots of boiling water. The washed residue was returned to the original beaker and further digested by boiling in 200 ml of 1.25% NaOH for 30 minutes. The digest was filtered to obtain the residue. This was washed three times with 50 ml aliquots of boiling water and finally with 25 ml ethanol. The washed residue was dried in an oven at 130°C to constant weight and cooled in a dessicator. The residue was scraped into a pre-weighed porcelain crucible, weighed, ashed at 550°C for two hours, cooled in a dessicator and reweighed. Crude fibre content was expressed as percentage loss in weight on ignition, AOAC (1990).

7. Determination of nitrogen content and estimation of crude protein

Macro-Kjeldahl method was used to determine the nitrogen content of the stem. 2g of dried stem were digested in a 100 ml Kjeldahl digestion flask by boiling with 10 ml of concentrated tetraoxosulphate (VI) acid and a Kjeldahl digestion tablet (a catalyst) until the mixture was clear. The digest was filtered into a 100 ml volumetric flask and the solution made up to 100 ml with distilled water. Ammonia in the digest was steam distilled from 10 ml of the digest to which had been added 20 ml of 45% sodium hydroxide solution. The ammonia liberated was collected in 50 ml of 20% boric acid solution containing a mixed indicator. Ammonia was estimated by titrating with standard 0.01 mol L-1 HCl solution. Blank determination was carried out in a similar manner. Crude protein was estimated by multiplying the value obtained for percentage nitrogen content by a factor of 6.25, AOAC(1990).

8. Estimation of carbohydrates and energy values

Available carbohydrate was estimated by difference, by subtracting the total sum of percent crude protein, crude lipid, crude fibre and ash from 100% DW of the fruit The plant calorific value (in kJ) was estimated by multiplying the percentages of crude protein, crude lipid and carbohydrate by the factors 16.7, 37.7 and 16.7 respectively, AOAC(1990).

9. Mineral analysis

The mineral elements Na, K, Ca, Fe, and Zn were determined on 0.3g fruits powder by the methods of Funtua, ,Funtua and Trace (1999); Funtua (2004). using Energy Dispersive X-ray Fluorescence (EDXRF) transmission emission spectrometer carrying an annuar 25 mCi 109Cd isotopic excitation source that emits Ag-K X-ray (22.1 keV) and a Mo X-ray tube (50KV, 5mA) with thick foil of pure Mo used as target material for absorption correction. The system had a Canberra Si (Li) detector with a resolution of 170eV at 5.9keV line and was coupled to a computer controlled ADCCard (Trump 8K). Measurements were carried out in duplicate. Na was analyzed after wet digestion of one gr. of the fruits powder with nitric/perchloric/sulphuric acid (9:2:1 v/v/v) mixture. Sodium was analyzed with a Corning 400 flame photometer,AOAC (1990).
Proximate analyses were performed in triplicate according to standard methods 44-19, 46-13, 30-25 and 08-16 of the AACC (1984), using a Goldfisch (Labconco Corp., Kansas City, MO) apparatus for fat extraction with hexane and total lipid extraction with methanol:chloroform (2:1, v/v), and a nitrogen to protein conversion factor of 6.25. Total carbohydrate content was determined by the phenol-sulfuric acid method described by Dubois et al. (1956), using raffinose as a standard. Low molecular weight sugars were analyzed by high resolution gas chromatography (Karoutis et al., 1992). Total starch was determined as glucose after hydrolysis of starch with amyloglucosidase (1,600 activity unit/g, from Rhizopus) (Sigma-Aldrich Canada Ltd., Oakville, ON). The reaction of the resultant glucose with *o*-toluidine was then colourimetrically measured (Chiang and Johnson, 1977). Total dietary fibre (TDF) was determined according to the AOAC (1985) procedure using Sigma total dietary fibre assay kit TDF-C10 (Sigma Chemical Co., St. Louis, MO). Colour was evaluated with a HunterLab Colour Difference Meter (Colour QUEST, Hunter Associates Laboratory, Inc., Reston, VA) equipped with Illuminant D65

10. Analysis of antinutritional factors

Trypsin inhibitor activity (TIA) was determined by a modification of the procedure of Kakade et al. (1974) as described by Smith et al. (1980) and Hamerstrand et al. (1981). All samples were defatted at room temperature (approximately 23°C) for 9 h using a wrist-action shaker with three solvent replacements in order to avoid any destructive effect of heat on the TIA of the samples.
Total phenolic assay: phenolic compounds were analyzed accordance standard method.

Samples	Protein (%)	Fat(%)	Total Ash(%)	Fiber %	Fructose g/100g	Glucose g/100g	Sucrose g/100g	Starch g/100g	Total sugarg/ 100g
Alocacia indica Sch	5.7	3.29	7.3	11.05	8.06	2.1	2.09	60.41	72.66
Asparagus officinalis DC	32.69	3.44	10.7	18.5	6.86	1.53	N.D	26.28	34.67
Portulaca oleracia Linn	23.47	5.26	22.6	8.0	0.86	0.01	N.D	39.8	40.67
Momordica dioicia Roxb	19.38	4.7	6.7	21.3	3.97	1.47	0.23	42.25	47.92
Eulophia ochreata Lindl	5.44	3.25	9.1	22.9	1.62	1.48	0.46	55.75	59.31
Solanum indicum Linn	12.85	13.76	11.0	23.9	5.21	3.19	0.59	29.5	38.49
Cordia myxa Roxb	8.32	2.2	6.7	25.7	9.38	12.75	29.09	5.86	57.08
Chlorophytum comosum Linn	4.54	2.0	10.38	17.24	7.82	3.41	3.07	51.54	65.84

Table 2. Amounts of protein, fat, ash, fiber, fructose, glucose, sucrose and starch of eight edible plants obtained from India and Iran.

Samples	Phytic acid mg/100g	Trypsin Inhibator (TIU/g)
Alocacia indica Sch	312.4	7.9
Asparagus officinalis DC	340.8	0.8
Portulaca oleracia Linn	823.6	16.9
Momordica dioicia Roxb	284.2	9.3
Eulophia ochreata Lindl	255.6	3.1
Solanum indicum Linn	695.8	10.6
Cordia myxa Roxb	248.0	1.39
Chlorophytum comosum Linn	468.8	4.7

Table 3. Total Phytic acid inhibitor compound and amount of Tripsin inhibitor of eight edible plants obtained from India and Iran.

Samples	Total phenolic compound mg/g	Vitamin E mg/100g
Alocacia indica Sch	0.87	N.D
Asparagus officinalis DC	3.17	6.56
Portulaca oleracia Linn	5.86	11.6
Momordica dioicia Roxb	3.69	4.5
Eulophia ochreata Lindl	2.43	6.32
Solanum indicum Linn	7.02	N.D
Cordia myxa Roxb	4.02	2.2
Chlorophytum comosum Linn	1.36	N.D

Table 4. Total phenolic compound(Antioxidant) and amount of Vitamin E(Antioxidant) of eight edible plants obtained from India and Iran.

Samples	Total Ash(%)	Sodium (Na) mg/g	Potassium(K) mg/g	Calcium(Ca) mg/g	Fe mg/g	Zn mg/g
Alocacia indica Sch.	7.3	4.4	3.4	0.88	0.48	1.21
Asparagus officinalis DC.	10.7	1.84	10.94	0.67	0.19	2.60
Portulaca oleracia Linn.	22.6	7.17	14.71	18.71	0.48	3.02
Momordica dioicia Roxb.	6.7	1.51	8.25	0.46	0.14	1.34
Eulophia ochreata Lindl.	9.1	1.62	4.63	7.37	5.04	3.83
Solanum indicum Linn.	11.0	1.51	8.32	4.48	10.56	0.95
Cordia myxa Roxb.	6.7	1.62	7.83	0.46	0.51	0.35
Chlorophytum comosum Linn.	10.38	3.95	4.29	13.14	1.89	0.76

Table 5. Amounts of macro and trace elements and ash of eight edible plants obtained from Iran and India

Many studies have been done by various research workers all over the world by selecting one or more plants particularly leaves, fruits, roots, stem, food plants and so on but rarely by selecting a particular family. In this investigation work seven families *(Araceae, Liliaceae, Boraginaceae, Orchidaceae, Cucurbitaceae, Portulacaceae* and *Solanaceae*) are selected.
Plant species selected were: Alocacia indica Sch.,Asparagus officinalis DC., Chlorophytum comosum Linn., Cordia Myxa Roxb., Eulophia Ochreata Lindl., Momordica dioicia Roxb., Portulaca oleracia Linn. and Solanum indicum Linn.Total ash values of eight samples of Alocacia indica Sch., Asparagus officinalis DC Chlorophytum comosum Linn.,Cordia myxa Roxb., Eulophia ochreata Lindl., Momordica dioicia Roxb., Portulaca oleracia Linn. and Solanum indicum Linn. were obtained 7.3%, 10.7%,10.38%, 6.7%, 9.1%, 6.7%, 22.6% and 11.0% respectively.The most of ash value and the least of ash value were for Portulaca oleracia Linn.and Momodica dioicia Roxb.or Cordia myxa Roxb. respectively. The ash medium value was obtained for Eulophia ochreata Lindl.(9.1%), If ash value in sample is more than others, it's mineral values is more than others. If mineral values to be high it is observe that plant have high nutritional value, because these mineral compounds are same mineral compounds of human body if theses edible plants is consumed by human in normal conditions. Minerals in the diet are required for proper growth and good health. Those needed in macro, or major quantities are calcium, phosphorus, magnesium, potassium, sulfur, sodium, and chlorine, and those needed in micro(trace) amounts are iron, iodine, copper, cobalt, chromium, manganese, selenium, zinc, fluorine, and molybdenum. The cruciferous and many other vegetables are excellent sources of minerals, particularly of calcium, phosphorus, magnesium, potassium, iron, sodium, and most of these minerals are present in the available form. The trace mineral content of fruits and vegetables depends on the amount present in the soil in which the plant was grown. The diverse geographical sources of fruits and vegetables and modern systems of transporting produce to market reduce the chance of a low intake. Calcium intake from fruits and

vegetables is small compared to that from the milk group but will assume more importance if milk intake is low. Vitamins and minerals present in the diet are necessary for normal growth and metabolism and influence the utilization of other nutrients such as protein. The deficiency of essential vitamins or minerals leads to several physiological disorders and diseases, slowed growth, and lack of deposition of proteins in tissues. An adequate supply of B- complex vitamins is necessary for critical protein utilization. The deficiency of minerals such as potassium, phosphorus, sodium, calcium, and magnesium also influences the capacity of the body to utilize amino acids and proteins.

Sodium values of eight samples above in this study in order to mg/g were obtained 4.4, 1.84, 3.95, 1.62, 1.62, 1.51, 7.17and1.51 respectively. *Portulaca oleracia Linn.*contains the highest value of sodium and *Momordica dioicia Roxb.*,or *Solanum indicum Linn.*contain the least values of sodium. *Alocacia indica Sch.* Contains sodium medium value(4.4mg/g).

Potassium values of eight samples above in this research in order to mg/g were obtained 3.4,10.94,4.29,7.83,4.63,8.25,14.71and 8.32 respectively. *Portulaca oleracia Linn.* contains the highest potassium value and *Alocacia indica Sch.*contains the least potassium value. *Cordia Myxa Roxb.* contains potassium medium value(7.83mg/g).

Calcium values of the samples above in order to mg/g were obtained 0.88, 0.67, 13.14, 0.46, 7.37,0.46, 18.17 and 4.48 respectively. *Portulaca oleracia Linn.*contains the highest calcium value and *Momordica dioicia Roxb.*or *Cordia myxa Roxb.* Contain the least calcium value. *Eulophia ochreata Lindl.* contains calcium medium value (7.37mg/g).

Iron values of eight samples in this research in order to mg/g were obtained 0.48, 0.19, 1.89, 0.51, 5.04, 0.14, 0.48 and 1.56 respectively. *Eulophia ochreata Lindl.* Contains highest iron value and *Momordica dioicia Roxb* contains the least iron value. *Chlorophytum comosum Linn.* contains iron medium value (1.89mg/g).

Zinc values of the samples above in this study in order to mg/g were obtained 1.21,2.60, 0.76, 0.35, 3.83, 1.34, 3.02 and 0.95 respectively. *Eulophia ochreata Lindl.* contains the highest zinc value and *Cordia myxa Roxb.* Contains the least zinc value. *Asparagus officinalis DC.* contains zinc medium value (2.60mg/g).

Therefore, it is observed that *Portulaca oleracia Linn.* contains the high value of macro-elements such as sodium, potassium, calcium and especially it have high ash value in comparison with others plants in this research. Therefore, *Portulaca oleracia Linn* has high nutritional value from standpoint of macro-elements. Because *Eulophia ochreata Lindl.* contains highest micro-elements such as iron and zinc in comparison with others plants in this study, it has high nutritional value from view of point of above trace(micro) elements. *Momordica dioicia Roxb. or Cordia myxa Roxb* have the minimum nutritional value, because they contain the least ash values and *Momordica dioicia Roxb.* has the least value of sodium and calcium, but *Cordia myxa Roxb.* has the least value of zinc. *Alocacia indica Sch.,Asparagus officinalis DC., Chlorophytum comosum Linn., Cordia Myxa Roxb., Eulophia Ochreata Lindl.*have nutritional medium values.

Protein, Fat, and calorie values of eight samples in this research were compared, it is observed that *Asparagus*(32.69%) and *Portulaca* (23.47%)have the highest protein values respectively, *Chlorophytum*(4.54%), *Eulophia*(5.44%) and *Alocacia*(5.7%) have the least protein values. *Momordica*(19.38%) have protein medium value.

Solanum(13.76%) has the highest Fat value and *Chlorophytum*(2%) has the least Fat value. *Portulaca*(5.26%) Fat value was approximately medium and the others samples have low fat values.

Momordica(with 4125/83Kcal/Kg) and *Cordia* (with 4067/94 Kcal/Kg) have the highest calorie values and *Portulaca*(with 2913/82 Kcal/Kg)has the least calorie value and the others samples have calorie medium values(with 3514/4Kcal/Kg- 3647/23Kcal/Kg). Therefore, *Asparagus* and *Portulaca* have the highest nutritional value from standpoint of proteins.

Plants such as vegetables and fruits have satisfactory edible proteins with high quality so that we can use them in food industries and as nutrition. Total proteins and nitrogen is related to Albumins, globulins, free Amino acids, enzymes, hormones, peptides and other nitrogen components. The most of these proteins have high nutritional values and contain all essential amino acids so that it is useful for our body cells and it is necessary that is consumed by human.

Total phenolic compounds of eight plants in this research were compared together, it is observed that *Solanum indicum Linn.*with 7.02mg/g has the highest phenolic compounds values and then *Portulaca oleracia Linn.* with 5.86mg/g contains high phenolic compounds. *Alocacia indica Sch.* with 0.87mg/g has the least phenolic compounds. *Cordia Myxa Roxb* with 4.02mg/g and *Momordica dioicia Roxb.* with 3.69mg/g and *Asparagus officinalis DC.* with 3.17mg/g contain phenolic compounds medium value.

Phytic acid contents of eight plants were compared in this research, it is reveal that *Portulaca oleracia Linn.* with 823.6mg/100g sample has maximum value and then *Solanum indicum* with 695.8 mg/100 g sample has high value and *Eulophia* with 255.6 mg/100g sample has minimum value and the others plants have less values.

Carbohydrates eight edible plants in this research were compared it is observed that fructose, glucose, sucrose and Fiber values of *Cordia myxa* Roxb. were 9.38%, 12.75%, 29.09% and 25.7% the highest values respectively, but it's starch (with 5.86%)value was the least value. Fructose, glucose, sucrose and fiber values of *Portulaca Oleracia* Linn. were the least values with values of 0.86%,0.01%, N.D.(Not detected) and 8% respectively, but it's starch value(with39.8%) was high. Starch value of *Alocacia indica* Sch. was maximum with 60.41%.*Alocacia indica* Sch. and *Asparagus officinalis* D.C. have maximum and minimum total carbohydrates with values of 72.66% and 34.67% respectively. Therefore energy value of obtained from total carbohydrates value in *Alocacia indica* Sch. was the highest value but energy values obtained from it's protein and fat were very low. Energy values of obtained from fat and protein in *Solanum indicum* and *Asparagus officinalis* D.C. were the highest values with 123.84kcal/100g and 130.76kcal/100g respectively.

Total energy values obtained from fat, protein and sugars in *Alocacia indica* Sch. and *Cordia myxa* Roxb.were 343.05kcal/100g and 281.4kcal/100g , the highest and the least values respectively.

Total sugar amounts of *Cordia* and *Asparagus* plants were compared with results of other researcher, it is showed that Parmar, C et, al (1982) reported that reducing and non-reducing sugars amounts in *Cordia* were 3.41% and 0.08 % respectively and Duke. J.A et al(1985) reported that carbohydrate and fiber values in *Asparagus* was 5% and 0.7% respectively. These comparison showed that sugar amounts of both plants in our research were very higher than them research results.

Trypsin inhibitor amounts of samples in this thesis is compared, it is observed that *portulaca* have the highest value(16.9TIU/g) and *Asparagus* have the least value(0.8TIU/g). *Solanum, Momordica* and *Alocacia* contain the high values of trypsin inhibitor respectively. trypsin inhibitor high values of samples are not relation with them protein high values. Asparagus have the most value of protein and the least value of this anti-nutrient(trypsin inhibitor).

Samples vitamin E amounts were compared, it is observed that *portulaca* have highest value (11.5 mg/100g), but vitamin E in *Solanum, Chlorophytum* and *Alocacia* are not detected. *Portulaca* have highest values phenolic compounds and vitamin E, therefore this plant have the highest antioxidant property. The antioxidant property give to plant high shelf-life then high consumption capacity in between of people, therefore this plant have high nutritional value.

There is currently much interest in phytochemicals as bioactive components of food. The roles of fruit, vegetables in disease prevention have been attributed, in part, to the antioxidant properties of their constituent polyphenols (vitamins E and C, and the carotenoids). Recent studies have shown that many dietary polyphenolic constituents derived from plants are more effective antioxidants *in vitro* than vitamins E or C, and thus might contribute significantly to the protective effects *in vivo*. It is now possible to establish the antioxidant activities of plant-derived flavonoids in the aqueous and lipophilic phases, and to assess the extent to which the total antioxidant potentials of wine and tea can be accounted for by the activities of individual polyphenols. because phenolic compounds have Antioxidant properties and to prevent from damage of plant tissues and all compounds that contain double bonds and aromatic structures especially to prevent from decomposition of fatty acids, vitamins, amino acids, flavours, and pigments in plants, therefore, *Solanum indicum Linn.* and then *Cordia Myxa Roxb* and *Momordica dioicia Roxb.* and *Asparagus officinalis DC.*have high nutritional values, because the most of them nutrients will be protected in harvest and post-harvest and in them storage during.

11. References

[1] Aberoumand, A. and Deokule, S.S.2008. Comparison of compounds of some edible plants of Iran and India, Pakistan J. Nutrition, 7 (4), 582-585.

[2] Abuye, C., Urga, K., Knapp, H., Selmar, D., Omwega, A., Imungi, J., & Winterhalter, P., (2003) A survey of wild, green, leafy vegetables and their potential in combating micronutrient deficiencies in rural populations, East African Medical Journal, 80, 247-252.

[3] Aletor, V., & Adeogun, O., (1995). Chemical analysis of the fruit of *Vitex doniana* (Verbenaceae). Food Chemistry, 53, 375-379.

[4] AOAC,(1990).Official methods of analysis, 14th edition, Association of Official Analytical Chemists, Washington DC. (pp.1137–1139). Arlington, Virginia, USA.

[5] Asibey-Berko, E. & Tayie, F., (1999). The antibacterial properties of some plants found in Hawaii, Ghana Journal Science, 39, 91-92.

[6] Edmonds, J., & Chweya, J., (1995). Black nightshades, *Solanum nigrum* L. and related species. Promoting the conservation and use of underutilized and neglected crops.(pp.221-234).Taylor & Francis, London.

[7] Faruq, U., Sani, A., & Hassan, L., (2002). Composition and distribution of deadly nightshade. Nigerian. Journal Basic Application Science, 11,157-164.

[8] Funtua, I., (2004). Minerals in foods: Dietary sources, chemical forms, interactions, bioavailability, Instrumentation Science. Technology, 32 , 529-536.

[9] Funtua, I., & Trace, J.,(1999). Quantitative variability in *Pisum* seed globulins: its assessment and significance. Plant Foods for Human Nutrition, 17, 293-297.

[10] Ifon, E.,& Bassir, O.,(1980). *Determination* of carbohydrates in foods. II—unavailable carbohydrates. Food Chemistry, 5, 231-235.

[11] Isong, E., & Idiong, U.,(1997). Nutrient content of the edible leaves of seven wild plants from Nigerian. Plant Foods for Human Nutrition, 51, 79-84.

[12] Nesamvuni, C., Steyn, N.,& Potgieter, M., (2001). nutrients analysis of selected western African foods, South African Journal of Science, 97, 51-54.

[13] Plessi, M., Bertelli, D., Phonzani, A., Simonetti, M., Neri, A., & Damiani, P.,(1999). Role of indigenous leafy vegetables in combating hunger and malnutrition, Food Composition Analalysis,12, 91-96.

[14] Sena, L., VanderJagt, D., Rivera, C., Tsin, A., Muhammadu, I., Mahamadou, O. ,Milson, M., Pastosyn, A., & Glew, R., (1998). Nutritional profile of some edible plants from Mexico, Plant Foods for Human Nutrition, 52, 17-30.

[15] Vadivel, V., & Janardhanan, K., (1999). Analysis of nutritional components of eight famine foods of the Republic of Nigerian. Plant Foods for Human Nutrition, 55, 369-381.

5

Technologies and Varieties of Fodder Beet in Organic Farming

Hana Honsová[1], František Hnilička[2], David Bečka[1] and Václav Hejnák[2]
Czech University of Life Sciences in Prague,
Faculty of Agrobiology, Food and Natural Resources,
[1]Department of Crop Production,
[2]Department of Botany and Plant Physiology, Prague
Czech Republic

1. Introduction

In the organic farming system where the concentrate feeds are purchased a crop rotation for producing none only forage has been found to be expensive in relation to forage production costs, fossil energy inputs and the loss of production while crops are being established. The aim of organic farming is to create coexistence of multilateral, biologically and ecologically balanced weeds with low biomass production and strong culture crop. In weeds regulation we use preventive measures (seed rotation, late sowing, parallel growing of covering under sowings etc.), but also direct regulation methods, i.e. harrowing and line weeding (Petr et al., 1992).

Fodder beet is a crop for which cultivation areas are reduced, since in 2000 the sown area of 7597 hectares, but in 2007 decreased to 807 ha in the Czech Republic. A slight increase can be recorded in the year 2008 - 845 ha. Even though the area of fodder beet reduced this crop has an irreplaceable role in maintaining biodiversity in agro ecosystems. Therefore, at present there is a new application in organic farming, which is among the good fore crop.

Fodder beet areas in all over the world are not great. But it is a pity, because this crop has very high feed quality. Nowadays fodder beet could find new use in organic farming, especially as excellent feed for dairy cattle and energy crops. In ecological production of fodder beet we have some unsolved questions concerning i.e. weeds reduction, beet competitiveness improvement and optimal stand density. Fodder beet is a wide-row crop with slow initial development, which decreases its competitiveness in relation to weeds.

This crop has very high feed quality. Fodder beet could find new use in ecological farming, especially as excellent feed for dairy cattle (Kodeš et al., 2001).

Energy crops with wide ratio of nutrients – fodder beet, semi-sugar beet and sugar beet – provide more energy in comparison with cereals or forage crops. Fodder beet provides maximum amount of energy per one hectare and presents easily digestible feed (Kosař, 1985).

The most important factor determining nutritional quality of feeds is digestibility. Its value significantly influences amount of nutrients and of energy available for animal (Mudřík et al., 2006).

In feed can be determined combustible heat (gross energy). Gross energy (BE) is determined in calorimeter by complete combustion of feed in oxygen atmosphere and is expressed in mega joules (MJ). Energy value of feed for cattle is determined in MJ as NELs (for lactation cattle) and NEVs (for growing cattle - weight gain above 800 g/day). For energy content determination it is also necessary to determine metabolized energy content for cattle (MEs) (Zeman, 2002).

Besides the traditional use of fodder beet as the dietary food new ways of use appear. It is the use in bioenergetics, such as the production of bioethanol (Reed et al., 1986; Mähnert and Linke, 2009; Chochola, 2007; Pulkrábek et al. 2007) and biogas (Scherer, et al., 2009; Klocke et al., 2007). Use of fodder beet as a source of renewable energy results from the fact that it provides more energy than cereals and fodder crops (Urban et al., 2005; Hnilička et al., 2009; Martínez-Pérez et al., 2007).

The aim of our research was to compare and to recommend chosen varieties of fodder beet organic growing based on production ability evaluation. In three years experiments (2005 - 2007) small-plot trials were established (in four repetitions on plots with harvest area of ten square meters) with fodder beet on certified and controlled ecological area.

2. Methodology

The aim of our research was to compare and recommend 1. various growing technologies and 2. chosen varieties of fodder beet for organic growing based on production ability evaluation and to compare their feed value. In three years experiments based in 2005 - 2007 small-plot trials were established with fodder beet on certified and controlled ecological area of Experimental station of Department of Crop Production of Czech University of Life Sciences in Prague - Uhříněves.

Six cultivars of fodder beet were used in experiment - especially volume types (Lenka, Hako, Jamon and Monro) and compromise type (Kostelecká Barres, Starmon) and sugar beet cultivar Merak (Table 1). Only in 2007 variety Bučanský žlutý válec (volume type) compensated variety Kostelecká Barres.

During vegetation stands were kept in non-weed state by inter-row hoeing and by manual hoeing and weeding in rows. No chemical protection against fungal diseases was used.

Number of plants per plot was determined before harvest. Harvest was performed by manual collection of roots, which were weighed in a field. Average weight of one root was determined and also total yield per hectare was recorded.

2.1 Growing technologies

In three-year trials various growing technologies of fodder beet differ with row distance (45 cm and 37.5 cm), plant distance in row (18 and 25 cm) and weed regulation were compared. Ranking with weeds, attack by leaf diseases, chlorophyll content and yield of roots were evaluated.

The aim of the project was to reach fodder beet stand structure optimization in ecologic growing regarding weed infestation, leaf diseases and production.

Weeds regulation problematics was solved by stand organization change. In order to achieve former rows covering we tested reduction of interrow distance from 45 cm to 37.5 cm. In our experiments changes caused by different stand organization and further treatments (Table 1) per number of vascular bundle circles and production indicators were evaluated. During vegetation weed infestation and degree of leaf diseases were evaluated.

Row distance	Plant distance in row	Canopy density	Weed regulation
45 cm	18 cm	100 thou.ha^{-1}	without weeds
45 cm	18 cm	100 thou.ha^{-1}	line weeding (as necessary) + 1x digging in row during singling
45 cm	18 cm	100 thou.ha^{-1}	line weeding (as necessary) + 1x digging in row before canopy connection
37.5 cm	18 cm	120 thou.ha^{-1}	without weeds
37.5 cm	18 cm	120 thou.ha^{-1}	line weeding (as necessary) + 1x digging in row during singling
37.5 cm	18 cm	120 thou.ha^{-1}	line weeding (as necessary) + 1x digging in row before canopy connection
37.5 cm	25 cm	100 thou.ha^{-1}	without weeds

Table 1. Canopy organization variants and weed regulation

2.2 Varieties and energy

Six fodder beet varieties and one sugar beet variety were compared in three-year experiments at ecological area (in 2005 and 2006 Lenka, Hako, Kostelecká Barres, Jamon, Monro, Starmon and sugar beet Merak, in 2007 Bučanský žlutý válec site of Kostelecká Barres) (Table 2).

Variety	Type	Rezistance	Properties
Merak	sugar beet N/S	rhisomania, cercospora	2003 – diploid
Lenka	cubical	-	1992 – 2n, monogerm, yellow bulb, cylindrical form with blunt root termination
Hako	cubical	-	1977 – 3n, multigerm, light yellow bulb with orange shade, cylindrical with sudden termination
Kostelecká Barres	compromise	-	1937 - multigerm, orange bulb with olive shape, 1/3 – ½ in ground
Jamon	cubical	-	1997 – 3n, monogerm, yellow bulb
Monro	cubical	-	1994 – 3n, monogerm, red bulb
Starmon	compromise	rhisomania	Monogerm, yellow bulb
Bučanský žlutý válec	cubical		multigerm, cylindrical bulb, yellow coloured with orange shade, 1/3 in ground

Table 2. Variants of variety experiment

The energy content was investigated office on the basis of combustion calorimetry methods. Combustion calorimetry as one of the many destructive biological method has a wide range of applications from production and environmental plant physiology, which can be evaluated not only individual products but also the vegetation and ecosystem. Its foundation is the stress physiology of plants to determine the effect of exposure to stressors plants and then to detect the resistance of plant species or varieties. Important place in the combustion calorimetry quickly evaluate alternative sources of renewable bio-energy. Nor can it ignore the question of the nutritional value of feed and thus the quality of feed and fodder (primary sources, but the final product).

Obtained values of gross and net energy serves as the basis for calculations of energy balance of plant breeding, feed livestock, but also for establishing the energy efficiency of production, since the units of energy are all the same in comparison with bank transfers, and therefore it is preferable to determine the efficiency of production of individual commodities or the whole enterprise just over the energy balance.

The results were evaluated by statistical program SAS using analysis of variance at significance level $\alpha = 0.05$. Confirmatively different values are marked with different letters (a, b, c, d).

3. Results and discussion

3.1 Technologies

Modification in stand organization (reduction of interrow distance and stand density increasement) did not bring confirmative changes in leaf diseases infestation of plants in 2005 (Table 5). During 2006 - 2007 stand organization and weeds regulation influenced plants infestation with leaf diseases.

Statistical evaluation of harvest results in 2005 did not prove influence of interrow distance change and stand density on roots yield (Table 4). Average weight of one root was influenced by stand organization (Graph 1) and weed infestation regulation (Table 3, graph 2). Number of vascular bundles was not influenced by stand organization.

Weeds regulation method confirmatively influenced plants infestation with leaf diseases in 2005. Variants, in which weeds in row were not regulated, but they were regulated only in interrow, have been during vegetation confirmatively more infested with leaf diseases. At the end of vegetation more infested were beet leaves in non-weed variants.

Before harvest in 2006 the least statistically confirmative infestation was found in non-weed variant with wider rows (34%) and the highest infestation was found in variant with narrow rows with line weeding and hoeing (39%). Diseases infestation in 2006 in all monitored variants at the end of vegetation reached in average only 35%.

In 2007 differences before harvest disappeared, leaf diseases infestation was non-confirmative among compared variants. In total average of all monitored variants diseases infestation reached 64% at the end of vegetation in 2007.

Roots production (graph 3 and 4) was during 2005 and 2006 significantly influenced by weeds regulation method (Table 4). In 2005 with both stand densities (determined by different interrow distances – 45 cm and 37.5 cm) the highest yield was reached by control variant without weeds.

In 2006 the highest yield was reached by variant with wider rows with hoeing (86.8 $t.ha^{-1}$), control variant with narrow rows without weeds (83.8 $t.ha^{-1}$). The worst were variants with narrow rows with line weeding, narrow rows with line weeding and hoeing and narrow rows without weeds with higher distance between plants in row.

Row distance (cm)	Technology	1 bulb average weight (g)			
		2005	2006	2007	average
45	without weeds	1095	1080	1042	1090
45	line weeding	204	1200	976	667
45	line weeding and digging	596	1300	964	982
37.5	without weeds	884	1330	842	806
37.5	line weeding	213	1120	918	739
37.5	line weeding and digging	586	1180	940	784
37.5 (25 cm in row)	without weeds	1051	1490	1157	1233

Table 3. One bulb average weight - technologies compare

Average weight of one root was the highest in 2006 in non-weed variant with narrow rows and higher distance of plants in row (1490 g). Number of vascular bundles was not influenced by stand organization (Table 4). Yield values, weight of one root and number of vascular bundles were not statistically confirmative in 2006.

Higher yields in 2007 were reached in variants with narrow rows in comparison with wider rows. The highest yield was reached by variant of narrow rows with hoeing. Differences among obtained yields were not confirmative.

In 2007 average weight of one root was the highest in non-weed variant with narrow rows and higher distance between plants in row (1160 g). Number of vascular bundles was not influenced by stand organization. Values of one root weight were not statistically confirmative among compared variants.

Row distance (cm)	Technology	Yield ($t.ha^{-1}$)			
		2005	2006	2007	average
45	without weeds	114.0^{c}	79.1	87.9	93.7
45	line weeding	17.2^{a}	74.4	87.2	59.6
45	line weeding and digging	59.4^{b}	86.8	79.6	75.3
37.5	without weeds	102.5^{c}	83.8	94.8	93.7
37.5	line weeding	23.9^{a}	70.7	94.9	63.2
37.5	line weeding and digging	66.5^{b}	72.5	97.0	78.7
37.5 (25 cm in row)	without weeds	108.9^{c}	72.8^{ns}	92.3^{ns}	91.3

Table 4. Yield of bulbs - technologies compare

Regarding relatively small weed infestation, roots production was more influenced by stand organization than by weeds regulation method. Generally higher yield was reached by variants with narrow rows in comparison with wide-rows variants. Nor can it ignore the question of the nutritional value of feed and thus the quality of feed and fodder (primary sources, but the final product).

Row distance (cm)	Technology	% of attacked leaves before harvest					
		2005	significancy	2006	significancy	2007	significancy
45	without weeds	99	*c*	34	*c*	65	*a*
45	line weeding	94	*bc*	37	*abc*	65	*a*
45	line weeding and digging	85	*ab*	35	*abc*	65	*a*
37.5	without weeds	82	*ab*	35	*b*	64	*a*
37.5	line weeding	92	*abc*	38	*ab*	63	*a*
37.5	line weeding and digging	89	*abc*	39	*a*	66	*a*
37.5 (25 cm in row)	without weeds	80	*a*	33	*c*	64	*a*
						ns	

Table 5. Plant attack by leaf diseases – technologies compare

In case of fodder beet organically growing it is possible to achieve high yields, but only with a thorough weeding throughout the vegetation. Row spacing or pitch variation in weed-free yield of roots was not much influenced.

All compared variants without weeds reached in the three-year average high yields of roots above ninety tonnes per hectare. This indicates the need for weeding during the growing period.

Weed infestation significantly reduced root yields. In average of three years provided the lowest yields income variations, where only line weeding were done. Weed infestation not only reduced yields but also decreased the weight of the tubers.

Significant influence of year was discovered. In 2005 exchange of canopy organization did not exchange plant attack by leaf diseases and bulb yield and way of weed regulation had significant influence to plant attack by leaf diseases and bulb production. In 2006 exchange of canopy organization exchanged plant attack by leaf diseases. Bulb yield was influenced by way of weed regulation. In 2007 exchange of canopy organization did not influence to plant attack by leaf diseases but it influenced the bulb production. Higher yield were reached at the variants of narrower rows.

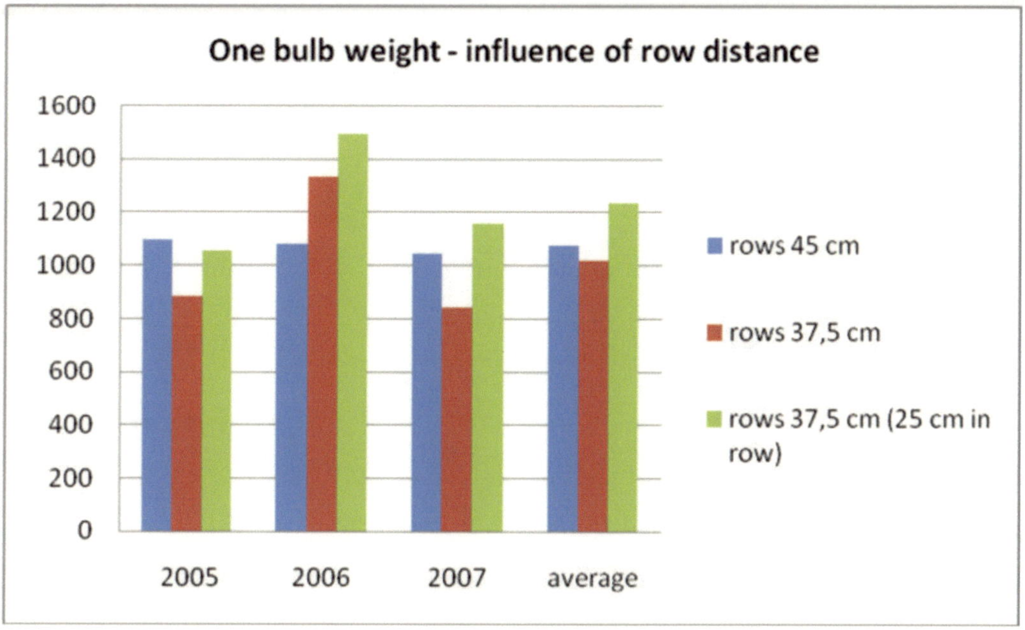

Fig. 1. One bulb weight (g) – influence of row distance

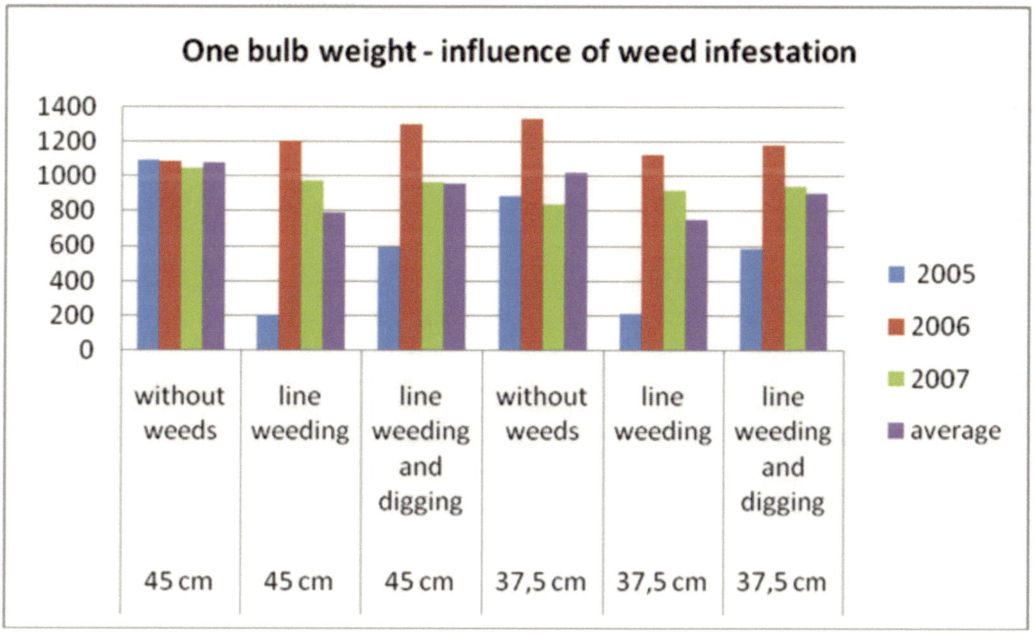

Fig. 2. One bulb weight (g) – influence of weed infestation

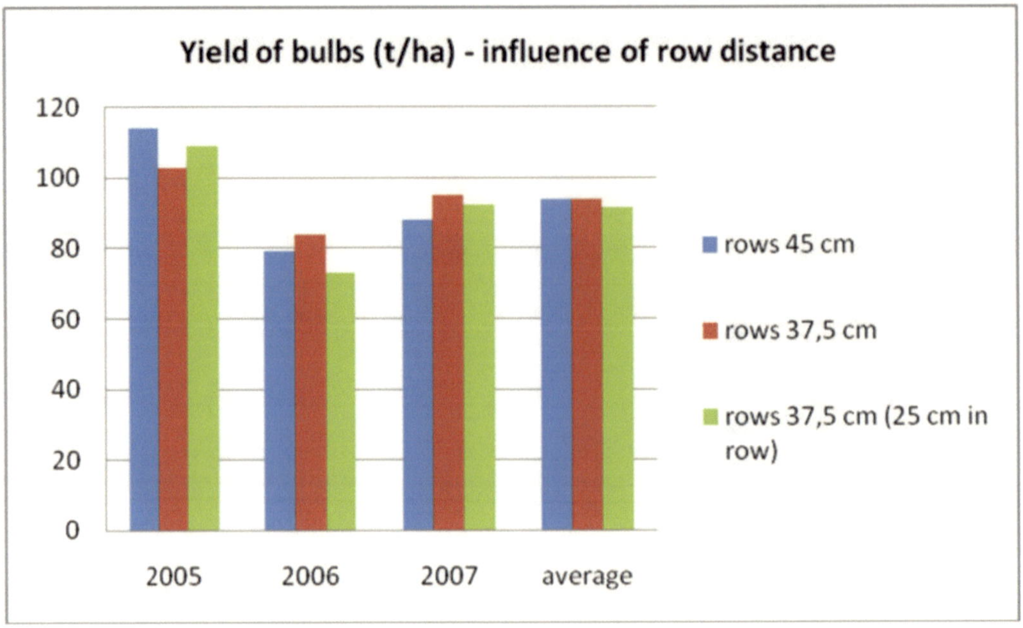

Fig. 3. Yield of bulbs – influence of row distance

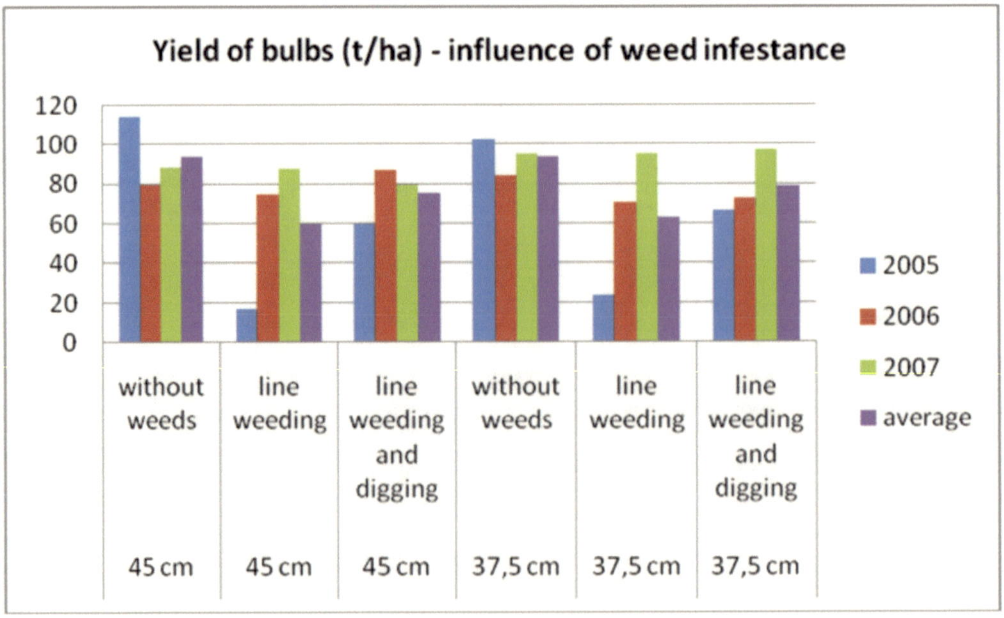

Fig. 4. Yield of bulbs – influence of weed infestation

3.2 Varieties and energy
3.2.1 Varieties
Yields of roots were strongly influenced by year of growing and by number of plants in harvest (Table 6, graph 5). Due to timely sowing and favourable weather conditions in 2005 beet emerged well. In 2005 after singling we obtained balanced and high numbers of plants at individual plots. Long winter, late start of spring and drought in the period after sowing in 2006 caused lower emergence. In 2006 total numbers in individual variants were relatively low in order to achieve relative uniformity between plots. In 2007 due to rainfall deficiency in period after sowing the plants emerged slowly and the canopy was off balance.
In 2005 cultivars Monro, Starmon, Hako and Kostelecká Barres reached yields of roots above one hundred tons per hectare, while in 2006 and 2007 none of varieties exceeded this level (Table 8). In 2006 the highest yields were reached in cultivars Hako and Jamon. In 2006 the highest yield of roots reached varieties Hako and Jamon, in 2007 Bučanský žlutý válec and Hako. In average of three years the most yielding cultivar was Hako (graph 7).

Variety	Plant number in harvest in thousands per hectar		
	2005	2006	2007
Merak	106	41	100
Lenka	85	49	77
Hako	102	64	74
Kostelecká Barres	110	38	
Bučanský žlutý válec			80
Jamon	94	64	93
Monro	104	65	92
Starmon	101	64	46

Table 6. Plant number in harvest – varieties compare

Weight of one root (Table 7, graph 6) was determined so by genetic dispositions of varieties and the canopy density and weather conditions. In average of three years varieties Lenka, Kostelecká Barres and Hako were the highest weight of one root.

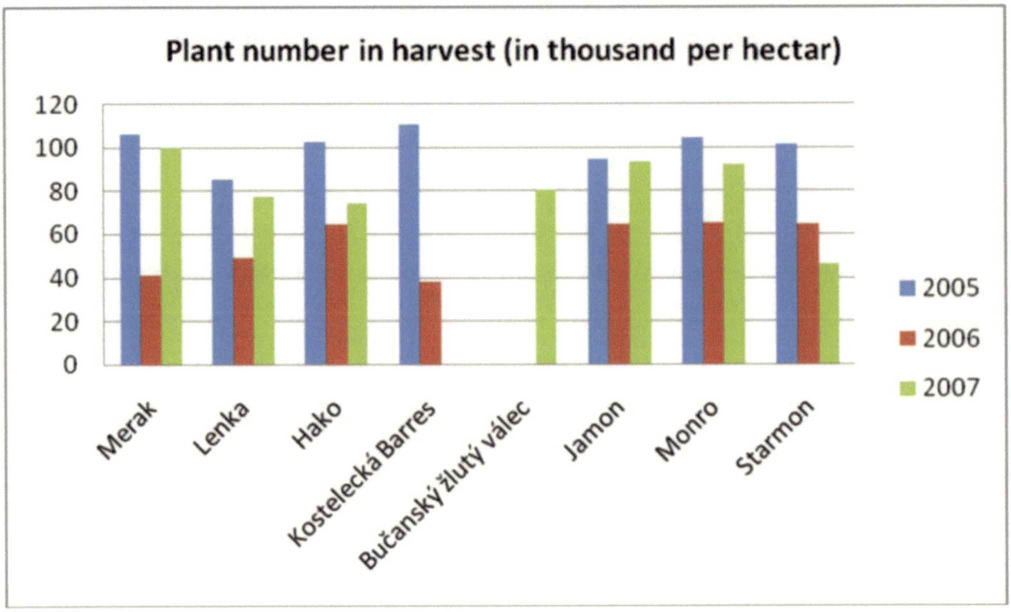

Fig. 5. Plant number in harvest - variety comparison

Variety	Average weight of one bulb (g)			
	2005	2006	2007	average
Merak	790	930	701	807
Lenka	1078	1640	1133	1284
Hako	1047	1430	1215	1231
Kostelecká Barres	955	1570		1263
Bučanský žlutý válec			1177	1177
Jamon	944	1420	914	1093
Monro	1051	1160	945	1052
Starmon	1055	1120	1287	1154

Table 7. One bulb average weight - varieties compare

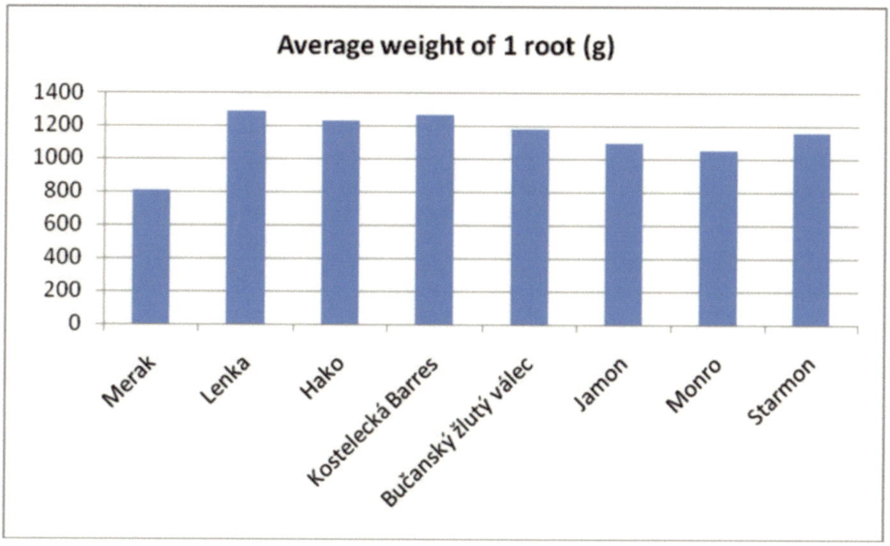

Fig. 6. Average weight of 1 root – variety comparison

Variety	Yield of bulbs (t.ha-1)						
	2005	significancy	2006	significancy	2007	significancy	average
Merak	83.3	*a*	37.6	*c*	69.2	*bc*	63.4
Lenka	90.9	*abc*	79	*ab*	86.3	*a*	85.4
Hako	106	*cd*	91.5	*a*	89.4	*a*	95.6
Kostelecká Barres	104.3	*bcd*	61.8	*bc*			83.1
Bučanský žlutý válec					91.3	*a*	91.3
Jamon	88.6	*ab*	87.5	*ab*	84.2	*ab*	86.8
Monro	108.9	*d*	74.6	*ab*	86.4	*a*	90.0
Starmon	106.3	*cd*	70.1	*ab*	71.0	*c*	82.5

Table 8. Yield of bulbs – varieties compare

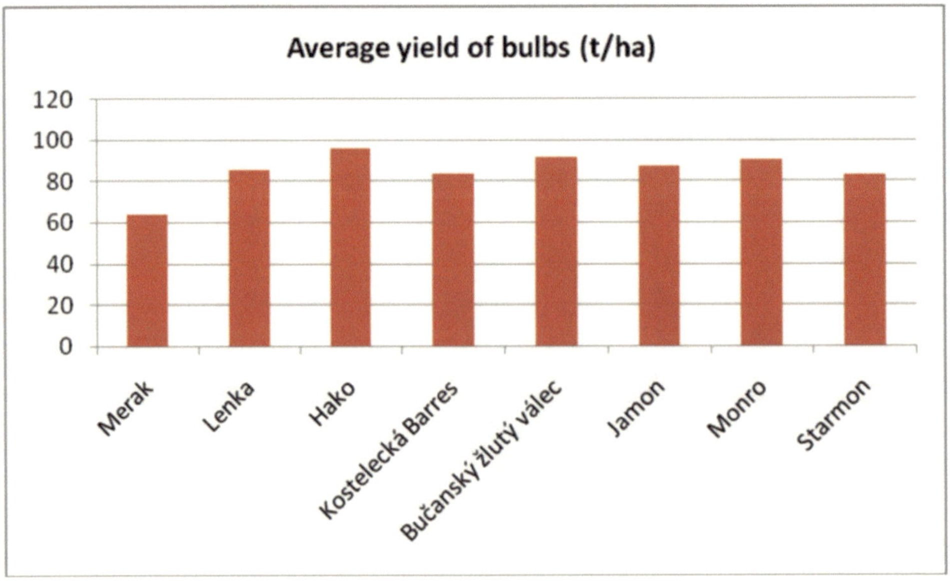

Fig. 7. Average yield of bulbs - variety comparison

	% of attacked leaves before harvest					
Variety	2005	significancy	2006	significancy	2007	significancy
	59	*a*	2	*c*	5	*b*
	89	*b*	22	*c*	45	*a*
Hako	99	*b*	26	*ab*	46	*a*
Kostelecká Barres	94	*b*	30	*ab*		
Bučanský žlutý válec					46	*a*
Jamon	91	*b*	29	*a*	43	*a*
Monro	94	*b*	36	*a*	60	*a*
Starmon	90	*b*	28	*ab*	56	*a*

Table 9. Plant attack by leaf diseases – varieties compare

3.2.2 Energy

3.2.2.1 The energy content of fodder beet

The content of energy in bulb of beet has been investigated by combustion calorimetry. The method is based on a complete burning of plant material in 100% oxygen atmosphere. The burning of the sample was used parabolic calorimeter IKA C200 (company IKA, Germany). To determine the net energy (energy content of ash-free) on the dry matter of sample.

From the experimental genotypes showed a variety Jamon, Lenka and Starmon lower energy content than the average value was calculated net energy of all observed varieties, which was 16.93 kJ.g-1. From Figure 1 shows that the lowest energy content showed a variety Jamon (16.54 kJ.g-1) and the highest variety Lenka (16.87 kJ.g-1). On the other hand, higher energy content in comparison with the average variety, should Monro (17.17 kJ.g-1) and Hako (17.28 kJ.g-1). The results obtained are in contradiction with the conclusions (Golley, 1961; Novák and Hnilička, 1996; Hnilička, 1999; Bláha et al., 2003; Hnilička et al., 2010). The authors note that monitored between genotypes of wheat, corn, but in general there are differences in energy content. Consistent with these findings indicates Honsová et al. (2007) that among the genotypes of fodder beet there are conclusive difference in energy content. In contrast, according Hnilička et al. (2005) and Urban et al. (2005) were surveyed between beet genotypes found conclusive difference.

Besides the variety in energy content was influenced by vintage bulb beet growing, as documented by graph 9. Based on the results of statistical analysis by Tukey HSD test was taken on a significance level α = 0.05 alternative hypothesis statistically conclusive differences between the years of cultivation. The above analysis shows conclusively that statistically the lowest average net energy content was obtained in 2007 in comparison with other experimental years. This year, the average energy content of 16.71 kJ.g-1, as documented in graph 8. On the other hand, the highest gross calorific value were measured in 2006, when the average net energy of bulb was 17.12 kJ.g-1. Effect of volume on the energy content of corn is confirmed as working (Fuksa et al., 2006), beet (Urban et al., 2005; Hnilička et al., 2005) and fodder beet (Honsová et al., 2007).

year	Energy content (kJ.g-1)	Yield of bulb (t.ha-1)	Energy yield (GJ.t-1)
2005	16.72 a. b	80.52 a	1345.54 a
2006	16.95 b	89.12 b	1511.83 b
2007	17.12 a. b	94.50 c	1617.09 c
average	16.93	88.05	1491.49

Legend: a, b, c - statistically significant difference on the border

Table 10. Plant a Statistical analysis by Tukey HSD test the impact of volume on observed characteristics.

Table 10 shows the results of statistical analysis of genotype and response to the annual energy content. From the statistical analysis at a significance level α = 0.05 shows conclusively that the lowest energy content was found in 2007 in a variety Starmon (16.38 kJ.g-1), while the highest value of net energy this year was found in a variety Hako (17.62 kJ.g-1). Similarly, the lowest energy content in 2005 was set at a variety Starmon (16.47 kJ.g-1) and highest for variety Hako (17.61 kJ.g-1). In 2006, the interval of the measured values of net energy from 16.53 kJ.g-1 (Jamon) to 17.53 kJ.g-1 (Monro).

3.2.2.2 The energy yield of fodder beet

The values for the energy contained in the unit of dry matter and economic yield of the main product is possible to calculate the energy yield.

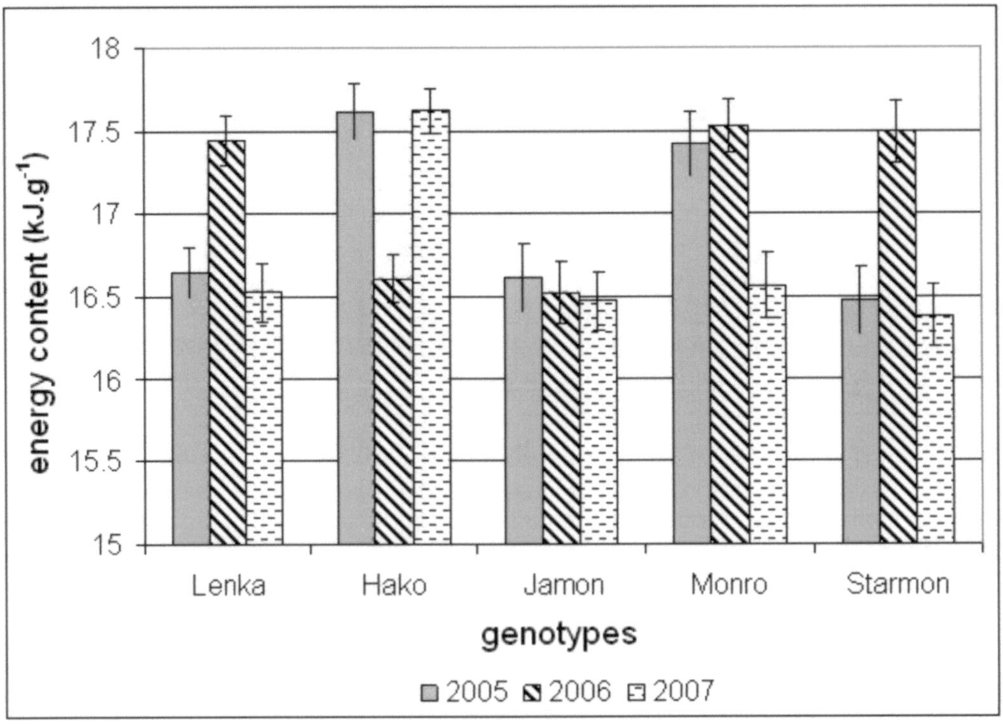

Fig. 8. The influence of genotypes and year onto energy content by bulb of beet (kJ.g^{-1})

Based on the results of statistical analysis by Tukey HSD test was taken on a significance level α = 0.05 alternative hypothesis statistically conclusive differences calculated values of energy yield between genotypes observed varieties, as documented in graph 4. From this graph it is clear that the observed varieties had the lowest yield variety Starmon (1354 GJ.ha^{-1}), while the highest variety Hako (1697.97 GJ.ha^{-1}).
The results of these statistical methods are also evident that the varieties Starmon, Jamon and Monro were lower than the average yield, which was within the tested varieties 1491.48 GJ.ha^{-1}. On the other hand, the variety Hako and Lenka should yield higher than average. The lower yield of varieties Starmon is due not only to low energy, but also statistically proven to yield of bulb the lowest. The Hako variety was found completely opposite trend is the highest yield of bulb and the highest content of energy-rich substances in bulb. According Hnilička et al. (2001) and Honsová et al. (2007) is the energy yield of wheat and fodder beet also influenced by genotype. This conclusion was confirmed also in the case of fodder beet.
Yield was also as its basic ingredients influenced by vintage, the statistically significant lowest average yield was calculated in 2007, which amounted to 1345.54 GJ.ha^{-1}. Conclusively highest yield of bulb was in 2006 (1617.09 GJ.ha^{-1}), see Figure 5. These differences are mainly due to the fact that in 2006 he was demonstrably the highest energy content, but the lowest yield. Low energy yield value determined in 2007 is mainly due to conclusively lowest calorific value, expressed as net energy.
According to Austin et al. (1979) is the gross energy yield of biomass to sugar beet in Great Britain around 222 GJ.ha^{-1} and the sugar cane fields of Queensland and the Transvaal 682

GJ.ha-1. Similarly, the results were not confirmed by Mohammedi et al. (2008), who observed the yield of potatoes in Iran and provides its value 20.81 GJ.ha^{-1}. Energy output was also higher than in their work shows Koga (2009). The author states that energy sugar beet production is 346.1 GJ.ha^{-1}. This difference is probably due not only to the amount of revenue the main product, but also the energy content per unit of dry matter and its conversion from gross energy to net energy. The energy yield of fodder beet is located in the interval of values for sugar beet states (Hnilička et al., 2009).

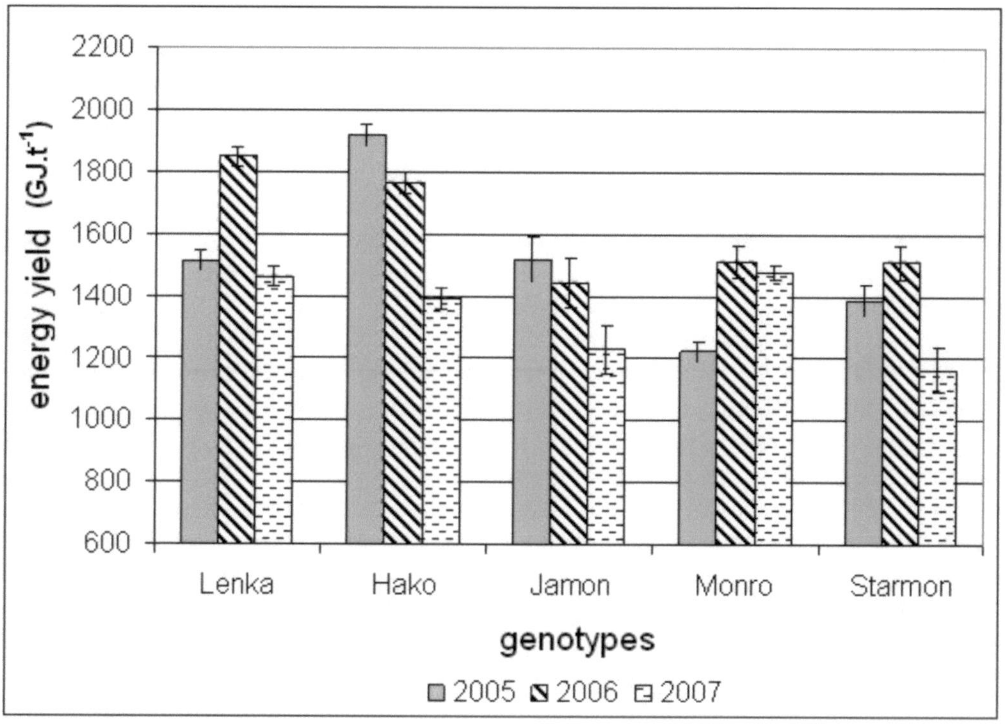

Fig. 9. The influence of genotypes and year onto energy yield by bulb of beet (GJ.t^{-1})

Table II shows the results of statistical analysis of genotype and response to the annual energy yield. From the statistical analysis by Tukey at a significance level α = 0.05 shows conclusively that the lowest yield was recorded in 2007 for a variety Starmon (1162.41 GJ.ha-1), where also was the value of all monitored years and varieties lowest. The highest energy yield this year was found in a variety Monro (1480.05 GJ.ha^{-1}). In 2005 was set at the lowest yield varieties of Monro (1221.19 GJ.t^{-1}) and highest for variety Hako (1917.68 GJ.ha^{-1}). This value was also the maximum value. In 2006, the interval of the energy yield of bulb by fodder beet 1445.52 GJ.ha^{-1} (Jamon) to 1849.18 GJ.ha^{-1} (Lenka).

The levels of energy production of the main product in the range of values for vegetation such as grass state Hirata et al. (1989). Energy production of the main product of sugar beet is higher than for wheat, winter barley and rape (Przybyl, 1994) and also higher than two to eight cuts fescue by Spasov and Kornyšev (1989).

Relationship of dependent variables (yield) on the used independent variables (yield and energy content) is a multidimensional linear regression model described in 99.9%, as evidenced by fully determinant coefficient (multipl. R^2). The calculated regression characteristics show statistical significance of all the variables (yield, energy content and an absolute member of regression equation). Given a regression model can therefore be described by the equation:

$$\text{Yield} = -1500.51 + 87.88 \,.\, 17.08 + \text{energy content} \,.\, \text{yield} \quad (1)$$

Based on the calculated values of energy yield, we can say that there are genotypic differences in this characteristic, because the varieties Starmon, Jamon and Monro had lower yield compared to varieties Lenka and Hako. Lower yield of bulb varieties Starmon is due not only to low energy, but also low-yield of bulb. In contrast, the Hako variety was found completely opposite trend. Organic farming methods it is possible to achieve high yield of energy from both monogerm, so at polygerm varieties.

In all three years (2005 – 2007) high yields of fodder beet roots were reached. In average of three years the most yielding cultivar was Hako (95,6 $t.ha^{-1}$). It confirmed that French cultivars Monro, Starmon and Jamon are very yielding and regarding quality of seed they are suitable also for modern technologies of growing. Evaluated cultivars of fodder beet are suitable also for growing in organic farming. Yields of roots were strongly influenced by year of growing and by number of plants in harvest.

To the most yielding varieties belonged variety Hako, which in 2005 and 2006 gave the highest yield of bulbs and in 2007 it was the second belong Bučanský žlutý válec. High yield in 2005 had varieties Monro, Hako and Kostelecká Barres, in 2006 Hako and Jamon and in 2007 Bučanský žlutý válec and Hako. Statistically significant differences were determined among years of growing and among varieties.

Energetic value in dry matter was detected. The differences among years of growing and varieties were detected. Energy value of fodder beet bulbs was statistically significant to the variety and year of growing. In comparison of the varieties the highest energetic value had varieties of fodder beet Starmon and Jamon. The variety of sugar beet Merak had higher energetic value of one kilogram roots than the fodder beet.

Based on calculated values of energy yield of forage beet growing in ecological technology we can state, that we can reach higher energy yield of root in both of tested cultivars. The influence of year was evidenced.

4. Conclusion

4.1 Technologies

In case of fodder beet organically growing it is possible to achieve high yields, but only with a thorough weeding throughout the vegetation. Row spacing or pitch variation in weed-free yield of roots was not much influenced.

All compared variants without weeds reached in the three-year average high yields of roots above ninety tonnes per hectare. This indicates the need for weeding during the growing period.

Weed infestation significantly reduced root yields. In average of three years provided the lowest yields income variations, where only line weeding were done. Weed infestation not only reduced yields but also decreased the weight of the tubers.

Significant influence of year was discovered. In 2005 exchange of canopy organization did not exchange plant attack by leaf diseases and bulb yield and way of weed regulation had significant influence to plant attack by leaf diseases and bulb production. In 2006 exchange of canopy organization exchanged plant attack by leaf diseases. Bulb yield was influenced by way of weed regulation. In 2007 exchange of canopy organization did not influence to plant attack by leaf diseases but it influenced the bulb production. Higher yield were reached at the variants of narrower rows.

4.2 Varieties and energy

In all three years (2005 - 2007) high yields of fodder beet roots were reached. In average of three years the most yielding cultivar was Hako (95,6 t.ha-1). It confirmed that French cultivars Monro, Starmon and Jamon are very yielding and regarding quality of seed they are suitable also for modern technologies of growing. Evaluated cultivars of fodder beet are suitable also for growing in organic farming. Yields of roots were strongly influenced by year of growing and by number of plants in harvest.

To the most yielding varieties belonged variety Hako, which in 2005 and 2006 gave the highest yield of bulbs and in 2007 it was the second belong Bučanský žlutý válec. High yield in 2005 had varieties Monro, Hako and Kostelecká Barres, in 2006 Hako and Jamon and in 2007 Bučanský žlutý válec and Hako. Statistically significant differences were determined among years of growing and among varieties.

Energetic value in dry matter was detected. The differences among years of growing and varieties were detected. Energy value of fodder beet bulbs was statistically significant to the variety and year of growing. In comparison of the varieties the highest energetic value had varieties of fodder beet Starmon and Jamon. The variety of sugar beet Merak had higher energetic value of one kilogram roots than the fodder beet.

Based on calculated values of energy yield of forage beet growing in ecological technology we can state, that we can reach higher energy yield of root in both of tested cultivars. The influence of year was evidenced.

5. Acknowledgment

The research was supported by programme MSM 6046070901 - Sustainable Agriculture, Quality of Agricultural Production, Landscape and Nature Resources and Grants VaV 1C/4/8/04 and Q 650034.

6. References

Lima, P.; Bonarini, A. & Mataric, M. (2004). *Application of Machine Learning*, InTech, ISBN 978-953-7619-34-3, Vienna, Austria

Li, B.; Xu, Y. & Choi, J. (1996). Applying Machine Learning Techniques, *Proceedings of ASME 2010 4th International Conference on Energy Sustainability*, pp. 14-17, ISBN 842-6508-23-3, Phoenix, Arizona, USA, May 17-22, 2010

Siegwart, R. (2001). Indirect Manipulation of a Sphere on a Flat Disk Using Force Information. *International Journal of Advanced Robotic Systems*, Vol.6, No.4, (December 2009), pp. 12-16, ISSN 1729-8806

Arai, T. & Kragic, D. (1999). Variability of Wind and Wind Power, In: *Wind Power*, S.M. Muyeen, (Ed.), 289-321, Scyio, ISBN 978-953-7619-81-7, Vukovar, Croatia

Van der Linden, S. (June 2010). Integrating Wind Turbine Generators (WTG's) with Energy Storage, In: *Wind Power*, 17.06.2010, Available from http://sciyo.com/articles/show/title/wind-power-integrating-wind-turbine-generators-wtg-s-with-energy-storage

Austin, R. B., Kingstona, G., Longdena, P. C. & Donovana, P. A. (1978). Gross energy yields and the support energy requirements for the production of sugar from beet and cane; a study of four production areas. *The Journal of Agricultural Science*, Vol. 91 , No. 3, (December 1978), p. 667-675. ISSN 0021-8596

Bláha, L., Hnilička, F., Hořejš, P. & Novák, V. (2003). Influence of abiotic stresses on the yield, seed and root traits at winter wheat *(Triticum aestivum* L.). *Scientia Agriculturae Bohemica*, Vol. 34, No. 1, (March 2003), p. 1-7. ISSN 0582-2343

Curtis, G. J. & Hornsey, K. G. (1972). Competition and yield compensation in relation to breeding sugar beet. The Journal of Agricultural Science, *Vol. 79, No. 1, (August 1972), p. 115-119. ISSN 0021-8596*

Fuksa, P., Kocourková, D., Hakl, J. & Kalista, J. 2006. Influence of weed infestation on the calorific value and chemical composition of maize (*Zea mays* L.). *Journal of Plant Diseases Protection*, Vol. 20, No. Sp. Iss., (October 2006), p. 823-830. ISSN 1861-830

Golley, F. B. (1961). Energy valorous of ecological materials. *Ecology*, Vol. 42, No. 3, (March 1961), s. 581-584. ISSN 0012-9658

Hirata M.; Sugimoto Y. & Ueno M. (1989). Productivity and energy efficiency of Bahiagrass (*Paspalum notatum* Flugge) pasture. I. Energy mass of plant and later, net primary production, and efficiency for solar energy utilisation. *Bulletin of the Faculty of Agriculture, University of Miyazaki*, Vol. 36, No. 1 (December 1989), p. 231-237. ISSN 0370-940X

Hnilička, F., Urban, J., Pulkrábek, J. & Hniličková, H. (2009). Energetická bilance pěstování cukrové řepy. *Listy cukrovarnické a řepařské*, Vol. 129, No. 9, (September 2009), p. 260-266. ISSN 1210-3306

Hnilička, F., Hniličková, H., Holá, D., Kočová, M. & Rothová, O. (2010). Shor-term effect of drought on the photosynthetic accumulation energy in maize. *Növénytermelés*, Vol. 59, No. Suppl. 4, (July 2010), s. 489-492. ISSN 0546-8191

Hnilička, F.: *Vliv dusíkaté výživy na fyziologické charakteristiky a obsah energie u pšenice ozimé.* Prague, 1999, 94 p. Disertační práce na Katedře botaniky a fyziologie rostlin FAPPZ ČZU v Praze.

Hnilička, F., Bláha, L. & Novák, V. (2001): Vliv abiotických stresů na energetický výnos pšenice ozimé (*Triticum aestivum* L.). *Proceedings of Mezinárodní slovenský a český kalorimetrický seminář 2001.* ISBN 80-7042-803-1, Račkova Dolina, May 2001.

Hnilička, F.; Urban, J. & Pulkrábek, J.: Obsah netto energie v jednotlivých orgánech cukrové řepy. *Proceedings of 27. Mezinárodní český a slovenský kalorimetrický seminář. ISBN 80-7194-764-4,* Svratka, May 2005

Hoffmann, Ch. M., Huijbregts, T., van Swaaij, N. & Jansen, R. (2009). Impact of different environments in Europe on yield and quality of sugar beet genotypes. *European Journal of Agronomy.* Vol. 30, No. 1, (January 2009), p. 17-26. ISSN 1161-0301

Honsová, H.; Bečková, L. & Pulkrábek, J.: Roots and energy yield of fodder beet in organic farming. *Scientia Agriculturae Bohemica.* Vol. 38, No. 4, (December 2007), p 157-161. ISSN 0582-2343

Chochola, J. (2007). Ekonomické aspekty pěstování řepy na bioetanol. *Listy cukrovarnické a řepařské.* Vol. 123, No. 7/8, (August 2007), p. 211-215. ISSN 1210-3306

Klocke, M., Mahnert, P., Mundt, K., Souidi, K. & Limke, B. (2007). Microbial community analysis of a biogas-producing completely stirred tank reactor fed continuously with fodder beet silage as mono-substrate. *Systematic and applied microbiology,* Vol. 30, No. 2 (February 2007), p. 139-151. ISSN 0723-2020

Kodeš, A., Mudřík, Z., Hučko, B. & Kacerovská, L. (2001): *Základy moderní výživy prasat,* CULS in Prague, ISBN 80-213-0786-2, Prague

Koga, N. (2008). An energy balance under a conventional crop rotation system in northern Japan: Perspectives on fuel ethanol production from sugar beet. *Agriculture, Ecosystems and Environment.* Vol. 125, No. 1-4 (May 2008), p. 101-110. ISSN 0167-8809

Kosař, J. (Eds.) (1985): Krmná řepa, SZN Prague, Prague.

Luković, J., Zorić, L., Nagl, N., Perčić, M., Polić, D. & Putnik-Delić, M. (2009). Histological characteristics of sugar beet leaves potentially linked to drought tolerance. *Industrial Crops and Products,* Vol. 30, No. 2, (February 2009), p. 281-286. ISSN 0926-6690

Mähnert, P.; Linke, B. (2009). Kinetic study of biogas production from energy crops and animal waste slurry: Effect of organic loading rate and reactor size. *Environmental Technology,* Vol. 30, No. 1, (December 2008), p. 93-99. ISSN 0959-3330

Martínez-Pérez, N., Cherryman, S. J., Premier, G. C., Dinsdale, R. M., Hawkes, F. R., Kyazze, G. & Guwy, A. J. (2007). The potential for hydrogen-enriched biogas production from crops: Scenarios in the UK. *Biomass and Bioenergy,* Vol. 31, No. 2-3, (February-March 2007), p. 95-104. ISSN 0961-9534

Mohammadian, R. Abd Elahian Noughabi, M., Baghani, J. & Haghayeghi, A.A.GH. (2009). The relationship of morphological trakte at early growth stage of three sugar beet genotypes with final root yield and white sugar yield under different drought stress conditions. *Journal of Sugar Beet,* Vol. 25, No. 1, (January 2009), p. 23-38. ISSN #0899-1502

Mohammedi, A., Tabatabaeefar, A., Shahin, S., Rafiee, S. & Keyhani, A. (2008). Energy use and economical analysis of potato production in Iran a case study: Ardabil province. *Energy Conversion and Management.* Vol. 49, No. 12, (December 2008), p. 3566-3570. ISSN 0196-8904

Mudřík, Z., Doležal, P. & Koukal, P. (2006). *Základy moderní výživy skotu,* CULS in Prague, ISBN 80-213-1559-8, Prague.

Novák, V. & Hnilička, F. (1996). Vliv rozdílného přihnojení dusíkem na akumulaci energie u rostlin pšenice ozimé. *Proceedings of Kalorimetrický seminář 1996.* Trojanovice v Beskydech, Mai 1996.

Petr, J. & Dlouhý, J. (1992). *Ekologické zemědělství,* Zemědělské nakladatelství Brázda, Prague, ISBN 80-209-0233-3, Prague

Przybyl J. (1994). Porownanie technologii zbioru burakow cukrowych w aspekcie sposobu wykorzystania lisci. Zeszyty Problemowe Postepow Nauk Rolniczych. Vol. 416, No. 416, (Jun 1994), p. 125-130. ISSN 0084-5477

Pulkrábek, J., Peterová, J., Řezbová, H. & Urban, J. (2007). Konkurenceschopnost produkce a ekonomika plodin využitelných pro výrobu bioetanolu. *Listy cukrovarnické a řepařské,* Vol. 123, No. 7/8, (August 2007), p 216-220. ISSN 1210-3306

Reed, W.; Geng, S.; Hills, F. J. (1986). Energy Input and Output Analysis of four Field Crops in California. *Journal of Agronomy and Crop Science*, Vol. 157, No. 2, (August 1986), s. 99-104. ISSN 09312250

Shrestha, N., Geerts, S., Raes, D., Horemans, S., Soentjens, S., Maupas, F. & Clouet, P. (2010). Yield response of sugar beets to water stress under Western European conditions, *Agricultural Water Management*, Vol. 97, No. 2, (February 2010), p. 346-350. ISSN 0378-3774

Scherer, P., Neumann, L., Demirel, B., Schnidt, O. & Unbehauen, M. (2009). Long term fermentation studies about the nutritional requirements for biogasification of fodder beet silage as mono-substrate. *Biomass and Bioenergy*, Vol. 33, No. 5, (May 2009), p. 873-881. ISSN 0961-9534.

Spasov V. P. & Kornyšev D. S. (1989): Accumulation of solar energy by plants and energetic nutritive value of tall fescue (*Festuca arundinacea* Schreb.) at different cutting frequencies. *Proceedings of the XVI International Grassland Congress*. ISBN 2950411002, Nice, France, October 1989.

Šroller J. & Pulkrábek J. (1993). *Základy pěstování krmné řepy*, Institut výchovy a vzdělávání, Ministry of agriculture CR, Prague, ISBN 80-7105-036-9 Prague

Urban, J., Hnilička, F. & Pulkrábek, J. (2005). Obsah energie v bulvách a chrástu cukrové řepy. *Listy cukrovarnické a řepařské*, Vol. 121, No. 9/10, (October 2005), p. 282-285. ISSN 1210-3306

Zeman, L. (1995). *Katalog krmiv: Tabulky výživné hodnoty krmiv*, ČAZV Prague, ISBN 80-901598-3-4 , Prague

Zeman, L. (2002): *Výživa a krmení hospodářských zvířat*, July 29th 2011, Available from: <www.premianti.cz/storage/vyziva.doc>

6

Seed and Crop Production of Yardlong Bean Under Organic Farming System

Raumjit Nokkoul[1], Quanchit Santipracha[1,2] and Wullop Santipracha[2]
[1]Department of Agricultural Technology,
King Mongkut's Institute of Technology Ladkrabang, Chumphorn Campus,
[2]Department of Plant Science, Faculty of Natural Resources,
Prince of Songkla University, Hat Yai, Songkhla
Thailand

1. Introduction

Yardlong beans (Vigna sesquipedalis (L.) Fruw) is an economic crop in the leguminosae. It has potential for export both fresh and frozen and can be grown all year round and in every part of Thailand. However, the problem of pests occurs all through its growing life, prompting farmers to use chemicals to control it. The use of chemicals without considerations of their impacts and safety have induced various problems such as dangers to farmers themselves, ecological balance disturbance and effects on environment through food chain and then to the consumers. The deposit in soil, water contamination and residues in plants are all dangerous to living things and human health.

Yardlong bean production using reduced amount of chemicals or organic farming system, hence, has become important and increasingly wanted. Organic farming system is the production system which avoids the use of synthetic fertilizers, insecticides and plant growth regulators. The standard requirement of organic plant production is that the seeds used for growing must be from organic farming production that has been approved. This is especially true for the Common European Market Council which requires farmers operating under the organic farming system to use the seeds produced via organic farming system since January 1, 2004. Thailand has also adopted that approach.

However, there are many factors involving the production of seeds under the organic farming system, making the yield low. Hence, in producing organic seeds, suitable varieties should be selected to suit each area and they should be the open-pollinated varieties with regular quality high yield. It should be able to grow in low fertile soil, resist pests and diseases, and compete with weeds. The suitable season should be selected for the production of seeds and the planting areas should not be repeated. Rotation corps such as the bean family should be emphasized. Compost, farm manure, green manure, wastes from other materials, organic and inorganic matters from nature should be used as nutrients.

The use of bio-extract solution and gypsum mixture is an alternative in the organic farming system because bio-extract solution is made from nature and can be used instead of chemical fertilizers as plant growth regulators and can be used for disease and pest prevention and elimination. It is easy to produce and safe for the users, consumers and environment. It can be used in producing various kinds of vegetable for consumption such as cabbage, broccoli, lettuce, Chinese cabbage, Chinese turnip, carrot, chili, egg plant, cucumber, kale, yardlong bean crops and seeds. As for Gypsum, likewise, is a natural mineral, a source for calcium and sulfur which can help boost the ability of the bean family plants to create more root nodule, improve soil physical structure and increase seed yields of Chinese turnip, wheat, bean family plant and peanut. Hence, the study about the use of bio-extract solution and gypsum mixture in the production of yardlong bean under the organic farming system which will help perfect the process and reduce the negative effects and dangers in using chemicals

The aim to study the yield, seed quality and the selected PSU yardlong bean produced under the organic farming system in comparison with those produced using chemicals.

2. Materials and methods

The first trial studied types and quantity of bio-extract solution in producing yardlong bean seeds using 3 formulas: 1) Water Convolvulous bio-extract solution, made from 3 kilograms of Water Convolvulous, 1 kilogram of molasses, 100 grams of microorganism/1 liter of water, 2) fruit bio-extract solution, from 3 kilograms of papaya, 3 kilograms of pumpkins, 3 kilograms of bananas, 3 kilogram of molasses, 300 grams of microorganism/1 liter of water, and 3) sea fish bio-extract solution, from 6 kilograms of ground sea fish, 3 kilograms of molasses, 200 grams of microorganism/1 liter of water. These were kept in covered bins for 45 days. The 3 formulas of bio-extract solutions at 1:500 and 1:1000 were used to water the Yearlong beans in the trial beds. Tobacco extract solution was used for the first three treatments while chemical insecticides. In comparison, the use of chemicals were done by bedding each planting hole with 1 gram of Carbofuran, applying 15-15-15 formula fertilizer at the rate of 20 kilograms/rai at the age of 2, 5 and 7 weeks after planting. Phriphonil solution at 20 cc./1 liter was sprayed to prevent and eliminate pests every 7 days.

The second trial was to study the effect of bio-extract solution and gypsum mixture on yields and quality of yardlong bean seeds. The water convolvulus bio-extract solution at 1:1.000 to water the plant every 4 days gained from the first trail was used in the preparation of the trial beds with 50 kilograms of gypsum/rai, and a bio-extract solution from water convolvulus rated 1:1.000 + gypsum rated 50 kilograms/rai., compared with a conventional method (chemicals application) for control. Tobacco extract solution was used for the first three treatments while chemical insecticides were used with the fourth treatment to control major insect pests when necessary.

The third trial studied the effects of methods in increasing the amount of bio-extract solution to produce seeds under the organic farming method. The water convolvulus bio-extract solution at 1:1.000 was used to bio-extract solution watering once for 4 days, bio-extract solution watering once for 7 days alternated with spraying once for 4 days, bio-extract solution spraying once for 3 days were compared with conventional method (chemical application).

The fourth trial studied the production of fresh crop production from organically produced seeds and the use of chemicals. The seeds from the 2nd and 3rd trials were planted to produce crop. The trial was done at the Department of Plant Science, Faculty of Natural Resources, Prince of Songkla University, Hat Yai, Songkhla, Thailand.

3. Results and discussion

The first trial studied types and quantity of bio-extract solution in growing yardlong bean seeds (Table 1, 2 and 3). It was found that the suitable bio-extract solution for producing yardlong bean seeds was the water convolvulus bio-extract solution at 1:1.000. The seed yield was 49.81 kilograms/rai which were higher than the production using other types and ratios of bio-extract solution but lower than growing by using chemicals with the yield of 52.17 kilogram/rai. The germination rate of the seeds produced by any method was higher than 89% whereas the use of water convolvulus bio-extract solution yielded seeds stronger than any other methods. Hence, water convolvulus bio-extract solution at 1:1.000 was used in the second trial.

Treatment	Days to flowering 50% (days)	Days to harvested seed (days)	No. of harvested plants (%)	Seed yield (kg/rai)
Chemical method	40	53	88	52.17a
Water convolvulus bio-extract solution at 1:500.	40	53	86	37.55ab
Water convolvulus bio-extract solution at 1:1.000.	40	54	91	49.81a
Fruit (namva, pumpkin, papaya) bio-extract solution at 1:500.	41	54	85	42.39ab
Fruit (namva, pumpkin, papaya) bio-extract solution at 1: 1.000.	41	54	88	33.55b
Sea fish bio-extract solution at 1:500.	40	53	88	40.48ab
Sea fish bio-extract solution at 1: 1.000.	41	54	90	37.59ab
F-test	ns	ns	ns	*
C.V. (%)	3.59	2.41	5.96	21.47

ns = non-significant * = significant different at $P \leq 0.05$
Within each column, means not followed by the same letter are significantly different at the 5% level of probability as determined by DMRT

Table 1. Days to flowering 50%, days to harvested seed, no. of harvested plants and yield of yardlong bean seed by application of bio-extract solution compared with chemical method

The second trial studied the effects of bio-extract solution and gypsum on yields and quality of yardlong bean seeds (Table 4, 5 and 6). It was found that the use of water convolvulus bio-extract solution at 1:1,000 yielded 40 kilograms of yardlong bean seeds /rai which was higher than the production using gypsum and bio-extract solution + gypsum but lower than the production using chemicals (90 kilograms/rai). As for quality, the seeds produced using bio-extract solution had more seed size and seed dry weight than seeds produced by any other methods. However, standard germination and seeds vigor were not different no matter what method was used (97-98%).

Treatment	Seed size (cm)		Seed dry weight (mg/seed)	Standard germination (%)	Field emergence (%)
	width	Length			
Chemical method	0.52	1.07b	127.50	91.50	92.50
Water convolvulus bio-extract solution at 1:500.	0.55	1.12a	127.50	91.50	93.50
Water convolvulus bio-extract solution at 1:1.000.	0.53	1.08b	125.00	92.00	95.50
Fruit (namva, pumpkin, papaya) bio-extract solution at 1:500.	0.53	1.07b	130.00	89.50	87.00
Fruit (namva, pumpkin, papaya) bio-extract solution at 1: 1.000.	0.54	1.06b	120.00	90.00	89.50
Sea fish bio-extract solution at 1:500.	0.53	1.07b	130.00	89.00	93.50
Sea fish bio-extract solution at 1: 1.000.	0.53	1.05b	130.00	90.00	93.00
F-test	ns	*	ns	ns	ns
C.V. (%)	2.60	2.41	3.21	3.87	4.78

ns = non-significant * = significant different at $P \leq 0.05$
Within each column, means not followed by the same letter are significantly different at the 5% level of probability as determined by DMRT

Table 2. Seed size, seed dry weight, standard germination and field emergence of yardlong bean seed by application of bio-extract solution compared with chemical method

When the seeds age were accelerated to study their ability storage, it was found that seeds produced using bio-extract solution + gypsum had the highest germination rate of 98% whereas the production using bio-extract solution and gypsum had the germination rates of 92.50% and 90.50%, respectively. On the other hand the production using chemicals had the germination rate after the age acceleration of 93.50%. This meant that the seeds produced using bio-extract solution + gypsum could be storage longer than the seeds produced by other methods. However, the production of seeds using convolvulus bio-extract solution at 1:1,000 to water the plants every 7 days might not give them enough nutrients for growth and seed production because they took a long time—20 days after the flowers started to bloom, or the pods had to become brown—before they could be harvested. It could be seen that the leaves turned yellow during the flowering and yielding, on the fifth day after the application of bio-extract solution. Some of the plants yielded at least 10 pods each. The calculation of the amount of bio-extract solution used to water the plants all through the season revealed that there were 192.00, 19.55 and 640.44 gram of N, P, and K respectively/rai only. Yardlong beans usually needed 1.6-3.2 kilogram of Nitrogen/rai and 8.0-9.6 of Phosphorus and Potassium/rai to be sufficient for growth and yield. Hence, more bio-extract solution was needed in the seed production.

Treatments	Speed of germination index	Seedling dry weight (mg/seedling)	Conductivity (µmho/cm/gm)	AA germination (%)
Chemical method	14.01ab	67.50	13.57	84.00
Water convolvulus bio-extract solution at 1:500.	14.43a	61.50	14.82	82.50
Water convolvulus bio-extract solution at 1:1.000.	14.47a	69.50	14.98	83.00
Fruit (namva, pumpkin, papaya) bio-extract solution at 1:500.	12.18c	63.75	15.77	87.00
Fruit (namva, pumpkin, papaya) bio-extract solution at 1: 1.000.	13.23b	63.00	15.40	83.00
Sea fish bio-extract solution at 1:500.	14.05ab	68.00	15.99	80.00
Sea fish bio-extract solution at 1: 1.000.	13.69ab	66.50	14.71	73.00
F-test	*	ns	ns	ns
C.V. (%)	5.03	5.03	13.30	6.79

ns = non-significant * = significant different at $P \leq 0.05$
Within each column, means not followed by the same letter are significantly different at the 5% level of probability as determined by DMRT

Table 3. Speed of germination index, seedling dry weight, conductivity and AA germination of yardlong bean seed by application of bio-extract solution compared with chemical method

Treatment	Days to flowering 50% (days)	Days to harvested seed (days)	No. of harvested plants (%)	Seed yield (kg/rai)
Chemical method	41.25	52.83	71.46	89.78 a
Bio-extract	40.50	52.75	75.83	40.06 b
Gypsum	41.41	52.99	73.96	31.41 b
Bio-extract + Gypsum	40.99	53.17	70.21	29.55 b
F-test	ns	ns	ns	*
C.V. (%)	1.79	1.03	18.18	29.66

ns = non-significant * = significant different at $P \leq 0.05$
Within each column, means not followed by the same letter are significantly different at the 5% level of probability as determined by DMRT

Table 4. Days to flowering 50%, days to harvested seed, no. of harvested plants and yield of yardlong bean seed by application of bio-extract solution, gypsum and mixture of bio-extract solution and gypsum compared with chemical method

Treatment	Seed size (cm)		Seed dry weight (mg/seed)	Standard germination (%)	Field emergence (%)
	width	Length			
Chemical method	0.55	1.05	128.54	97.00	100.00
Bio-extract	0.56	1.08	131.90	97.50	100.00
Gypsum	0.53	1.06	130.41	98.00	99.50
Bio-extract + Gypsum	0.54	1.04	130.39	98.00	99.50
F-test	ns	ns	ns	ns	ns
C.V. (%)	3.08	10.77	1.69	2.03	0.71

ns = non-significant

Table 5. Seed size, seed dry weight, standard germination and field emergence of yardlong bean seed by application of bio-extract solution, gypsum and mixture of bio-extract solution and gypsum compared with chemical method

Treatments	Speed of germination index	Seedling dry weight (mg/seedling)	Conductivity (µmho/cm/gm)	AA germination (%)
Chemical method	33.33	73.21 a	28.21	93.50 ab
Bio-extract	33.33	76.00 a	28.31	92.50 b
Gypsum	33.16	67.98 b	27.92	90.50 b
Bio-extract + Gypsum	33.20	74.25 a	28.22	98.00 a
F-test	ns	*	ns	*
C.V. (%)	0.63	3.33	6.67	3.50

ns = non-significant * = significant different at $P \leq 0.05$
Within each column, means not followed by the same letter are significantly different at the 5% level of probability as determined by DMRT

Table 6. Speed of germination index, seedling dry weight, conductivity and AA germination of yardlong bean seed by application of bio-extract solution, gypsum and mixture of bio-extract solution and gypsum compared with chemical method

The third trial studied the effects of methods in increasing the amount of bio-extract solution in the production of seeds under the organic farming system (Table 7, 8, 9 and 10). It was found that the production using chemicals gave the highest yield of 160 kilograms/rai, not significantly different from watering bio-extract solution every 4 days, watering every 7 days together with spraying every 4 days, and spraying every 3 days, which gave the seeds yields at 146, 138 and 133 kilograms/rai respectively. Using bio-extract solution every 4 days was the most effective way.

The seeds produced by watering bio-extract solution every 4 days had more seed dry weight than seeds produced by other methods. However, their germination rate was not different from those of the seeds produced by other methods (95.50-97.25%). Seed age acceleration to find out their potential in storage time revealed that the seeds produced by watering bio-extract solution every 4 days had the highest germination rate (96%), which was different from the seeds produced using chemicals and watering bio-extract solution every 7 days together with spraying at every 4 days, which had the germination rates after age acceleration of 90.00 and 94.00% respectively.

Treatment	Days to flowering 50%(days)	Days to harvested seed (days)	No. of harvested plants (%)
chemical method	45.00	61.00	87.81
bio-extract solution watering once for 4 days	45.00	61.00	85.94
bio-extract solution watering once for 7 days alternated with spraying once for 4 days	45.00	60.00	90.63
bio- bio-extract solution spraying once for 3 days	44.00	60.00	91.81
F-test	ns	ns	ns
C.V. (%)	3.22	0.87	13.81

ns = non-significant

Table 7. Days to flowering 50%, days to harvested seed and no. of harvested plants of yardlong bean seed by application of bio-extract solution compared with chemical method

Treatment	Seed yield (kg/rai)	Seed size (cm)		Seed dry weight (mg/seed)
		width	Length	
chemical method	160	0.54	1.00	131.58
bio-extract solution watering once for 4 days	146	0.55	1.00	132.01
bio-extract solution watering once for 7 days alternated with spraying once for 4 days	138	0.55	1.16	131.35
bio- bio-extract solution spraying once for 3 days	133	0.55	1.16	131.40
F-test	ns	ns	ns	ns
C.V. (%)	13.31	1.53	1.30	0.77

ns = non-significant

Table 8. Seed yield , seed size and seed dry weight of yardlong bean seed by application of bio-extract solution compared with chemical method

Treatment	Standard germination (%)	Field emergence (%)	Speed of germination index
chemical method	96.50	98.50	32.70
bio-extract solution watering once for 4 days	97.25	99.50	33.24
bio-extract solution watering once for 7 days alternated with spraying once for 4 days	96.75	100.00	33.16
bio- bio-extract solution spraying once for 3 days	95.50	100.00	33.32
F-test	ns	ns	ns
C.V. (%)	1.32	1.58	1.25

ns = non-significant

Table 9. Standard germination, field emergence and speed of germination index, of yardlong bean seed by application of bio-extract solution compared with chemical method

Treatment	Seedling dry weight (mg/seedling)	Conductivity (μmho/cm/gm)	AA germination (%)
chemical method	65.00	25.32 ab	90.00 b
bio-extract solution watering once for 4 days	62.50	30.16 a	96.00 a
bio-extract solution watering once for 7 days alternated with spraying once for 4 days	67.50	20.77 b	94.00 b
bio- bio-extract solution spraying once for 3 days	65.00	24.53 ab	94.50 ab
F-test	ns	*	*
C.V. (%)	10.41	13.93	3.41

ns = non-significant * = significant different at $P \leq 0.05$
Within each column, means not followed by the same letter are significantly different at the 5% level of probability as determined by DMRT

Table 10. Seedling dry weight, conductivity and AA germination of yardlong bean seed by application of bio-extract solution compared with chemical method

However, the method of using bio-extract solution to water the plants every 4 days yielded only 14 kilograms of produce less than the yield produced using chemicals. This was probably because the plants received more nutrients as bio-extract solution was given more frequently (from every 7 days to every 4 days). The nutrients received were sufficient for growth and seed production as could be seen that the plants did not show the sign of nutrients lacking. The stems were healthy and the number of pods/plant was more than those produced using bio-extract solution to water every 7 days. The calculation of the amount of bio-extract solution used to water the plants every 4 days all through the planting season revealed that there were 266.76, 33.35 and 964.00 grams of N, P, and K respectively/rai which was higher than applying it every 7 days. This was also because the bio-extract solution also had secondary nutrients which were Ca, Mg, and S at 1111.50, 166.72 and 144.49 grams/rai and also carbohydrate, protein, enzyme, organic acid and plant hormones which were important factors enhancing biochemical reaction leading to cell division and reproduction cell production, making the plants strong and finally yield flowers and seeds. Apart from that, bio-extract solution had micro-organism with the ability to decompose organic matters in the soil so that more nutrients were released into the soil for the plants to use.

Treatments	Days to indeterminate 50% (days)	Days to flowering 50% (days)	Days to harvested (days)	No. of harvested plants (%)
Chemical method	20.00	40.00	48.00	96.88
Bio-extract	20.00	40.00	48.00	94.06
Gypsum	20.00	40.00	48.00	94.06
Bio-extract + Gypsum	20.00	40.00	48.00	96.88
F-test	ns	ns	ns	ns
C.V. (%)	1.93	1.43	1.00	3.00

ns = non-significant.

Table 11. Days to indeterminate 50%, days to flowering 50%, days to harvested , and no. of harvested plants of yardlong bean seed by application of bio-extract solution, gypsum and mixture of bio-extract solution and gypsum compared with chemical method

Treatments	Wilted disease and death rate (%)	Marketable yield (kg/rai)	Non-marketable yield (kg/rai)
Chemical method	2.19	2,079	275
Bio-extract	5.31	2,171	255
Gypsum	5.00	1,894	281
Bio-extract + Gypsum	2.50	1,846	273
F-test	ns	ns	ns
C.V. (%)	89.58	12.82	19.33

ns = non-significant.

Table 12. Wilted disease and death rate, Marketable yield and Non-marketable yield of yardlong bean seed by application of bio-extract solution, gypsum and mixture of bio-extract solution and gypsum compared with chemical method

The fourth trial studied fresh crop production from organic seeds and the use of chemicals (Table 11, 12 and 13). The seeds gained from the 2nd and 3rd trials were planted for crops. To be specific, the seeds produced in the trial to study the effects of using bio-extract solution and gypsum on yields and quality of seeds were used. All methods yielded non-significantly different amounts of fresh pods. The use of bio-extract solution yielded 2,171 kilograms/rai of marketable yields, higher than those produced by using chemicals, gypsum and bio-extract solution + gypsum which yielded 2,079, 1,894, and 1,846 kilograms/rai, respectively. Production using bio-extract solution to water the plants every 7 days could have given sufficient nutrients for growth and pod production since the plants did not reveal the symptoms of nutrients deficiency. The plants were healthy and yielded many pods/plant. In addition to that, the beans were creeping plants and their flowers bloomed in succession so the pods could be harvested everyday. The needs for nutrients to feed the plants and pods, hence, were less than those in producing seeds because the pods had to be left on the plants until the time to harvest the seeds.

Treatments	Pod length (cm)	Pod weight (g)	Pod color
Chemical method	63.08 a	24.46	143C
Bio-extract	63.49 a	22.71	143C
Gypsum	61.31 b	20.89	143C
Bio-extract + Gypsum	61.51 b	21.38	143C
F-test	*	ns	-
C.V. (%)	1.11	11.28	-

ns = non-significant * = significant different at $P \leq 0.05$
Within each column, means not followed by the same letter are significantly different at the 5% level of probability as determined by DMRT

Table 13. Pod length, pod weight and pod color of yardlong bean seed by application of bio-extract solution, gypsum and mixture of bio-extract solution and gypsum compared with chemical method

When the seeds from the study of the effects of the methods in increasing the amount of bio-extract solution in the production under organic farming method were used to produce fresh pods (Table 14, 15 and 16), it was found that the seeds produced by using organic farming method and using chemicals yielded no differences in fresh crop production. The crops were possible to harvest after the flowers had bloomed for 10 days and could be harvested for 25 days with marketable yields. The seeds produced using bio-extract solution to water every 4 days gave the highest yield of 1,606 kilograms/rai of marketable yields, higher than the yields from the production using bio-extract solution to water every 7 days together with spraying every 4 days, spraying every 3 days and using chemicals which gave the yields of 1,414, 1,285, and 1,587 kilograms/rai respectively. However, the yields in this production were smaller than the production using bio-extract solution to water every 7 days, probably because the environment during the planting time was different. In this planting time, during the time from stem growing to flowering to pod producing, there were continuous rains with high amount of water, a lot of clouds and hence little light, resulting in the significant growth in the stem but less flowering.

Treatment	Days to flowering 50%(days)	Days to harvested (days)	No. of harvested plants (%)
chemical method	40.00	48.00	93.75 a
bio-extract solution watering once for 4 days	40.00	47.00	84.69 ab
bio-extract solution watering once for 7 days alternated with spraying once for 4 days	40.00	48.00	82.19 ab
bio- bio-extract solution spraying once for 3 days	40.00	47.00	77.81 b
F-test	ns	ns	*
C.V. (%)	1.76	1.40	10.35

ns = non-significant * = significant different at P ≤ 0.05
Within each column, means not followed by the same letter are significantly different at the 5% level of probability as determined by DMRT

Table 14. Days to flowering 50%, days to harvested and no. of harvested plants of yardlong bean seed by application of bio-extract solution compared with chemical method

Treatments	Wilted disease and death rate (%)	Marketable yield (kg/rai)	Non-marketable yield (kg/rai)
chemical method	9.41	1,578	129 a
bio-extract solution watering once for 4 days	10.00	1,606	122 a
bio-extract solution watering once for 7 days alternated with spraying once for 4 days	15.69	1,414	90 b
bio- bio-extract solution spraying once for 3 days	13.13	1,285	87 b
F-test	ns	ns	*
C.V. (%)	61.92	16.29	10.47

ns = non-significant * = significant different at P ≤ 0.05
Within each column, means not followed by the same letter are significantly different at the 5% level of probability as determined by DMRT

Table 15. Wilted disease and death rate, Marketable yield and Non-marketable yield of yardlong bean seed by application of bio-extract solution compared with chemical method

It can be concluded from all the trials in producing yardlong bean seeds and fresh crops under the organic farming system that the production of seeds using the increased amount of convolvulus bio-extract solution at 1:1,000 to water the plants every 4 days, using 40 liters each time in the 1x5 meter beds was the method that gave the highest yield, as high as the production using chemicals both in terms of amount and quality. The production of fresh crops using the morning glory water convolvulus bio-extract solution at 1:1,000 to water the plants every 7 days, using 40 liters each time in the 1x5 meter beds was the method that gave the highest yield, as high as the production using chemicals. Hence in the use of bio-extract solution in producing seeds and fresh pods under the organic farming method, the yardlong bean plants must be observed closely. If the leaves turn yellow and the plants are not healthy, it means that the nutrients are not sufficient. Hence, bio-extract solution should be added more frequently. Besides, the production of seeds and fresh crops under the organic farming method needs more meticulous care and attention in tending to the plants all through the planting season than the use of chemicals. Farmers need to have knowledge, experience and understanding about the production under the organic farming method.

Treatments	Pod length (cm)	Pod weight (g)	Pod color
chemical method	61.40 b	22.05 a	143C
bio-extract solution watering once for 4 days	62.47 a	22.09 a	143C
bio-extract solution watering once for 7 days alternated with spraying once for 4 days	61.63 b	21.31 b	143C
bio- bio-extract solution spraying once for 3 days	61.53 b	21.35 b	143C
F-test	*	*	-
C.V. (%)	0.69	1.28	-

* = significant different at $P \leq 0.05$
Within each column, means not followed by the same letter are significantly different at the 5% level of probability as determined by DMRT

Table 16. Pod length, pod weight and pod color of yardlong bean seed by application of bio-extract solution compared with chemical method

4. References

AOAC. 1990. Official Method of Analysis. Virginia: The Association of Official Analytical Chemists, INC.

AOSA. 2002. Seed Vigor Testing Handbook. Contribution No. 32 to the Handbook on Seed Testing. Washington: the Association of Official Seed Analysts.

Ara, N., All, M. O., All, M. M. and Basher, M. K. 1999. Effects of spacing and fertilizer levels on yield and quality of radish seed. Journal of Scientific and Industrial Research 34: 174-178.

Boelt, B., Deleuran, L. C. and. Gislum, R. 2002. Organic Forage Seed Production in Denmark. Slagelse: Department of Plant Biology, Danish Institute of Agricultural Sciences Research Centre Flakkebjierg.

Borgen, A. 2002. Organic Seed Production and Seed Regulation. http://www. grologica.dk/LatviaSEED2002.final.htm. 8/12/2547.

Finch, S. and Collier, R. H. 2000. Intergrated pest management in field vegetable crop in northern Europe-with focus on two key pests. Crop Protection 19: 817-824.

Guan, P. C., Liu, H. C. and Chen, Y. D. 2000. Studies on characteristics of NPK absorption by asparagus bean (*Vigna unguiculata* W. ssp. sesquipedalis (L.) Verd.). China-Vegetables 5: 12-15.

Gundogmus, E. 2006. Energy use on organic farming: A comparative analysis on organic versus conventional apricot production on small holdings in Turkey. Energy Conversion and Management 47: 3351-3359.

Hamza, M. A. and Anderson, W. K. 2003. Responses of soil and grain yields to deep ripping and gypsum application in a compacted loamy of sand soil contrasted with a sandy clay loam soil in Western Australia. Journal of Agricultural Research 54: 273-282.

Hardarson, G. and Atkins, C. 2003. Optimising biological N_2 fixation by legumes in farming systems. Plant and Soil 252: 41-54.

Hellou, G. C. and Crozat, Y. 2005. N_2 fixation and N supply in organic pea (*Pisum sativum* L.) cropping systems as affected by weeds and peaweevil (*Sitona lineatus* L.). Europian Journal of Agronomy 22: 449-458. ISTA. 2003. International Rules for Seed Testing. Rules 2003. Basserdorft: International Seed Testing Association.

Kaute, W. V. 2003. Crop Breeding for Organic Agriculture. http:// www.w.vogt-kaute naturland.de. 5/12/2547.

Lammerts van Bueren, E. T., Struik, P. C and Jacobsen, E. 2003. Organic propagation of seed and planting material: an overview of problems and challenges for research. Journal of Agricultural Science 51: 263-277.

Lampkin, N. H. and Padel, S. 1994. The Economics of Organic Farming an International Perspective. Bristol: Department of Agricultural Sciences, University of Wales, Aberystwyth.

Lane, G. and Steve, D. 2000. Organic Greenhouse Vegetable Production. Horticulture System Guide. Rural Business-Cooperative Service. http:// www.attra.ncat.org. 10/7/2546.

Langer, V. and Rohde, B. 2005. Factors reducing yield of organic white clover seed production in Denmark. Grass and Forage Science 60: 168-174.

Marinari, S., Mancinelli, R., Campiglia, E. and Grego, S. 2006. Chemical and biological indicators of soil quality in organic and conventional farming systems in central Italy. Ecologial Indicators 6: 701-711.

Martini, E. A., Jeffrey, S. B., Dennis, C. B., Timothy, K. H. and Denison, R. F. 2004. Yield increase during the organic transition: improving soil quality or increasing experience?. Field Crop Research 86: 255-266.

Nadia, E. S. and Caroline, H. 2002. Organic Agriculture, Environment and Food Security. Rome: FAO. OECD. 2003. Organic Agriculture: Sustainability, Markets and Policies. Danvers: CABI.

Peoples, M. B., Ladha, J. K. and Herridge, D. F. 1995. Enhancing legume N_2 fixation through plant and soil management. Plant and Soil 174: 83 -101.

Porter, P. M., Huggins, C. A., Perillo, S. R., Quiring and Crookston, R. K. 2003. Organic and other management strategies with two- and four-year crop rotations in Minnesota. Agronomy Journal 95: 233-244.

Raumjit Nokkoul, Quanchit Santipracha, and Wullop Santipracha. 2007. Bio-extracts Solution on Yield, Quality and Storability of Yardlong Bean Seed. Songklanakarin. Journal of science and technology 29(3) 637-646.

Raumjit Nokkoul, Quanchit Santipracha, and Wullop Santipracha. 2008. Method Use of Bio-extract Solution in Seed Production of Yardlong Bean Under Organic Farming System. Thai Science and Technology Journal 6(2) 59-67

Raumjit Nokkoul, Quanchit Santipracha, and Wullop Santipracha. 2009. Crop Production of Yardlong Bean from Organic Seed. Thai Science and Technology Journal 17(1) 87-95.

Raumjit Nokkoul, Quanchit Santipracha, and Wullop Santipracha. 2010. Method Use of Bio-extract Solution in Yardlong Bean Production. King Mongkut's agricultural journal. 28(2) 37-44.

Robin, G. B., Arbindra, R. and Steve, R. 2000. Comparative cost analyses of conventional, integrated crop management, and organic methods. Hortechnology 4: 785-793.

Sorensen, C. G., Madsen, N. A. and Jacobsen, B.H. 2005. Organic farming scenarios: Operational analysis and costs of implementing innovative technologies. Biosystems Engineering 91: 127-137.

Steve, D., George, K. and Holly, B. 1999. Organic Tomato Production. Horticulture Production Guide. Rural Business-Cooperative Service. http://www.attra.ncat. org. 10/7/2546.

Stout, W. L. and Priddy, W. E. 1996. Use of fuel gas desulfurization (FGD) by -product gypsum on alfalfa. Soil Science Society of America 27: 2419-2432.

Sumner, M. E., Shahandeh, H., Bouton, J. and Hammel, J. 1986. Amelioration of an acid soil profile through deep liming and surface application of gypsum. Soil Science Society of America 50: 1254-1258.

Teasdale, J. R., Mangum, R. W., Radhakrishnan, J. and Cavigelli, M. A. 2004. Weed seedbank dynamics in three organic farming crop rotations. Agronomy Journal 96: 1429-1435.

Toma, M., Sumner, M. E., Weeks, G. and Saigusa. M. 1999. Long-term effects of gypsum on crop yield and subsoil chemical properties. Soil Science Society of America 63: 891-895.

7

Wheat Growing and Quality in Organic Farming

Petr Konvalina[1], Zdeněk Stehno[2], Ivana Capouchová[3] and Jan Moudrý[1]
[1]*University of South Bohemia in České Budějovice,*
[2]*Crop Research Institute in Prague,*
[3]*Czech University of Live Sciences in Prague,*
Czech Republic

1. Introduction

Agricultural crop species represent a negligible part of the existing biodiversity. Over 50 percent of the daily global requirement of proteins and calories is met by just three crops - maize, wheat and rice (FAO, 1996) - and only 150 crops are commercialised on a significant global scale. On the other hand, ethnobotanic surveys indicate that, worldwide, more than 7,000 plant species are cultivated or harvested from the wild (Wilson, 1992). The composition of crops has significantly changed in farming history. Introducing new more efficient crops has jeopardized obsolete landraces being important genetic resources, serving for the breeding process (Collins & Hawtin, 1999). At present, genetic diversity in agriculture as well as in nature is often seriously endangered (Dotlačil et al., 2002).

At least 1.8 million hectares of main cereal species in the world are under organic management (including in-conversion areas). As some of the world's large cereal producers (such as India, China and the Russian Federation) did not provide land use details, it can be assumed that the area is larger than shown here (Willer & Kilcher, 2009). Comparing this figure with FAO's figure for the world's harvested cereal area of 384 million hectares (FAOSTAT, 2011), 0.5 percent of the total cereal area is under organic management. *Triticum* L., and bread wheat (*Triticum aestivum* L.) in particular, is the most frequent crop in organic farming, the same as in conventional farming. It is grown in organic system on a total surface of more than 700 000 ha (Willer & Kilcher, 2009).

2. Grown wheat species and their suitability for the organic farming system

Wheat species are the most frequently grown crops in the organic farming system. However, not all of them are suitable for organic farming, the ones grown in marginal regions in particular. Currently, a lot of alternative crops, including the marginal wheat species, have become attractive too. Such species have been bred neither in order to increase the yield rate nor for the intensive farming system. Although the baking quality is not high from the conventional point of view, these species have a lot of specific characteristics (e.g. a higher proportion of proteins, a favourable composition of amino acids, and a high proportion of mineral elements). Products made of such wheat species are considered specialities with a higher added value at the market and they may be applied well.

2.1 Grown wheat species

Bread wheat (*Triticum aestivum* L.) is a traditionally grown species in all farming systems in the Czech Republic. It is a species that began to be domesticated 10,000 years ago in the Levant region (Iraq, Iran, Syria and Jordan). As it has been brought closer to Central Europe, it has significantly changed and adapted to farming technologies. The selection of this species had been unconscious at first, nevertheless, it started to be conscious later. The continuity of the development of landraces has been maintained, the same as the interaction between these species and agrotechnological conditions of a particular farm. The first breeding farms had been established just after the industrial revolution and the breeding process had been converted from the field conditions to the sterile laboratory ones. Therefore, the profitable conventional varieties were created, whose ideotypes are not suitable for the low-input farming systems.

The landraces and obsolete cultivars of bread wheat (*Triticum aestivum* L.) contained in the gene bank collection at the Crop Research Institute in Prague (CRI) deserve particular care and attention, and a number of authors - e.g. Gregova et al (2006) - in pointing this out, have also referred us to the high level of proteins contained in the grains - much higher than in the modern wheat varieties. The landraces are not able to compete with the modern bred varieties from the point of view of the yield level, but they have many valuable characteristics, which make them very interesting. They are characterised by high nutritive and dietetic values (Marconi & Cubadda, 2005). They have been selected by the natural and environmental conditions of a particular region (Belay et al. 1995) and thus the material is very well adapted to the domestic environment and conditions and it is very variable from the point of view of genetics (Hammer et al., 2003).

Durum wheat (*Triticum durum* Desf.) is the second most important species of *Triticum* genus It is a tetraploid wheat species that comes from the Mediterranean. It represents about 9% of the wheat surface worldwide. It requires high temperatures, it grows especially in the regions characterised by long warm and dry summers. It is mostly used in the production of pasta and non-yeasty baked goods (biscuits). Caryopsis are naked, and have a glassy, amber colour, which is related to a higher proportion of carotenoids in their endosperm and it influences the semolina's colour too, which is yellowish.

Einkorn (*Triticum monococcum* L.) is an old cereal known to have been grown 9,000 years ago, and its use had extended to the Balkans and Central Europe in the neolithic period. It has attracted farmers because of such valuable characteristics as resistance to diseases and the quality of its grain, which contains 17.0 – 22.5 % protein, a good supply of carotenoides and perfect characteristics for the production of biscuits and bakery products without the use of yeast (Frégeau-Reid & Abdel-Aal, 2005).

Emmer wheat [*Triticum dicoccum* Schrank (Schuebl)] has been traditionally grown and used as a part of the human diet (Marconi & Cubadda, 2005). As requirements for the diversity and quality of food products becoming more demanding, interest in this wheat variety is increasing (Hammer & Perinno, 1995). The grains contain more crude protein than the grains of modern varieties (Marconi *et al.*, 1999); wholemeal flour is a valuable source of dietary fibre, in its insoluble forms, cellulose and hemicellulose, and it contains high quantities of P, Zn, Cu, K, Mg and Mn (Marconi & Cubadda, 2005).

Spelta wheat (*Triticum spelta* L.) is thought to be an old European cultural wheat, interest in which has been prompted by the development of organic farming. It contains more proteins, mineral elements, lipids, fibre and vitamins than bread wheat and it also has a more suitable composition of amino acids. The breeding process would aim to eliminate the particularly unfavourable characteristics of the spelt, by increasing spike productivity or resistance to lodging (Abdel-Aal & Hucl, 2005). Spelt wheat is a suitable crop for organic farming systems (Moudrý & Dvořáček, 1999).

2.2 Can the ideotype of 'the conventional variety' be suitable for the organic farming system?

Concerning the critical points of conventional and certified bred varieties of wheat, there are 4 groups of problems (Wolfe, 2006) and they are interconnected. They are: the efficiency of absorption and use of nutrients, competitiveness against weeds, resistance to diseases and pests, degree and stability of the yield and the qualitative parameters of production (See Table 1).

Criteria	Desirable Variety Characteristics
Nutrient Uptake and Use:	Adaptation to low, organic inputs and fluctuating nutrient dynamics, efficient in capturing water and nutrients, their uptake and their use; deep, intensive root architecture; ability to interact with beneficial soil microorganisms.
Weed Competiveness:	Plant architecture for early soil cover and more light-competitiveness.
Crop Health:	Durable resistance, field tolerance, plant morphology, combining ability for crop or variety mixtures, capable of interaction with beneficial microorganisms.
Yield and Yield Stability:	Maximum yield level and yield stability under low, organic input.
Product Quality:	High processing/baking quality, good taste, high storage potential.

Table 1. Criteria for organic plant breeding and propagation strategies derived from the non-chemical and agro-ecological approach) (according to Lammerts van Bueren, 2002)

2.2.1 Nutrient uptake and utilization efficiency

Organic farming is a system using a limited quantity of nutrients (especially nitrogen) and serial applications of nitrogen (Köpke, 2005). The possession or non possession of the ability to absorb nitrogen in early spring is an important issue in the growing of winter varieties of cereals in an organic farming system; cold wet soil is characterized by a low degree of microbial activity. The mineralization of nutrients (especially of nitrogen) is limited in this period (Moudrý, 2003). The efficient absorption of nitrogen is also an important factor; it provides good-quality production and development of plants in the early stages of growth. (Steinberger, 2002). Varieties must be adapted to the lower inputs of nutrition into the agroecosystem (Lammerts van Bueren, 2002).

A wide range of studies has been carried out in the last few years; their common purpose has been to determine the changes in efficiency of varieties during the breeding process, and changes in the efficiency of the exploitation of nutrients. Muurinen et al. (2006) studied the efficiency of the exploitation of nitrogen in wheat, oat and barley, bred in Finland between 1909 and 2002. Modern varieties of wheat and oat were more efficient, they absorbed more nitrogen and were able to use it more efficiently than the older ones. It was different in the case of barley. They also point out that the improvement in the efficiency of absorption and use of nitrogen was caused by the more efficient use of the absorbed nutrients in a plant, not the increased ability of absorption of nutritions by the root system.

Ericson (2006) states that modern varieties provide a higher efficiency in absorption and use of nutrients than landraces (various amounts of industrial fertilizers). This is valid for conventional farming systems. However, this statement is not so unambiguous for natural low-input farming systems. Gorny (2001) states in his study that landraces of baking wheat provide a higher efficiency in the absorption and use of nitrogen than modern European varieties in low-input farming systems. He clarifies the reason for this in his study. Slafer et al. (1990) studied 6 varieties of baking wheat which had been bred between 1912 and 1980 and found out that the ability of the root system to absorb nitrogen did not improve during the growing and flowering season of the breeding process. The breeding caused an increase in the grain yield thanks to a change of the harvest index, the harvest index of nitrogen and the increasing number of grains. The change in the harvest index was greater than the change in the harvest index of nitrogen; it led to a 'dilution' of nitrogen and a lower concentration of nitrogen in the grain. Because of that, the varieties being bred in conditions with an abundance of soluble nutrients (especially nitrogen) are not able to absorb nutrients from less accessible bonds and use the accessible nutrients more efficiently, and thus need less accessible nutrients. This fact supports the carrying out of the breeding process in the conditions of the organic farming system, and the selection of tribes with greater potential.

Baresel et al. (2005) also support this idea in their work. They were studying the varieties of wheat and found the conditions of organic farming very varied and dissimilar to the conditions of conventional farming. The varieties adapted to the conditions of conventional farms may not have been adapted to the conditions of low-input farming. The efficient genotypes (those able to absorb and use nitrogen in the first stages of their growth) are more suitable for the organic farming system. Most modern varieties are well used and applied in farming systems which are characterized by high inputs of nutrients. They provide a low degree of interaction between- genotype and the environment. They do not achieve the required baking quality in low-input conditions. On the other hand, old cultivars and biological varieties contain more protein in grains (in both organic farming and conventional systems). The higher proportion of protein is usually connected with a lower level of yield (Ericson, 2006).

A well-developed root system, responsive to the interaction with the soil edaphone in a positive way, is a very important aspect of the efficient absorption of nutrients (Lammerts van Bueren, 2002). The growth of roots is more important than the growth of upper phytomass in a soil characterized by a lower concentration of accessible nitrogen. On the other hand, the shape of the root system is influenced not only by the soil structure, but by the proportion of nutrients and water in the soil, by a genetic factor (Fitter, 1991, Fitter & Stickland, 1991) and by the selection of varieties which provide a high level of yield in the conditions of conventional farming, but with negative consequences (Siddique et al., 1990). This means that the selection of suitable varieties for the low-input farming system should be applied to the conditions of organic farming (Lammerts van Bueren, 2002).

The selection of an efficient root system, adapted to the absorption of nutrients from the soil, should take into account the limited competitiveness of varieties for the assimilates and a good position of the roots. A long and deep root system with a lot of small young roots forms a better and richer branching with more capillary roots. The deep roots assure the sufficient absorption of water and nutrients from the deeper layers of the soil profile (Köpke, 2005).

The interaction between the root system and the other soil organisms (bacteria, fungi) is a very important aspect of the agroecosystem; it increases the extent of mineralization of nutrients (Lee & Pankhurst, 1992; Mäder et al., 2000). Hetrick et al. (1993) realised that modern varieties of wheat responded less to mycorrhizal symbiosis. The interaction between microorganisms and roots is determined by genetic factors; nowadays, this factor is not taken into consideration in the breeding process.

2.2.2 Weed suppression

Weed plants are one of the main factors limiting the level of agricultural yield. Because of the availability of herbicides in the last 50 years, the competitiveness of field crops to weeds has been overlooked. The relationship between the crops and the weed plant was supposed to be negative. However this relationship could contribute to the formation of a stable agroecosystem (Lammerts van Bueren, 2002) as the weeds can play a positive role in the agroecosystem (Wolfe, 2002). We cannot consider the cultured plant as naturally competitive to weed plants, because it has not confronted any important competitive weed plants during the breeding process. Modern conventional varieties are not selected in accordance with their indirect morphological or biological features; however, these features - the shape of a tuft, the length of a plant or the position of leaves - contribute to an increase in competitiveness. Nevertheless, the competitiveness of the currently bred conventional varieties can be tested in the conditions of an organic farming system. Sufficient tillering is one of the complex characteristics responsible for high competitiveness against weeds (Kruepl et al., 2006). Selection is also one of the main parameters in this respect (Köpke, 2005). The architecture of a plant also has an important effect (length of stalk, percentage of leaves, position, compactness and shape of leaves) (Regnier & Ranke, 1990). Medium to tall varieties are the most suitable in this respect (Moudrý, 2003). Kunz & Karutz (1991); Eisele & Köpke (1997); Müller (1998) and Köpke (2005) also point to the higher competitiveness of the taller varieties. However, the taller varieties also cause such problems as lodging (Kruepl et al., 2006). Fast growth of the plant in the first stages of life is a very important aspect as it allows an early achievement of a high LAI value. A planofile position of leaves (>45°) in the first stages of growth assures a higher degree of coverage of the soil surface, and a deterioration in the growing conditions for weeds, although in the worse nutritive stations this can also lead to slower development of the plants. An erectofile position of leaves is a more favourable feature for the later stages of the plant's growth (Hoad et al., 2005). The competitiveness of plants also depends on the speed of collumning, LAI, capacity of the upper phytomass and the tallness of plants in the DC 31-75 stage (Köpke, 2005).

A number of authors also point out that competitiveness is determined by a good ability to absorb nutrients in low-input farming conditions. Varieties must be adapted to the negligible use of nitrogenous fertilizers and be able to cover the soil as fast as possible (Kunz & Karutz, 1991; Eisele & Köpke, 1997; Müller, 1998). Alleopathic secretions may also influence the growth of other crops. However, according to studies, alleopathic secretions play an important role in the growing system of rye and oat, but not wheat (Köpke, 2005). Nevertheless, research results also rebut this fact; they point out that the aleopatic potential may lead to a reduction in yield and quality (Regnier & Ranke, 1990).

2.2.3 Disease resistance

A plant's health depends primarily on preventive measures, which can mean the creation of optimum conditions for growth, prevention against stressors, and the taking into account of the natural tolerance to plant competitors. Several diseases occur not because of poor growing conditions, but because of an imbalance between the plant and the environmental conditions; this can lead to an imbalance in the metabolism processes, and the attraction of insects, fungal and bacterial diseases (Tamis & Van den Brink, 1999).

The main selection criterion for good breeding is not the level of resistance; it is rather the ability of a specific plant to create a certain level of yield and quality in spite of the pressure of infectious diseases (Lammerts van Bueren, 2002). The resistant plant should not be just resistant, but its morphological features should also guarantee its resistance in conditions of higher infection. This fact is not taken into consideration in the selection process of conventional varieties. However, it is one of the reasons for the reduced resistance of conventional varieties, which are without any chemical protection against fungal diseases, as the following examples show: the occurrence of *Septoria nodorum* is influenced by a plant's architecture (Kunz, 1983), in that the transfer of spores from leaves to spikes by raindrops may be reduced by a longer distance between spike and flag leaf (Köpke, 2005); high plants are more resistant (Kunz, 1983) and *Fusarium* spp, an infection of spikes, is influenced by the distance between spike and flag leaf (Engelke, 1992).

2.2.4 Yield stability and product quality

Organic yield is in the case of the best organic farms about 20-30 % lower than the conventional (Mäder et al., 2002; Lammerts van Bueren et al., 2002; Konvalina et al., 2009). The quality and stability of the yield are the main priorities for organic farming which does not lay stress on the quantity of production. Farmers usually need to grow 'reliable' and 'solid' varieties which are able to tolerate potential fluctuations in the weather and the potential pressure of diseases; they must in any case be able to provide sufficient yield of grains and straw. The target variety should be bred to provide a lower, but stable yield. The selection of the conventional varieties is based on the yield level and it is carried out in uniform conditions. According to the results of tests carried out by organic farmers, conventional varieties which provide a high yield are not as efficient as organic varieties in marginal areas. The suitability of the conventional varieties may be tested in the conditions of the organic farming system where relatively stable varieties providing a high yield can be selected.

A variety may be characterized by specific features due to the interaction between genotype and environment; a favourable factor may be that such varieties can be marketed as a regional product. This aspect is based on the fact that its flavour adds special features and character to the variety (Lammerts van Bueren & Hulscher et al., 1999).

The high baking quality of the organic varieties is characterized by the proportion and total content of crude protein, high value of the Zeleny - sedimentation, flour binding capacity and flour yield, falling number and test weight. The baking quality of wheat is a complex feature; the breeding of such varieties (to a high quality) is a long and difficult process (Fossati et al., 2005).

Organic methods of farming may have negative effects on the technological value, especially in the case of crucial crude protein content (Moudrý & Prugar, 2002). The proportion of crude protein in grain is reduced because of the reduced availability of soluble nitrogen

(Krejčířová et al., 2006). The composition of storage proteins also changes, there are more protoplastic proteins (albumins and globulins) (Krejčířová et al., 2007), and this increases the nutritive value of grain.

2.3 Suitability of wheat species for organic farming

Exact small-plot trials with particular selected varieties (bread and durum wheat) and genetic resources of hulled wheat species (einkorn, emmer wheat, spelt wheat) were established at the authors' working places between 2005 and 2010. Significant and important characteristics for organic farming (morphological, biological characteristics, yield formation and structure of yield, qualitative parametres of the production) were evaluated.

2.3.1 Bread wheat (modern winter varieties)

In the experimental years 2006-2008, 10 varieties and strains of bread wheat (Capo, Eriwan, Element, Eurofit, Clever, Ludwig, Epsilon, Element, SE 304/05, SE 320/05), coming from the conventional and organic breeding programmes of Austrian breeding stations, were grown in small plot trials (10 m2) with two replications at the location of South Bohemia, experimental fields of the University of South Bohemia in České Budějovice.

Grain yield was strictly dependent on the year, analysis of the variation (ANOVA) punctuated the dominating effect of the year on the grain yield (93%). The average yield was highest in 2008. There were observed significant differences between the varieties. The Clever variety belonged to the least profitable ones (2,52 - 6,1 $t.ha^{-1}$). On the other hand, the Eurofit (4,21 - 7,2 $t.ha^{-1}$) and the Capo (4,47 - 7,40 $t.ha^{-1}$) varieties belonged to the most profitable (Table 2). Lack of available nitrogen proved to be the most limiting factor of the yield formation. The inflow of such nitogen depends on the total degree of absorption from the soil, translocation of assimilates into the grain and losses of the absorbed nitrogen (Papakosta, 1994; Bertholdsson & Stoy, 1995; Barbottin et al., 2005). The detailed analysis of crude protein yield ($t.ha^{-1}$) provides interesting results; it makes the positive correlation with the grain yield (r=0,96) (Table 3). The year had an even more significant and dominating effect (96%) (Table 3) than the grain yield. Crude protein yield is a more stable feature than the total grain yield. The cultivars reached 52 % of the grain yield level and 58 % of the crude protein yield level in 2006 (compared to 2008). It means the cultivars provide higher grain yield, but lower crude protein content in grain in more favourable years for the creation of the yield. Slafer et al. (1990) presents a possible explanation; he quotes the ability to absorb nitrogen from the soil, and this did not improve during the breeding process of modern cultivars; nevertheless, the distribution of the assimilate in a plant did improve - it leads to the dillution of the concentration of nitrogenous elements in grain, which is connected with the increase of the grain yield.

Table 2 shows the stability of the selected parametres of the baking quality, produced in the low-input farming system. Starch content is the most stable feature (CV = 1 in all the studied years). On the other hand, Zeleny sedimentation value is the least stable indicator of the baking quality in the nitrogen low-input farming system. The crude protein content and wet gluten content did not fluctuate.

Weather progress was favourable for the crude protein content in 2006 (Burešová & Palík, 2006); the average crude protein content amounted to 12.6 %. It reached 9.7 % in 2007 and 10.8 % in 2008. There were some cultivars exceeding the average values, e.g. Element (14.5%

- 2006; 11.2% - 2007; 11.6 - 2008), and some subnormal cultivars, e.g. Clever (10.6% - 2006; 8.7% - 2007; 10.7 – 2008). These examples show how the selection of an unsuitable variety may cause a significant negative difference in the crude protein content (up to 3.9% (2006); 2.4% (2007) or 1.7% (2008). Considering the close relationship (r=0.93) between the crude protein content and wet gluten content (Table 3), Element variety had the highest wet gluten content value (2006, 2007) and the second highest wet gluten content value in 2008. The relationship between the crude protein content and wet gluten content is in accordance with the results of Krejčířová et al. (2006) who quotes that there is an even closer relationship between these two idnicators in the low-input farming system than in the conventional one. Starch content increased in less favourable years for the protein formation (2007, 2008) (a negative relationship between the protein content and starch content, r=-0.37). In 2006, the Clever cultivar was characterised by the highest starch content, whereas it was characterised by the lowest crude protein content at the same time (Clever).

Variety	Yield Parametres		Selected Parametres of the Baking Quality			
	Grain Yield (t/ha)	Crude Protein Yield (t/ha)	Crude Protein Content (%)	Wet Gluten Content (%)	Zeleny Test (ml)	Starch Content (%)
Ludwig	5.32	0.57	10.8	20.4	39	67.7
Eurofit	5.27	0.57	11.0	19.1	38	67.2
Erivan	4.80	0.49	10.4	18.1	41	66.8
Element	4.50	0.54	12.4	23.6	50	66.3
Clever	4.42	0.45	10.0	19.5	30	67.3
Capo	5.60	0.63	11.3	21.9	47	67.5
408/04	5.02	0.53	10.3	19.6	37	67.2
322/04	5.60	0.59	10.6	20.0	36	67.0
320/05	5.85	0.60	10.4	19.2	37	67.6
304/05	5.29	0.60	11.3	20.8	42	66.1
Mean	5.2	0.6	10.9	20.2	39.7	67.1
SD	0.83	0.09	0.75	1.83	7.00	0.82
CV (%)	18	18	7	9	21	1

Table 2. Yeld and quality of winter wheat varieties (mean of 2006-2008)

Zeleny sedimentation value characterises the viscoelastic features and quality of the proteins, it allows the fermentation process in dough (Zimolka et al., 2005). Positive middle correlation was observed between the crude protein content and Zeleny sedimentation value (r=0.44). Element seems to be better from the perspective of protein quality (51 ml – 2006; 38 ml – 2007; 62 ml - 2008). On the other hand, the Clever variety proved the lowest values (24 ml – 2006 and 12 ml – 2007). In 2008, the values of Zeleny sedimentation increased in the cases of all the varieties (by 20 ml in comparison with 2006; by 32 ml in comparison with 2007).

Iendicator		1	2	3	4	5	6
Crude Protein Yield	1	1.00					
Grain Yield	2	0.96	1.00				
Crude Protein Content in Grain	3	-0.13	0.14	1.00			
Wet Gluten Content	4	-0.12	0.13	0.93*	1.00		
Zeleny Sedimentation Value	5	0.65*	0.78*	0.44*	0.41*	1.00	
Starch Content	6	0.81*	0.71*	-0.37*	-0.36*	0.56*	1.0

* statistically significant $p<0.05$

Table 3. Correlation analysis of the yield level and quality parametres

The results of the analysis proved the low-input (organic) farming system is connected with the reduction of the yield level and technological quality, expressed by the reduction of the crude protein content in grain and reduction of the protein swelling (Zelehy sedimentation values). The dominating effect of the yearly progress on these factors was also confirmed. According to the results of the analysis, a selection of „elite varieties" is recommended for the low-input farming systems – the varieties with high crude protein content and high Zeleny sedimentation values (e.g. Element). "Elite varieties" also respond to the absence of supporting elements (easily soluble nitrogenous fertilizers) by a reduction of the crude protein content in grain. Such a reduction is usually smaller than in worse-quality varieties, grown in the same conditions. On the other hand, „elite varieties" provide grains, characterised by better baking quality, but they provide lower yield than worse-quality varieties. This fact has to be taken into account when selecting suitable cultivars for food and feed processing.

2.3.2 Bread wheat (comparison of modern spring varieties and old varieties)

Tested varieties come from the Gene Bank of the Research Institute of Crop Production in Prague. Four old varieties of bread wheat and two top bread wheat modern cultivars, Vanek (German origin) and SW Kadrilj (Swedish origin), have been used as control varieties there. Varieties were sown in a randomized, complete block design on experimental parcels in Prague and Ceské Budejovice during 2007, 2008 and 2010.

We have evaluated particular agronomically significant characteristics influencing the total yield rate of the old and modern bread wheat varieties. Table 4 presents the results of the research from the point of view of a comparison of all the tested varieties. All the bread wheat varieties were affected by powdery mildew and rust. Especially the intermediate form of bread wheat (Rosamova přesívka) was less resistant to rust. Modern varieties of bread wheat were characterised by better and more efficient nutrient-management at the station that was supplied better with nitrogen. Correlation analysis (Table 5) has also proven a relationship between the quantity of nitrogen in the plant fytomass in the flowering period and the total quantity of nitrogen in the grains of bread wheat ($r = 0.77$). Old wheat varieties have also been characterised by a relatively low weight of one thousand grains (TGW) (39.55 g) in comparison to control (43.12 g) bread wheat varieties. The tested and evaluated old wheat varieties have achieved 69 % of the yield level control cultivars (SW Kadrilj, Vanek). Concerning the total hectare crude protein yield, the difference between the cultivars was at the same level. On the other hand, the old wheat varieties were characterised by higher crude protein content in grain (15.08 %) than the control (13.73 %) bread wheat varieties. The grain and protein yield were more stable in the case of the old wheat cultivars (Table 4). These results have indicated the fact that the old bread wheat landraces are more adaptable to different runs of the year and different nutritive states of different localities than the modern bread wheat varieties. However, the main disadvantage of its growing is lower productivity in comparison with modern bread wheat varieties.

Parameter	Old Varieties	New Varieties
Powdery Mildew Resistance (0-9 = resistant)	7.24±0.77[c]	8.03±0.89[b]
Rust Resistance (0-9 = resistant)	7.02±1.27[b]	7.33±1.01[b]
Plant Length (cm)	99.67±18.07[b]	89.42±13.14[c]
Index of Lodging	8.14±1.01[a]	8.81±0.45[a]
Number of Tillers	1.62±0.51[b]	1.52±0.49[b]
N Content in Plant (%)	1.72±0.42[a]	1.77±0.55[a]
N Content in Grain (%)	15.08±1.66[b]	13.73±1.22[c]
Yield (t/ha)	4.24±1.74[b]	5.02±2.29[a]
Yield of Dehulled Grain (t/ha)	4.24±1.74[b]	5.02±2.29[a]
Yield of Protein (t/ha)	0.629±0.24[a]	0.682±0.31[a]
Harvest Index	0.40±0.05[b]	0.46±0.03[a]
Thousand Grain Weight (g)	39.55±7.51[b]	43.13±4.70[a]

Different letters document statistical differences between varieties for theTukey HSD test, P < 0.05

Table 4. Differences in Selected Agronomically Important Traits in Different Groups of Varieties (mean + SD of three years, two localities)

Parameter	Bread Wheat – Old Varieties			Bread wheat – Modern Varieties		
	Protein Content	Grain Yield	Protein Yield	Protein Content	Grain Yield	Protein yield
Powdery Mildew Resistance	-0.40[ns]	-0.53*	-0.68**	-0.20[ns]	-0.77*	-0.30[ns]
Rust Resistance	0.15[ns]	0.02[ns]	0.03[ns]	0,42 [ns]	-0.81*	-0.24[ns]
Plant Length	-0.48[ns]	0.63**	0.56*	-0.56[ns]	0.81*	0.74*
Index of Lodging	-0.26[ns]	-0.62*	-0.75*	-0.20[ns]	-0.68*	-0.73*
Number of Tillers	0.15[ns]	0.07[ns]	0.10[ns]	0.12[ns]	0.21[ns]	0.23[ns]
N content in plant	0.40*	0.41[ns]	0.54*	0.77*	0.26[ns]	0.39[ns]
Harvest index	-0.23[ns]	0.25[ns]	0.20[ns]	0.78*	-0.54[ns]	-0.43[ns]
TGW	-0.06[ns]	0.22[ns]	0.18[ns]	-0.15[ns]	0.54[ns]	0.53[ns]

statistically significant P < 0.05; ** highly statistically significant P < 0.01; nsnot significant

Table 5. Correlation Between Selected Agronomically Important Traits

2.3.3 Hulled wheat species

Competitiveness against weeds and resistance to lodging are the essential factors influencing the productivity of wheat growing. Longer plants are more resistant and competitive with weeds (Cudney et al., 1991). Plants must be resistant to lodging (Konvalina et al., 2010). As for the studied and evaluated wheat species, spelt and emmer wheat plants were longest (127 cm) (Table 6). On the other hand, SW Kadrilj, a control variety, had short stalks (88.7 cm). It may be a cause of danger if this cultivar is grown in an overweeded crop stand. Resistance to lodging was an important factor too. Short plants do not have to be automatically more resistant to lodging (Pagnotta et al., 2005). SW Kadrilj, a control variety, did not inclinate to lodging at all. As for the hulled wheat species, all of them attained a similar rate of resistance to lodging.

The good disease resistance of plants is extremely important in nature-friendly farming systems because they perform under limited chemical treatment and protection of plants (Wolfe et al., 2008). Our research assessed the resistance to mildew and brown rust attacks. Genetic resources are usually considered as originators and carriers of such resistance (Heisey et al., 1997). All einkorn varieties were resistant to brown rust and powdery mildew as well and most of emmer wheat varieties were also resistant (Table 6). Spring spelt wheat varieties were not greatly infested with powdery mildew. All the varieties were, nevertheless, less resistant to brown rust; it might cause serious problems if a strong brown rust infection attacked the crop stand. Brown rust is considered as one of the most serious wheat diseases in developing countries (Heisey et al., 1997). Health and wholesomeness of farm products have to be guaranteed in the sustainable farming system. If the cropping is neither suitable nor well compiled (Vogelgsang et al., 2008) or if less resistant varieties are grown (Ittu et al., 2010), the crop stands may be attacked by *Fusarium* spp. Such infections can result in yield losses, but more important in contamination of the grain with mycotoxins produced by the pathogens (Köhl et al., 2007). Harvested products are contaminated due to the accumulation of toxins such as deoxynivalenol (DON) produced by *Fusarium* spp. (Nedělník et al., 2007). Mean grain contamination rates did not exceed the permitted limit norms (1.25 mg/kg = limit for contamination according to EC Regulation No. 1126/2007). Spelt wheat grains contained a low proportion of DON (0.11 mg/kg) and there were minimum differences between spelt wheat varieties. Most emmer wheat varieties were also very minimally contaminated with DON (Rudico, Weiser sommer, May emmer). Triticum dicoccon (Tapioszele) was, on the other hand, a problematic variety (0.79 mg/kg). Its grains would be greatly contaminated with DON if this variety was grown after an unsuitable forgoing crop or if the crop stand was lodged (Vogelgsang et al., 2008). Such grains would not be good for consumption by people. Hulls may highly contribute to a reduction of the DON grain contamination rate. They protect grains and they are peeled away from grains just before the final processing of grains (Buerstmayr et al., 2003).

Mean world wheat yield rates attain 3 t/ha at maximum (Mitchell & Mielke, 2004). The yield rate is lower in organic farming systems as supporting instruments are limited in such farming systems (mineral fertilizers, pesticides) (Neascu et al., 2010). A stable (even if it is lower) yield rate is the most important aspect (Wolfe et al., 2008). As for our research, control varieties attained a mean yield rate of 3.0 t/ha (SW Kadrilj - 3.7 t/ha). Hulled wheat species attained lower yield rates (Table 6). Einkorn varieties attained the lowest yield rates which were not very variable. As for emmer wheat varieties, Rudico attained the highest yield rate (2.8 t/ha) and Triticum dicoccon (Tapioszele) attained the lowest yield rate (1.5

t/ha). Concerning spring spelt wheat varieties, the yield rates varied from 2.5 to 2.7 t/ha. The hulled wheat usually attain lower values of the harvest index (Marconi & Cubadda, 2005). Therefore, some of the wheat landraces may be grown in farming systems working with less nutrients in the soil (organic farming) (Trčková et al., 2005) or on less fertile parcels (Marconi & Cubadda, 2005).

Comparison of the per hectare crude protein yield showed an interesting fact. It attained a mean value of 389.3 kg/ha in the control varieties (SW Kadrilj - 450.1 kg.ha), whereas it was lower in einkorn varieties where it varied from 301.4 to 346.8 kg/ha. Emmer wheat varieties attained similar values too, except from Rudico (432.3 kg/ha). Two spelt wheat varieties attained higher values of the per hectare crude protein yield than the control ones (Triticum spelta Tabor 22 – 453.2 kg/ha; Triticum spelta No. 8930 – 475.0 kg/ha).

Many literary sources present specific parametres of the production as a frequent reason for the growing of the hulled wheat species (Suchowilska et al., 2009). The proportion of proteins in grain is the crucial wheat quality indicator (Shewry, 2009). The control varieties attained the lowest values in our research (SW Kadrilj – 12.3%). Muurinen et al., 2006, explain it in such a way that the modern breeding process should provoke an increase of the yield rate by "grain dilution." Emmer wheat varieties attained the highest proportion of proteins in grain – a mean value of 16.8% (Triticum dicoccon Tapioszele – 17.4%), whereas spelt wheat varieties attained a mean value of 16.5% (Triticum spelta No. 8930 – 17.5%) and einkorn varieties attained a mean value of 15.8%n (Triticum monococum 44 – 16.9%).

The hulled wheat varieties contained more wet gluten than the control wheat varieties. The technological quality of the wheat species was very different. Generally said, the wheat species may be divided into two different groups: the first one involves the varieties suitable for baking (production of yeasty goods) and the second category involves the varieties suitable for other sorts of production (Shewry, 2009). The varieties suitable for baking should attain high gluten index values (70) and high sedimentation values (50 ml). Einkorn and emmer wheat varieties attained very low gluten index values (12.7 – 20.7 ml) which was caused by an absence of the D genome (Marconi & Cubadda, 2005). Such gluten is weak and is not good for the production of yeasty goods. Einkorn and emmer wheat varieties also attained low values on the SDS test (einkorn – a mean value of 29.9 ml; emmer wheat – mean value of 31.8 ml). The sedimentation test values are reflected in a volume of bakery products, which means that einkorn or emmer wheat bakery products are not too yeasty and they are flat. Spelt wheat attained higher gluten index values (28.2 – 44.5) and higher sedimentation values (46.2 – 70.2 ml), which were close to the values attained by the control bread wheat varieties like SW Kadrilj (gluten index = 75.0; SDS test = 74.7 ml).

Resistance to diseases (powdery mildew and brown rust) is the crucial advantage of einkorn and emmer wheat varieties (it has been confirmed by our research and trials). They have been also characterised by a lower DON grain contamination rate than bread wheat varieties. Some of the spelt wheat varieties have been infested and damaged by brown rust, but the DON grain contamination rates have been lowest there. Particular varieties have been less resistant to lodging. The selection of suitable and resistant varieties should be, therefore, done very carefully. Concerning the total yield rate, the studied hulled wheat varieties have attained lower yield rate values. Higher per hectare crude protein yield has been an important advantage of particular varieties (spelt wheat, emmer wheat) (being compared to SW Kadrilj, a control bread wheat variety). As for the yield formation, the hulled wheat varieties are suitable for growing in less favourable conditions (montane areas, dry regions) or in low-input and organic farming systems.

Parameter	Einkorn	Emmer	Spelt	Bread Wheat Control
Plant Length (cm)	114.1±10.6	127.0±15.6	126.8±10.4	103.4±22.0
Lodging (0-9)	5.6±2.9	6.0±2.1	5.9±2.6	7.6±2.0
Mildew (0-9)	8.9±0.1	8.8±0.3	8.5±0.6	8.4±0.6
Rust (0-9)	8.8±0.2	8.5±0.6	6.8±1.0	6.2±1.9
DON (ppb)	168.8±321.1	192.7±696.3	110.6±253.1	234.2±314.1
Yield (t/ha)	2.1±1.3	2.1±1.2	2.6±1.4	3.0±1.7
Protein Yield (kg/ha)	324.1±210.8	348.0±195.3	422.6±238.6	389.3±228.9
Protein Content (%)	15.8±2.4	16.8±2.4	16.5±2.0	13.2±2.2
Wet Gluten (%)	38.5±9.8	41.4±8.3	44.4±7.7	31.6±8.6
Gluten Index	15.0±4.9	15.2±9.9	36.4±14.7	66.0±15.5
SDS (ml)	29.9±9.6	31.8±12.8	59.6±13.5	66.9±15.6

Table 6. Agronomic and Quality Parameters of Hulled Wheat Species

Concerning the quality, the hulled wheat varieties have contained a higher proportion of proteins in grain. Spelt wheat is suitable for direct baking (the selection of varieties has to be done, however, very carefully). On the other hand, einkorn and emmer wheat varieties are suitable for production of unyeasty goods (e.g. pasta, biscuits, etc.) as they have attained low sedimentation values and gluten index values. All the hulled wheat species are good for the production of traditional food goods or they may be processed in so called craft bakery machines. Growing and processing of the hulled wheat species as organic products would bring higher added value to farmers.

3. Conclusion

More than 50 % of a acreage of organic arable land is cropped with cereals. Bread wheat (*Triticum aestivum* L.) is the most important market cereal species. As organic farming has undergone a significant development and it is still unevenly set up in various countries, there is a deficiency of suitable varieties for the sustainable farming systems. High costs for breeding, weak and uneven representation of the organic farming are the main reasons of such a state. Almost any modern bred varieties of bread wheat which are conventionally grown are not suitable for organic farming. Different selective criteria from the ones applied to the selection of varieties for organic farming are among the main reasons. E.g. less efficient root system, low competitiveness to weeds, low resistance to usual diseases or reduced baking quality provoked by a reduction of the proportion of nitrogen in the soil. Organic farmers have several options when selecting suitable varieties for organic farming:

1. Selection of a conventional bred variety - almost no conventional varieties of bread wheat (*Triticum aestivum* L.) and durum wheat (*Triticum durum* Desf.) have been tested in organic farming conditions. Organic farmers may base the selection of varieties on results of official trials that were carried out in the conventional farming system, they may follow the advice of advisors, distributors of seeds, research and their own experience and knowledge.
2. Selection of organic bred varieties of wheat – very narrow and an unsufficient range of available varieties, just in a small number of countries.

3. Application of a wide diversity of species and growing of various wheat species (not only bread wheat), e. g. einkorn (*Triticum monococum* L.), emmer wheat (*Triticum diccocum* Schrank) or spelt wheat (*Triticum spelta* L.). A competitiveness to weeds, efficient root systems and resistance to usual wheat diseases are the main advantages of the above-mentioned wheat species. Concerning the production marketing, a grain with a specific quality is an important advantage too.

4. Acknowledgment

Supported by the Ministry of Agriculture of the Czech Republic - NAZV, Grant No. QH 82272 and Grant No. QI 91C123

5. References

Abdel-Aal, E-S.M. & Hucl, P. (2005). Spelt: A speciality wheat for emerging food uses. In *Speciality Grains for Food and Feed*. E-S.M. Abdel-Aal; P. Wood (Eds.), Minnesota, American Association of Cereal Chemists Inc., p. 109-142

Barbotin, A.; Lecomte, C.; Bouchard, C. & Jeuffroy, M. H. (2005): Nitrogen remobilisation during grain filling in wheat: genotypic and environmental effects. *Crop Sciences*, Vol.45, pp. 1141-1150

Baresel, J.P.; Reents, H.J & Zimmermann, G. (2005). Field evaluation criteria for nitrogen uptake and nitrogen efficiency. In: E.T. Lammerts van Bueren; I. Goldringer & Østergård, H. (Eds), *Organic plant breeding strategies and the use of molecular markers*. ECO PB, Driebergen, p. 49-54

Bertholdsson, N. O. & Stoy, V. (1995): Yields of dry matter and nitrogen in highly diverging genotypes of winter wheat in relation to N-uptake and N-utilisation. *Journal of Agronomy and Crop Sciences*, Vol.175, pp.285-295

Buerstmayr, H.; Stierschneider, M.; Steiner, B.; Lemmens, M.; Griesser, M.; Nevo, E & Fahima, T. (2003). Variation for resistance to head blight caused by Fusarium graminearum in wild emmer (Triticum dicoccoides) originating from Israel. *Euphytica*, Vol.130, pp.17-23

Burešová, I. & Palík, S., (2006). *Kvalita potravinářských obilovin ze sklizně 2006*. In: Sborník z konference Jakost obilovin 2006, 9.11.2006, Kroměříž, pp. 6-12 (In Czech)

Collins, W.W. & Hawtin, G.C. (1999). Conserving and using crop plant biodiversity in agroecosystems. In: W.W. Collins, C.O. Qualset (Eds.). *Biodiversity in agroecosystems*. CRC Press, Boca Raton, USA, pp. 267-282

Cudney, D.W.; Jordan, L.S. & Hall, A.E. (1991). Effect of wild oat (Avena fatua) infestations on light interception and growth rate of wheat (Triticum aestivum). *Weed Sciences*, Vol.39, pp.175-179

Dotlačil, L.; Stehno, Z.; Faberová, I. & Michalová, A. (2002). Research, Conservation and Utilisation of Plant Genetic Resources and Agro-Biodiversity Enhancement – Contribution of the Research Institute of Crop Production Prague-Ruzyně. *Czech Journal of Genetics and Plant Breeding*, Vol.38, pp.3-15

Eisele, J.A. & Köpke, U. (1997). Choice of cultivars in organic farming: new criteria for winter wheat ideotypes. *Pflanzenbauwissenschaften, Vol.2*, pp.84-89

Engelke, F. (1992). Ertrag und Ertragsbildung von Winterweizen, Winterrogen und Winteriticale im Organischen Landbau-Aswertung von Sortenversuchen in drei

Versuchenjahren. Thesis (Ph.D.) - Faculty of Agriculture, University of Bonn Bonn, 1992, 103 p. (in German).

Ericson, L. (2006). Nutrient use efficieny. In: D. Donner & A. Osman (Eds), *Handbook cereal variety testing for organic and low input agriculture*. Louis Bolk Institute, Driebergen, p.N1-N8

FAO (1996). Report on the State of the World's Plant Genetic Resources for Food and Agriculture, Rome, Italy, 511 p.

FAOSTAT (2011) FAOSTAT > Production > Prodstat > Crops. The FAOSTAT homepage at http://faostat.fao.org/site/567/DesktopDefault.aspx?PageID=567#ancor. Download of June 15, 2011.

Fitter, A.H. & Stickland, T.R. (1991). Architectural analysis of plant root systems - architectural correlates of exploitation efficiency. *New Phytology*, Vol.118, pp. 375-382

Fitter, A.H. & Stickland, T.R. (1991). Architectural analysis of plant root systems - influence of nutrient supply on architecture in contrasting plant species. *New Phytology*, Vol.119, pp. 383-389

Fossati, D.; Kleijer, G. & Brabant, C. (2005). Practical breeding for bread quality. In: E.T. Lammerts van Bueren, I. Goldringer & H. Østergård (Eds), *Organic plant breeding strategies and the use of molecular markers*. ECO PB, Driebergen, pp. 31-35

Frégaeu-Reid J. & Abdel-Aal E-S.M. (2005). Einkorn: A potential functional wheat and genetic resource. In: *Speciality Grains for Food and Feed*. E-S.M. Abdel-Aal & P. Wood (Eds.). Minnesota, American Association of Cereal Chemists Inc., pp. 37-62

Gorny, A.G. (2001). Variation in utilization efficincy and tolerance to reduce water and nitrogen supply among wild and cultivated barleys. *Euphytica*, Vol.117, pp. 59-66

Gregová E.; Hermuth J.; Kraic J. & Dotlačil L. (2006). Protein heterogeneity in European wheat landraces and obsolete cultivars: Additional information II. *Genetics Resources and Crop Evolution*, Vol.53, pp. 867-871

Hammer, K. & Perinno, P. (1995). Plant genetic resources in South Italy and Sicily: studies towards in situ and on farm conservation. *Plant Genetics Resources Newsletter*, Vol.103, pp. 19-23

Hammer, K.; Gladis, T. & Diederichsen, A. (2003). In situ and on-farm management of plant genetics resources. *European Journal of Agronomy*, Vol.19, pp. 509-517

Heisey, P.W.; Smale, M.; Byerlee, D. & Souza, E. (1997). Wheat rusts and the costs of genetic diversity in the Punjab of Pakistan. *American Journal of Agricultural Economics, Vol.79*: pp. 726-737

Hetrick, B.A.D. & Wilson, G.W.T. (1993). Mycorrhizal dependence of moder wheat cultivars and ancestors: a synthesis. *Canadian Journal of Botany*, Vol.71, pp. 512-518

Ittu, M.; Cana, L.; Banateanu, C.; Voica, M. & Lupu, C. (2010). Multi-Environment Evaluation of Disease Occurence, Aggressiveness and Wheat Resistance in Wheat/Fusarium Pathosystem. *Romanian Agricultural Research*, Vol.27: pp. 17-26

Köhl, J., Kastelein, P., & Groenenboom de Haas, L. (2007). Population dynamics of Fusarium spp. causing Fusarium head blight. In: *Proceedings of the COST 860 SUSVAR workshop "Fusarium diseases in cereals – potential impact from sustainable cropping systems"*, S. Vogelgsang, M. Jalli, G. Kovács & V. Gyula (Eds.), Velence, Hungary, 1-2 June 2007. pp. 6-10

Konvalina, P.; Capouchová, I.; Stehno, Z.; Moudrý, J. jr., & Moudrý, J. (2010). Weaknesses of emmer wheat genetic resources and possibilities of its improvement for low-input and organic farming systems. *Journal of Food, Agriculture and Environment*, Vol.8, pp. 376-382

Konvalina, P., Stehno, Z., Moudrý, J. (2009). The Critical Point of Conventionally Bred Soft Wheat Varieties in Organic Farming Systems. *Agronomy Research*, Vol.7, pp. 801-810, ISSN 1406-894X

Köpke, U. (2005). Crop ideotypes for organic cereal cropping systems. In: *Organic plant breeding strategies and the use of molecular markers*, E.T. Lammerts van Bueren, I. Goldringer & H. Østergård (Eds), ECO PB, Driebergen, p.13-16

Krejčířová, L.; Capouchová, I.; Petr, J.; Bicanová, E. & Kvapil, R. (2006). Protein composition and quality of winter wheat from organic and conventional farming. *Žembdirbysté*, Vol.93, pp. 285-296

Krejčířová, L.; Capouchová, I.; Petr, J. & Faměra, O. (2007). The effect of organic and conventional growing systems on quality and storage protein composition of winter wheat. *Plant Soil Environment*, Vol.53, pp. 499-505.

Kruepl, C.; Hoad, S.; Davies, K.; Bertholdsson, N. & Paolini, R. (2006). Weed competitivness. In: *Handbook cereal variety testing for organic and low input agriculture*, D, Donner & A. Osman (Eds), Louis Bolk Institute, Driebergen, p.N1-N8

Kunz, P. & Karutz, C. (1991). *Pflanzenzüchtung dynamisch.* Die Züchtung standortpflangepasster Weizen und Dinkelsorten. Erfahrungen, Ideen, Projekten. Forschungslabor an Goetheanum, Dornach, Switzerland, 164 pp.

Kunz, P. (1983). Entwickungsstufen bei Gerste und Weizen - ein Beitrag zu einem Leitbild für die Züchtung. *Naturwissenschaft*, Vol.39, pp. 23-37

Lammerts van Bueren, E.T.; Hulscher, M.; Jongerden, J.; Haring, M.; Hoogendoorn, J.; van Mansvelt, J.D. & Ruivenkamp, G.T.P. (1999). *Sustainable organic plant breeding*. Louis Bolk Instituut, Driebergen, 60 p.

Lammerts van Bueren, E. T. (2002). Organic Plant Breeding and Propagation: Concepts and Strategies. PhD Thesis, Wageningen University, The Netherland, 196 p.

Lee, K.E. & Pankhurst, C.E. (1992). Soil organism and sustainable productivity. *Australian Journal of Soil Research*, Vol.30, pp. 855-892

Mäder, P.; Edenholfer, T.; Bolter, A.; Wiemken, A. & Niggli, U. (2000). Arbscular mycorrhizae in a long-term field trial comparing low-input (organic, biological) and high-input (conventional) farming systems in a crop rotation. *Biology and fertility of Soils*, Vol.31, pp. 150-156

Mäder, P.; Fliessbach, A.; Dubois, D.; Gunst, L.; Fried, P. & Niggli, U. (2002). Soil fertility and biodiversity in organic farming. *Science*, Vol.296, pp. 1694-1697

Marconi, M. & Cubadda, R. (2005). Emmer wheat. In: *Speciality grains for food and feed*. E-SM, Abdel-Aal & P. Wood (Eds.), American Association of Cereal Chemists, St. Paul, USA, pp. 63-108

Marconi, E.; Carcea, M.; Graziano, M. & Cubadda R. (1999). Kernel properties and pasta-making quality of five European spelt wheat (Triticum spelta L.) cultivars. *Cereal Chemistry*, Vol.76, pp. 25-29

Mitchell, D.O. & Mielke, M. (2005). Wheat: The Global Market, Policies, and Priorities. In.: *Global Agricultural Trade and Developing Countries*, M A. Aksoy & J C. Beghim (Eds.), The World Bank, Washington, USA, pp. 195-214.

Moudrý, J. & Prugar, J. (2002). Biopotraviny - hodnocení kvality, zpracování a marketing (*Bioproducts*). MZe, Praha, 60 p. (In Czech)

Moudrý J. & Dvořáček V. (1999). Chemical composition of grain of differnt spelt (*Triticum spelta* L.) varieties. Rostlinná výroba 45: 533-538

Moudrý, J. (2003). *Polní produkce (Field production)*. In: Ekologické zemědělství. J. Urban & B. Šarapatka (Eds.): MŽP, Praha, pp. 103-126 (In Czech)

Müller, K. J. (1998). From word assortments to regional varieties. In: *Organic plant breeding and biodiversity of cultural plants*. C. Wiethaler & E. Wyss (Eds.), NABU/FiBL, Bonn, pp. 81-87

Muurinen, S., Slafer, G.A. & Peltonen-Sainio, P. (2006). Breeding effects on nitrogen use efficiency of spring cereals under northern conditions. *Crop Sciences*, Vol.46, pp. 561-568

Neacsu, A., Serban, G., Tuta, C., Toncea, I. (2010). Baking Quality of Wheat Cultivars, Grown in Organic, Conventional and Low Input Agricultural Systems. *Romanian Agricultural Research*, Vol.27, pp. 35-42

Nedělník, J.; Moravcová, H.; Hajšlová, J.; Lancová, K.; Váňová, M. & Salava, J. (2007). Fusarium spp. in wheat grain in the Czech Republic analysed by PCR method. *Plant Protection Sciences*, Vol.43, pp. 135-137

Pagnotta, M.A.; Mondini, L. & Atallah, M.F. (2005). Morphological and molecular characterization of Italian emmer wheat accessions. *Euphytica*, Vol.146, pp. 29-37

Papakosta, D.K. (1994). Analysis of wheat cultivar differences in grain yield, grain nitrogen yield and nitrogen utilization efficiency. *Journal of Agronomy and Crop Sciences*, Vol.172, pp. 305-316

Regnier, E.E. & Ranke, R.R. (1990). Evolving strategies for managing weeds. In: *Sustainable agricultural systems*, C.A. Edvars (Ed.), Soil and Water Conservation Society, Ankeny/Lowa, p. 174-203.

Shewry, P.R. (2009). Wheat – Darvin Review. *Journal of Experimental Botany*, Vol.60, pp. 1537-1553

Siddique, K.H.M., Belfort, R.K. & Tennant, D. (1990). Root-shoot rations of old and modern, tall and semidwarf wheats in a Mediterranean environment. *Plant and Soil*, Vol.121, pp. 89-98

Slafer, G. A., Andrade, F. H., & Feingold, S. E. (1990). Genetic improvement of bread wheat (Triticum aestivum L.) in Argentina: relationship between nitrogen and dry matter. Euphytica, Vol.50, pp. 63-71

Steinberger, J. (2002). Züchtung für den Ökolandbau. Bundessortenamt, Hannover, p. 142.

Suchowilska, E., Kandler, W., Sulyok, M., Wiwart, M. & Krska, R. (2009). Mycotoxins profiles in the grain of Triticum monococcum, Triticum diccocum and Triticum spelta after head infection with Fusarium culmorum. *Journal of the Science of Food and Agriculture*, Vol.90, pp. 556-565

Tamis, W.L.M. & van den Brink, W.J. (1999). Conventional, integrated and organic winterwheat production in the Netherlands in period 1993-1997. *Agriculture, Ecosystems and Environment*, Vol.76, pp. 47-59

Trčková, M., Raimanová, I. & Stehno, Z. (2005). Differences among *Triticum dicoccum*, *T. monococcum* and *T. spelta* in rate of nitrate uptake. *Czech Journal of Genetics and Plant Breeding*, Vol.41, pp. 322-324

Vogelgsang, S., Sulyok, M., Hecker, A., Jenny, E., Krska, R., Schuhmacher, R. & Forrer, H.R. (2008). Toxigenicity and pathogenicity of Fusarium poae and Fusarium avenaceum on wheat. *European Journal of Plant Pathology*, Vol.122, pp. 265-276

Willer, H. & Kilcher, L. (Eds.) (2009). The World of Organic Agriculture. Statistics and Emerging Trends 2009, IFOAM, Bonn, and FiBL, Frick, 309 p.

Wilson, E.O. (1992). The Diversity of Life. Penguin, London, UK. 432 pp.

Wolfe, M.S.; Baresel, J.P.; Deslaux, D.; Goldringer, I.; Hoad, S.; Kovacs, G.; Löschenberger, F.; Miedaner, T.; Ostergard, H. & Lammerts van Bueren, E.T. (2008). Developments in breeding cereals for organic agriculture. *Euphytica*, Vol.163, pp. 323-346

Zimolka, J. et al. (2005). Pšenice - pěstování, hodnocení a užití zrna (Wheat - growing and processing). Profi Press, s. r. o., Praha, 180 pp. (In Czech)

Evolution of Nitrogen Compounds During Grape Ripening from Organic and Non-Organic Monastrell – Nitrogen Consumption and Volatile Formation in Alcoholic Fermentation

Teresa Garde-Cerdán[1,2], Cándida Lorenzo[1], Ana M. Martínez-Gil[1], José F. Lara[1], Francisco Pardo[3] and M. Rosario Salinas[1]
[1]*Cátedra de Química Agrícola, E.T.S.I. Agrónomos, Universidad de Castilla-La Mancha, Campus Universitario, 02071 Albacete,*
[2]*Servicio de Investigación y Desarrollo Tecnológico Agroalimentario (CIDA) Instituto de Ciencias de la Vid y del Vino (CSIC-Universidad de La Rioja-Gobierno de La Rioja), La Rioja*
[3]*Bodega San Isidro (BSI), Murcia, Spain*

1. Introduction

Presently, the wine consumers are more and more worried about to choose aliments harmless for health. For this reason, ecological agriculture is incremented its popularity. Today, the legislation says that ecological wines are those elaborated with ecological or organic grapes, that is to say, from grapes cultivated with limitations in the use of chemical fertilizers, insecticides and other pest control synthetic substances, but using sustainable agricultural practices such as cover crops and natural products such as compost (Moyano et al., 2009). The Monastrell variety, also known as Mourvedre, is the second red grape variety most cultivated in Spain, although is also cultivated in France, Australia, Portugal and United States, among others.

The nitrogen compounds of must are essential for growth and development of yeasts during the wine alcoholic fermentation as nitrogen is, after carbon, the second element utilized during their growth. The ammonium and amino acids are the main sources of nitrogen for *Saccharomyces cerevisiae*. The content of these compounds affects the kinetics of fermentation, as nitrogen-deficient musts can cause slow, sluggish and stuck fermentations (Bisson, 1991; Arias-Gil et al., 2007). For this reason, in many wineries it is common practice to add diammonium phosphate (DAP) to the must before the fermentation. However, it is important that this addition follows some criterion, since if large amounts of ammonium are added to the must can result in problems later on, such as risk of microbiological instability, with formation of biogenic amines and ethyl carbamate, which are negative compounds for wine quality (Moreno-Arribas & Polo, 2009; Uthurry et al., 2007).

Moreover, the consumption of nitrogen compounds during alcoholic fermentation depends on the physicochemical properties of the must (pH, acidity, sugars, ...), on the grape variety, on the nitrogen composition of the must, on yeast and on the fermentation temperature, etc. (Barbosa et al., 2009; Bell & Henschke, 2005; Bouloumpasi et al., 2002; Garde-Cerdán et al., 2011; Héberger et al., 2003; Henschke & Jiranek, 1993; Valero et al., 2003). Although other factors as the cultivated systems (organic or non-organic) could also affect the nitrogen composition of must and their consumption during alcoholic fermentation and so, they could affect the formation of volatile compounds.

Higher alcohols, fatty acids, and esters are important compounds in the wine aroma, especially for grape neutral varieties. These varieties present low concentrations of varietal aromas, so their wine aroma quality is principally related to the volatile compounds produced during the alcoholic fermentation (Lambrechts & Pretorius, 2000). The fermentative volatile compounds mainly come from sugar and amino acids metabolism of yeasts. *S. cerevisiae* yeast produces different quantities of aroma compounds in relation with the fermentation conditions and must initial composition, for example, yeast strain, temperature, grape variety, micronutrients, vitamins, additives and nitrogen composition of must (Carrau et al., 2008; Garde-Cerdán & Ancín-Azpilicueta, 2008; Lorenzo et al., 2008; Ruiz-Larrea et al., 1998).

For all these reasons, the objectives of this work were: (a) to study the amino acid and ammonium evolution during ripening of grapes from organic and non-organic Monastrell variety. In this way, we could have information about the optimum harvest moment, in terms of nitrogen composition of the must, as this is a determinant factor to a proper development of alcoholic fermentation as well as to wine aroma quality; (b) to study the effect of the crop management in the consumption of nitrogen compounds during the alcoholic fermentation of the musts. The consumption of nitrogen compounds can be influenced, among other factors, by their initial concentration in the must, and in its turn can affect the formation of volatile compounds, and (c) to study the differences in the formation of volatile compounds during the alcoholic fermentation of organic and non-organic Monastrell grapes, because fermentative volatile compounds determine the aroma quality of young wines coming from neutral varieties.

2. Methodology

2.1 Grapes

Monastrell red grape variety cultivated in O.D. Jumilla (SE of Spain) under non-organic and organic agriculture was used. The plots had similar edaphoclimatic conditions as they are located in the same area. In the conventional agriculture system, Monastrell non-organic, the vineyards were cultivated in trellis and were fitted with a drip irrigation system. They were fertilized with liquid fertilizer NPK 8-4-10 (%, w/w) (Agribeco, Spain), applied in total 250 g per vine. In the case of Monastrell organic the vineyards were cultivated in glass and were treated with fertilizer "cultivit ecológico" (Agribeco), consisting of dried granulated sheep manure, the composition of which was NPK 1.55-1.21-2.35 (%, w/w), applying in total 200 g per vine. The organic system was not irrigated.

2.2 Samples

Samples from organic and non-organic Monastrell were collected during grape ripening. The sampling was carried out by choosing the first vine of the plot at random, of a row also chosen randomly, and then in the same row was collected one grape bunch out of every five vines, until completing ten samples. Bunches from north and south exposition, as well as to different height and depth within the same vine were selected, in order to ensure that the sampling was representative. Samples from organic and non-organic Monastrell were collected on August 8, August 23, September 5, September 19 and September 27 during the year 2007. To obtain the must samples, several grains of grapes were caught at random from bunches collected for each sample. The musts were obtained manually for further analysis of their contents in nitrogen compounds and oenological parameters.

2.3 Vinification

The grape was destemmed and crushed to obtain the must. For each sample (organic and non-organic Monastrell at September 27), 400 mL was used, which was divided into 2 aliquots as they were fermented-macerated in duplicate. Must were inoculated with active dry *S. cerevisiae* subsp. *cerevisiae* (U.C.L.M. S325, Springer Oenologie, France) in a proportion of 0.2 g/L according to commercial recommendations. For this, 0.65 g of dry yeast was rehydrated in a sterile flask in 7.5 mL of distilled water with 0.07 g of sucrose (number of viable cells/mL $\geq 2\times10^9$); it was kept in this medium for 30 min at 35°C. The musts were inoculated while being mixed to obtain a homogeneous distribution. Before fermentation, the musts were sulphited with potassium metabisulfite to a final total SO_2 concentration of 70 mg/L in non-organic samples, and of 20 mg/L in organic samples. The fermentations-macerations took place in glass fermenters with a capacity of 250 mL and with a lid with two outlets; one for sample extractions and the other with a CO_2 trap to allow its exit and prevent the entrance of air during the alcoholic fermentation. The orifice for sample extraction was covered with a septum during the fermentation. The fermenters were placed over magnetic stirrers, to ensure a homogenous fermentation. The fermentations were carried out in a hot incubator at a controlled temperature of 28°C. The evolution of the fermentation was followed by the daily measurement of sugars through the refraction index at 20°C, using a refractometer CT (Sopelem, France). The samples were taken when the alcoholic fermentation was finished (reducing sugars < 2.5 g/L).

2.4 Oenological parameters

°Baumé, total acidity, volatile acidity, pH, reducing sugars, and alcohol of different samples were measured using ECC (1990) methods. The color intensity was determined by sum of the absorbance at 420, 520, and 620 nm, being this parameter called "color index".

2.5 Analysis of amino acids and ammonium by HPLC

The analysis of ammonium and amino acids was made using the method described by Garde-Cerdán et al. (2009a). The derivatization of amino acids and ammonium was carried out by reaction of 1.75 mL of borate buffer 1 M (pH = 9), 750 μL of methanol (Merck, Darmstadt, Germany), 1 mL of sample (previously filtered), 20 μL of internal standard (2-aminoadipic acid, 1 g/L) (Aldrich, Gillingham, England) and 30 μL of derivatization reagent diethyl ethoxymethylenemalonate (DEEMM) (Aldrich). The reaction of derivatization was done in a screw-cap test tube over 30 min in an ultrasound bath. The sample was then heated at 70-80°C for 2 h to allow complete degradation of excess DEEMM and reagent by-products. The analyses were performed on an Agilent 1100 HPLC (Palo Alto, USA), with a photodiode array detector. Chromatographic separation was performed in an ACE HPLC column (C18-HL) (Aberdeen, Scotland) particle size 5 μm (250 mm x 4.6 mm). Amino acids were eluted under the following conditions: 0.9 mL/min flow rate, 10% B during 20 minutes, then elution with linear gradients from 10% to 17% B in 10 minutes, from 17% to 19% B in 0.01 minutes, maintained during 0.99 minutes, from 19% to 19.5% B in 0.01 minutes, from 19.5% to 23% B in 8.5 minutes, from 23% to 29.4% B in 20.6 minutes, from 29.4% to 72% B in 8 minutes, from 72% to 82% B in 5 minutes, from 82% to 100% B in 4 minutes, maintained during 3 minutes, followed by washing and reconditioning the column. Phase A, 25 mM acetate buffer, pH = 5.8, with 0.4 g of sodium azide; phase B, 80:20 (v/v) mixture of acetonitrile and methanol (Merck). A photodiode array detector monitored at 280, 269 and 300 nm was used to detection. The volume of sample injected was 50 µL. The target compounds were identified according to the retention times and the UV-vis spectral characteristics of corresponding standards (Aldrich) derivatizated. Quantification was done using the calibration graphs of the respective standards in 0.1 N HCl, which underwent the same process of derivatization that the samples. The analysis of amino acids and ammonium was done in duplicate, so the results showed for amino acids and ammonium in the grape samples were the mean of 2 analyses and the results for the wine samples were the mean of 4 analyses, as the fermentations were done in duplicate.

2.6 Analysis of volatile compounds by GC-MS

The fermentative volatile compounds were analysed following the method described by Garde-Cerdán et al. (2009b). Compounds were extracted by introducing the polydimethylsiloxane coated stir bar (0.5 mm film thickness, 10 mm length, Twister, Gerstel, Mülheim and der Ruhr, Germany) into 10 mL of sample, to which 100 µL of internal standards γ-hexalactone and 3-methyl-1-pentanol solution at 1 µL/mL, both in absolute ethanol (Merck) was added. Samples were stirred at 500 rpm at room temperature for 60 min. The stir bar was then removed from the sample, rinsed with distilled water and dried with a cellulose tissue, and later transferred into a thermal desorption tube for GC–MS analysis. In the thermal desorption tube, the volatile compounds were desorbed from the stir bar at the following conditions: oven temperature at 330°C; desorption time, 4 min; cold trap temperature, -30°C; helium inlet flow 45 mL/min. The compounds were transferred into the Hewlett-Packard LC 3D mass detector (Palo Alto, USA) with a fused silica capillary column (BP21 stationary phase 30 m length, 0.25 mm i.d., and 0.25 µm film thickness; SGE, Ringwood, Australia). The chromatographic program was set at 40°C (held for 5 min), raised to 230°C at 10°C/min (held for 15 min). The total time analysis was 36 minutes. For mass spectrometry analysis, electron impact mode (EI) at 70 eV was used. The mass range varied from 35 to 500 u and the detector temperature was 150°C. Identification was carried out using the NIST library and by comparison with the mass spectrum and retention index of chromatographic standards (Sigma-Aldrich, Madrid, Spain). Quantification was based on five-point calibration curves of respective standards in synthetic wine. The analysis of volatile compounds in the wines was done in duplicate, and as the fermentations were done in duplicate, the results shown for these compounds were the mean of 4 analyses.

2.7 Statistical analysis

The statistical analysis of the volatile compounds data was performed using SPSS Version 17.0 statistical package for Windows (SPSS, Chicago, USA), by means mainly of one-way analysis of varianza (ANOVA).

3. Results and discussion

3.1 Oenological parameters of grape samples during ripening

Table 1 shows the oenological parameters in Monastrell organic and non-organic grapes during ripening. At first, in Monastrell organic samples the weight of 100 berries was higher than in Monastrell non-organic, but from 12th September, Monastrell non-organic continued rising and Monastrell organic dismissed. Therefore in Monastrell non-organic the weight of 100 berries was higher at the end of ripening, probably due to the irrigation. ºBaumé/total acidity index is used as a tool to measuring the industrial maturity grape, indicating, in general, the highest index the best value for harvesting. As can be seen in Table 1, Monastrell organic samples showed higher values for this index than Monastrell non-organic, although at the end of ripening the differences dismissed. The pH of the grapes evolved in the same way in both types of Monastrell, showing a tendency to increase throughout the ripening until the last point, in which slightly decreased. Finally, the color index also showed similar evolution in both types of grapes, but with the highest values in Monastrell organic, which could be related to the weight of berries, which being higher for the Monastrell non-organic, resulted in a lower concentration of phenolic compounds.

Samples	Weight of 100 berries (g)	ºBaumé/total acidity[a]	pH	Color index
Monastrell non-organic				
08-aug	90	0.24	2.72	0.83
23-aug	131	1.17	2.96	1.66
05-sep	175	1.29	3.13	2.16
12-sep	146	1.51	3.28	2.17
19-sep	168	1.87	3.37	3.18
27-sep	188	2.14	3.28	2.78
Monastrell organic				
08-aug	102	0.56	2.96	2.01
23-aug	145	2.16	3.02	4.07
05-sep	182	2.32	3.21	5.86
12-sep	151	2.71	3.27	5.20
19-sep	138	3.09	3.40	8.72
27-sep	150	2.36	3.17	5.34

[a] Total acidity expressed as g/L tartaric acid.

Table 1. Oenological parameters of the different samples during grape ripening.

3.2 Nitrogenous fractions of grape samples during ripening

Table 2 shows the evolution of ammonium, amino and assimilable nitrogen concentrations, and total amino acids during grape ripening. The ammonium is the nitrogen source preferred by yeast, as it is the first nitrogen compound that they assimilate during alcoholic fermentation (Cooper, 1982). The ammonium nitrogen concentration decreased after veraison, which occurred in August, between 1 and 8 in Monastrell organic and between 8 and 23, in Monastrell non-organic grapes. Before veraison, approximately the half of nitrogen in the pulp is as ammonium nitrogen, but after veraison it is transformed in amino acids and its concentration dismissed (Blouin & Guimberteau, 2004). After veraison, ammonium concentration changed and at harvest moment (27-sep) was higher in Monastrell non-organic than in organic grapes (Table 2). Ammonium content in the lasts sampling was low in both types of Monastrell, but it was between the usual limits for this compound in grapes (5-325 mg N/L) (Bell & Henschke, 2005).

Samples	Ammonium nitrogen	Amino nitrogen	Assimilable nitrogen	Total amino acids
Monastrell non-organic				
08-aug	68.0 ± 1.0	85.0 ± 2.0	151.0 ± 4.0	501.0 ± 15.0
23-aug	48.0 ± 1.0	156.0 ± 6.0	199.0 ± 6.0	746.0 ± 27.0
05-sep	32.3 ± 0.4	141.0 ± 2.0	172.0 ± 2.0	645.0 ± 5.0
12-sep	34.0 ± 1.0	141.0 ± 4.0	174.0 ± 5.0	628.0 ± 19.0
19-sep	20.2 ± 0.3	62.1 ± 0.8	82.0 ±1.0	285.0 ± 4.0
27-sep	25.0 ± 1.0	123.0 ± 4.0	148.0 ± 5.0	557.0 ± 17.0
Monastrell organic				
08-aug	18.8 ± 0.4	61.0 ± 1.0	78.0 ± 2.0	333.0 ± 5.0
23-aug	14.9 ± 0.2	56.1 ± 0.5	69.9 ± 0.6	291.0 ± 3.0
05-sep	22.2 ± 0.6	85.0 ± 2.0	106.0 ± 3.0	408.0 ± 11.0
12-sep	15.6 ± 0.0	49.6 ± 0.0	65.1 ± 0.1	260.4 ± 0.2
19-sep	28.5 ± 0.4	155.0 ± 2.0	183.0 ± 2.0	720.0 ± 7.0
27-sep	15.7 ± 0.0	65.1 ± 0.1	78.8 ± 0.1	346.1 ± 0.2

Table 2. Nitrogenous fractions (mg N/L) and total amino acids (mg/L) of the different samples during grape ripening. All parameters are given with their standard deviation (n = 2).

The evolution of amino and assimilable nitrogen concentration was similar (Table 2). Both nitrogen fractions increased after veraison in Monastrell non-organic grapes. In both types of samples it was observed that amino and assimilable nitrogen decreased. This decreasing occurred in Monastrell organic grapes at the end of ripening and in Monastrell non-organic in September, between the 12 and the 19, and then increased at the end of ripening. At the harvest moment, amino and assimilable nitrogen concentration were far higher in Monastrell non-organic than in Monastrell organic grapes. These differences in nitrogen compound contents can be due to the different fertilizer and irrigation. The fertilization of Monastrell organic grapevines provided more nitrogen than that of Monastrell organic, and moreover the last grapes only received nitrogen once. The irrigation also helps to the nitrogen assimilation by the plant. In order to the alcoholic fermentation evolved properly, musts have to contain assimilable nitrogen concentration above 140 mg N/L (Bely et al., 1990). This did not occur in the case of Monastrell organic (Table 2), which could cause that its fermentation was slower than that of Monastrell non-organic, as lately will be discussed.
Both Monastrell, non-organic and organic, showed higher total amino acid concentration at the end of grape ripening than at the beginning, which indicates these compounds were accumulated throughout the ripening (Table 2). Monastrell non-organic grapes showed higher total amino acid concentration than Monastrell organic at harvest moment, probably due to the different irrigation and fertilization, as we write above. This is important as these compounds affect the fermentative kinetics (Bisson, 1991) and the formation of volatile compounds during alcoholic fermentation (Rapp & Versini, 1991). Amino acid concentration at harvest depends on edaphoclimatic conditions and agronomic practices, while amino acid

profile mainly depend on variety and zone (Garde-Cerdán et al., 2009a; Hernández-Orte et al., 1999; Huang & Ough, 1991).

3.3 Free amino acid content in the grape samples during ripening

Figure 1 shows the amino acid concentration in organic and non-organic samples during grape ripening. Monastrell non-organic grapes had higher concentration than Monastrell organic in all the amino acids at the harvest moment and, in general, during grape ripening, except one week before harvest, date in which Monastrell organic showed the highest concentration in many of them.

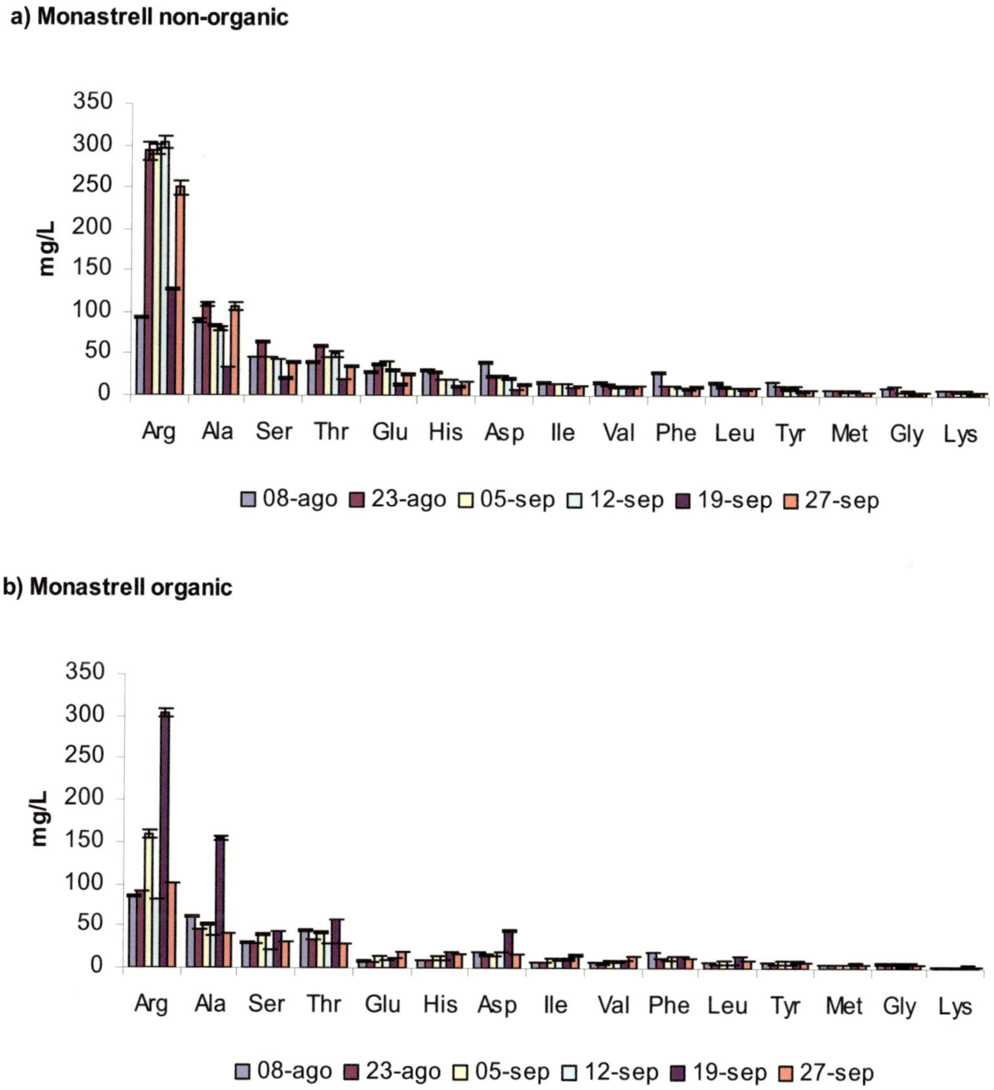

Fig. 1. Amino acid concentration (mg/L) in both types of samples during grape ripening. All parameters are given with their standard deviation (n = 2).

In both types of samples the majority and minority amino acids and so the qualitative composition was the same. Arginine was the most abundant amino acid in both types of samples, as other authors have shown (Garde-Cerdán et al., 2008; Henschke & Jiranek, 1993). This is important since arginine is one of the amino acids preferred by yeast as nitrogen source (Bell & Henschke, 2005; Cooper, 1982). The concentration of this amino acid in both types of Monastrell was higher at the end than at the beginning of ripening. Alanine, the second amino acid most abundant, also was higher at the end than at the beginning of ripening in Monastrell non-organic, but no in Monastrell organic. For some of the aroma compounds that are produced in the alcoholic fermentation, the precursor amino acids (threonine, isoleucine, leucine, valine, phenylalanine, tyrosine and methionine) showed lower concentrations at the end than at the beginning of ripening in Monastrell non-organic. However, in Monastrell organic, although threonine and phenylalanine also dismissed their concentration, the others showed concentration slightly higher at the end than at the beginning of ripening. These amino acids are very important since they can affect the aromatic quality of wines, because higher alcohols come from them directly (n-propanol from threonine, 2-methyl-1-butanol from isoleucine, 3-methyl-1-butanol from leucine, isobutanol from valine, 2-phenylethanol from phenylalanine, and 3-methylthio-1-propanol from methionine) and some of studied esters indirectly, as they come from these higher alcohols. The concentration of the rest of amino acids (serine, glutamic acid, histidine, aspartic acid, glycine and lysine) decreased or remained constant in both types of samples, except glutamic acid and histidine in Monastrell organic, concentrations of which increased at the end of ripening. All of these amino acids are considered good nitrogen sources for yeast (Garde-Cerdán et al., 2008; Henschke & Jiranek, 1993), except lysine and glycine, which are not considered good nitrogen sources for *S. cerevisiae,* although they could be metabolized by other microorganism, such as non-*Saccharomyces* yeast (Cooper, 1982).
The most abundant amino acid, arginine, was higher at the end of ripening than at the beginning. For this reason, as we write above, the total amount of amino acids in both types of samples -although slightly in Monastrell organic- was higher at the end of ripening than at the beginning, despite the rest of amino acids separately did not show this tendency.

3.4 Oenological parameters of wines and kinetics of fermentation

Wines from Monastrell non-organic grapes showed lower total and volatile acidity than those elaborated with Monastrell organic grapes (Table 3). In both types of samples volatile acidity was low and below levels detrimental to wine quality (Ribéreau-Gayon et al., 2006). The pH of wines was lower in Monastrell organic than in non-organic samples. At the end of fermentation almost all the sugars in the medium were consumed, remaining in both types of samples very low concentration of them.

Sample	Total acidity (g/L)[a]	Volatile acidity (g/L)[b]	pH	Reducing sugars (g/L)	Alcohol (v/v, %)	Color index
Monastrell non-organic	5.55	0.19	3.75	0.53	10.21	2.72
Monastrell organic	6.31	0.35	3.59	0.83	12.79	7.24

[a] As g/L tartaric acid. [b] As g/L acetic acid.

Table 3. Oenological parameters of the wines elaborated from the different grape samples.

Wines elaborated with Monastrell organic grapes had higher alcoholic degree than those from Monastrell non-organic (Table 3), as these grapes showed lower concentration of sugars in the initial musts (Monastrell non-organic: 161 g/L; Monastrell organic: 210 g/L). Likewise, color index was higher in wines from Monastrell organic than in those from Monastrell non-organic. This was due to grapes used to elaborate them showed the same trend (Table 1), and the higher color index in musts, the higher color index in wines (Franco & Iñiguez, 1999). Therefore, we can say that wines from Monastrell organic grapes will have the best color.

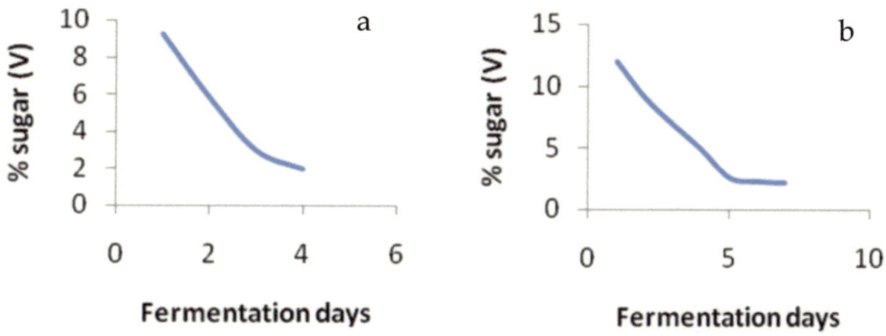

Fig. 2. Fermentation kinetics (a. Monastrell non-organic; b. Monastrell organic).

In Monastrell organic samples fermentation was slower (6 days) than in Monastrell non-organic (4 days) (Figure 2). This was due to nitrogen compounds content were higher in musts from Monastrell non-organic than in those from Monastrell organic (Table 2), and to Monastrell organic musts showed higher reducing sugars concentration than non-organic ones. Therefore, fermentation kinetic was favored when the medium showed higher nitrogen content and lower carbon content.

3.5 Nitrogenous fractions of the wines

Table 4 shows the nitrogen fraction of the wines from Monastrell organic and non-organic. As we write above, the ammonium is the first nitrogen source used by yeast. For this reason, in the fermentation carried out with Monastrell non-organic all the ammonium nitrogen had been consumed and in those from Monastrell organic only rested 1.6 mg/L in the wines. However, if we observed the Table 2, we can see that grapes from Monastrell organic presented at harvest moment lower content in ammonium nitrogen, so the yeast had consumed less quantity in this fermentation. Moreover, low concentrations of ammonium in the initial must could promote an increase of higher alcohols in the wines, because the yeasts are forced to use the amino acids of must as nitrogen source (Usseglio-Tomasset, 1998). Therefore, it would be expected that wines from Monastrell organic show higher quantity of higher alcohols than wines from Monastrell non-organic.

Sample	Ammonium nitrogen	Amino nitrogen	Assimilable nitrogen
Monastrell non-organic	-	58.5 ± 4.1	17.5 ± 0.4
Monastrell organic	1.6 ± 0.1	26.4 ± 1.6	16.1 ± 0.5

Table 4. Nitrogenous fractions (mg N/L) of the wines. All parameters are given with their standard deviation (n=4).

As we can calculate with data from Tables 2 and 4, the percentage of amino nitrogen consumed during the alcoholic fermentation carried out with Monastrell organic samples was slightly higher than those carried out with Monastrell non-organic (59.4% in the first and 52.4% in the last). However, the total consumption of assimilable nitrogen was far higher in the fermentation of Monastrell non-organic samples than in the fermentation carried out with organic samples.

3.6 Consumption of amino acids during the alcoholic fermentation

During the alcoholic fermentation, both in Monastrell non-organic and organic, the most consumed amino acids were arginine, alanine, serine, and threonine (Table 5), and these compounds showed also the highest concentration in the grapes at harvest (Figure 1). All of them are considered good nitrogen sources for *S. cerevisiae*, so this yeast consume them priority during alcoholic fermentation (Barrajón-Simancas et al., 2011; Garde-Cerdán et al., 2008). Regarding to amino acid precursors of higher alcohols (phenylalanine, leucine, isoleucine, valine, tyrosine and methionine), their consumption were higher in Monastrell organic fermentation, with exception of methionine and phenylalanine (Table 5). Glycine and lysine, which were the amino acids with the lowest concentration in grapes at harvest, were excreted or consumed at very small amounts during alcoholic fermentation, probably due to *S. cerevisiae* does not metabolize them.

Yeast, during the alcoholic fermentation, metabolized 78% of the amino acids presented in the initial Monastrell non-organic must and 71% of those in initial organic must. As yeast inoculated in both fermentations was the same, the different consumption of nitrogen compounds could be due to yeast adaptation to the initial medium conditions, that is to say, the higher amino acids quantity, the higher consumption (Garde-Cerdán et al., 2011).

	Monastrell non-organic	**Monastrell organic**
Aspartic acid	7 ± 2	6.2 ± 0.6
Glutamic acid	-2.9 ± 0.4	10.29 ± 0.03
Serine	35 ± 1	25.6 ± 0.1
Histidine	10.6 ± 0.2	11.2 ± 0.4
Glycine	-3.8 ± 0.8	-2.3 ± 0.4
Threonine	31 ± 1	28.6 ± 0.2
Arginine	240 ± 8	89.2 ± 0.8
Alanine	89 ± 5	27 ± 2
Tyrosine	2.2 ± 0.5	4.0 ± 0.2
Valine	-7 ± 3	16.1 ± 0.5
Methionine	1.68 ± 0.06	0.9 ± 0.3
Isoleucine	9.6 ± 0.1	13.1 ± 0.3
Leucine	6.0 ± 0.2	10.6 ± 0.5
Phenylalanine	6.0 ± 0.3	6.1 ± 0.5
Lysine	0.48 ± 0.02	-5.1 ± 0.6
Total amino acids	434 ± 18	245 ± 2

All parameters are given with their standard deviation (n = 4).

Table 5. Amino acid consumption (mg/L) during alcoholic fermentation of Monastrell non-organic and organic musts.

3.7 Formation of volatile compounds in the alcoholic fermentation

Figure 3 shows the concentration of higher alcohols in wines elaborated from organic and non-organic samples. Higher alcohols have not been considered as factors of wine quality, as they posses fusel-like odors (Mallouchos et al., 2002). However, they contribute to the wine aromatic complexity in moderate concentrations (<400 mg/L; Ribéreau-Gayon et al., 2006). Monastrell non-organic showed a quantity of total higher alcohols close to this limit, but the concentration of these in Monastrell organic were higher. As we write above, the great formation of higher alcohols in the alcoholic fermentation could be due to the low ammonium concentration in the initial musts, especially in Monastrell organic (Table 2). Monastrell organic showed higher concentration than non-organic in propanol, 2-hexen-1-ol and 2-phenylethanol, with this last compound being the only alcohol described at a sensory level in pleasant terms (Versini et al., 1994). In the case of isoamyl alcohols, 2-methyl-1-butanol and 3-methyl-1-butanol and isobutanol, their differences in both types of wine were not significant. The concentrations of 3-methylthio-1-propanol and 1-hexanol were lower in organic than in non-organic wines. Monastrell organic had higher concentration of total alcohols than non-organic, which may be related to the higher sugar content (Butzke, 1998; Marchetti & Guerzoni, 1987; Lorenzo et al., 2008). Moreover, Monastrell organic grapes were lower nitrogen content than non-organic grapes (Table 2), which can explain the less synthesis of alcohols in the fermentation of non-organic grapes. This is because, as we have written in the section 3.5., the higher nitrogen concentration in the initial must, the less alcohol synthesis during the alcoholic fermentation (Torrea et al., 2003; Ugliano & Henschke, 2009; Vilanova et al., 2007).

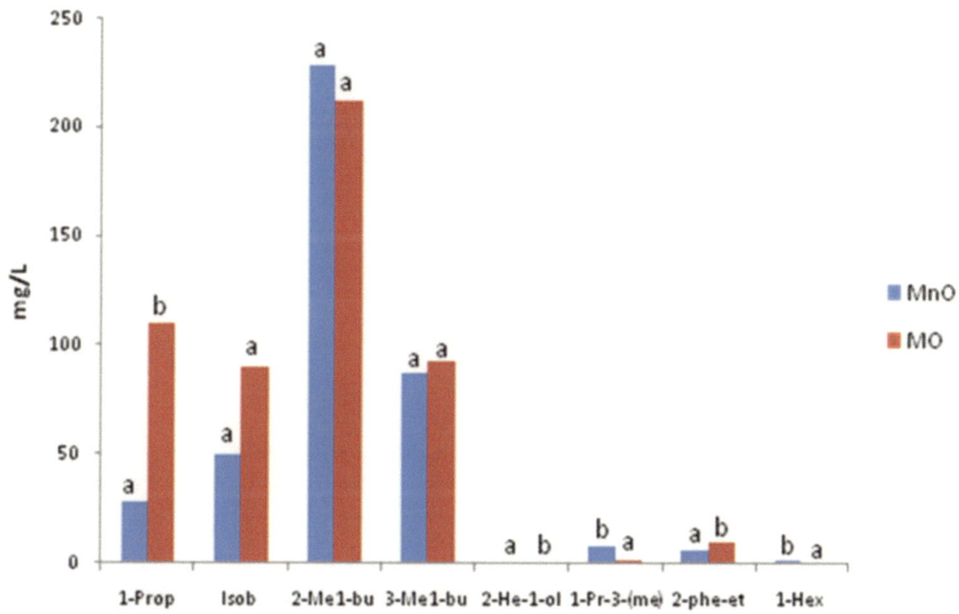

Fig. 3. Alcohol concentrations (mg/L) for Monastrell organic (MO) and Monastrell non-organic (MnO). For each compound, different letters indicate significant differences between the samples ($p < 0.05$).

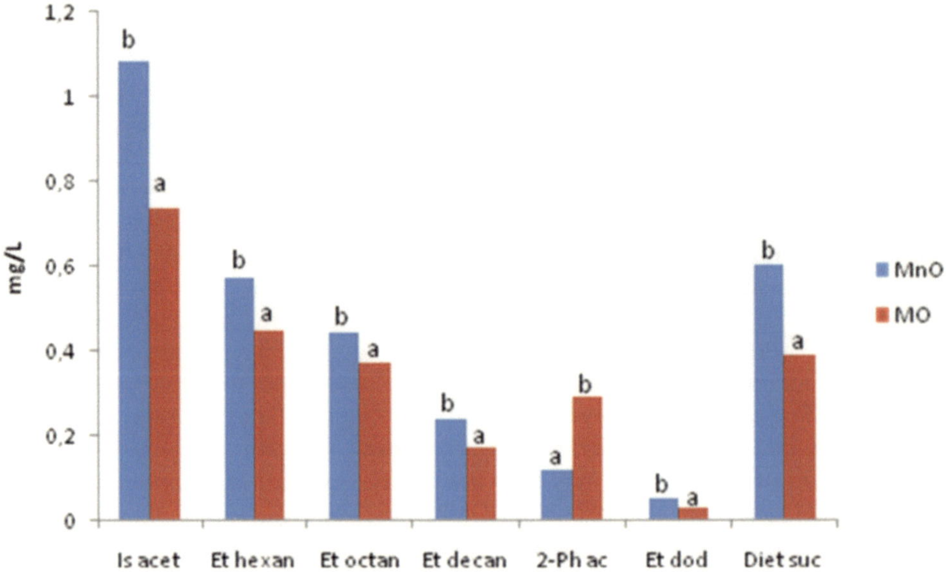

Fig. 4. Ester concentrations (mg/L) for Monastrell organic (MO) and Monastrell non-organic (MnO). For each compound, different letters indicate significant differences between the samples ($p < 0.05$).

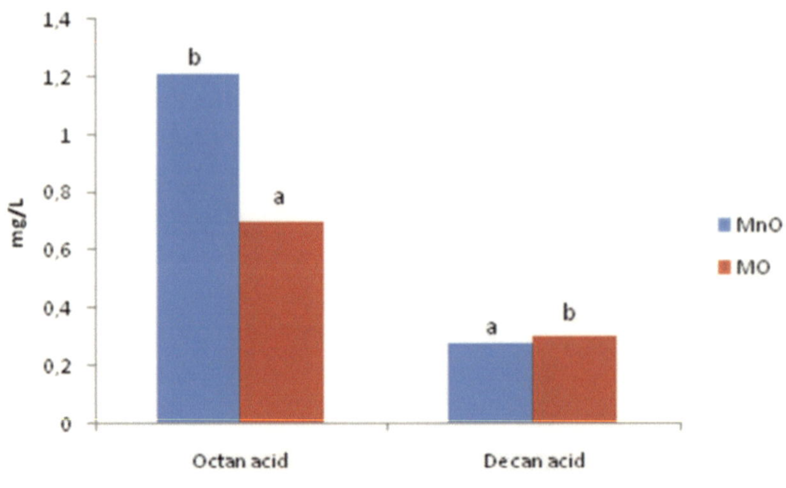

Fig. 5. Acid concentrations (mg/L) for Monastrell organic (MO) and Monastrell non-organic (MnO). For each compound, different letters indicate significant differences between the samples ($p < 0.05$).

Esters are very important compounds on wine quality, as they are the main compounds responsible for the fruity and floral character in wines (Ferreira et al., 1995; Franciolo et al., 2003). All the esters studied showed higher concentration for Monastrell non-organic wines,

except 2-phenylethyl acetate (Figure 4). Thus, the concentration of total esters was higher in non-organic than in organic samples. This is in accordance with the results obtained by Moyano et al. (2009) for Sherry wines, who explain the higher production of esters in non-organic due to the higher concentrations of SO_2 in this type of wines, like Shinohara (1986) and Valcarcel et al. (1990).
Figure 5 shows the concentration of acids in wines from organic and non-organic samples. In the same way that alcohols, although these compounds are not associated with wine quality, their presence plays an important role in the complexity of the aroma (Shinohara, 1985). Monastrell non-organic showed higher concentration of octanoic acid than organic samples, and the concentration of decanoic acid was slightly higher in Monastrell organic. Therefore, the concentrations of acids in these samples are also in accordance with Moyano et al. (2009).

4. Conclusion

The differences in irrigation and fertilization in Monastrell organic and non-organic grapes probably led to the different composition in nitrogen compounds and amino acids in both types of samples. And this, in its turn, carried out to the different kinetics of fermentation, being the alcoholic fermentation slower in Monastrell organic than in non-organic musts. According to this, the optimum harvest moment, in terms of nitrogen composition of the must, would be different in both types of samples, being later in Monastrell non-organic. The consumption of nitrogen compounds during the alcoholic fermentation by the yeasts was directly related with their initial concentration in the must. The amino acid profile and amino acids most consumed were the same in both types of samples. Finally, about the formation of volatile compounds, the concentration of total alcohols was higher in Monastrell organic wines, which could be due to the low ammonium concentration in the initial musts. However, the concentration of esters and acids was higher in Monastrell non-organic, which was related with the higher amino acid consumption in this type of sample.

5. Acknowledgment

Many thanks for the financial support given by the *Junta de Comunidades de Castilla-La Mancha* to the Project PII1I09-0157-9307 and to the FPI scholarship for A.M.M.-G. T.G.-C. thanks to the *Ministerio de Ciencia e Innovación* for the contract of the project AGL2009-08950 and also to the *Consejo Superior de Investigaciones Científicas (CSIC)* for the JAE-Doc contract. We wish to express our gratitude to Kathy Walsh for proofreading the English manuscript.

6. References

Arias-Gil, M., Garde-Cerdán, T. & Ancín-Azpilicueta, C. (2007). Influence of addition of ammonium and different amino acid concentrations on nitrogen metabolism in spontaneous must fermentation. *Food Chemistry*, Vol.103, pp. 1312-1318, ISSN 0308-8146

Barbosa, C., Falco, V., Mendes-Faia, A. & Mendes-Ferreira, A. (2009). Nitrogen addition influences formation of aroma compounds, volatile acidity and ethanol in nitrogen deficient media fermented by *Saccharomyces cerevisiae* wine strains. *Journal of Bioscience and Bioengineering*, Vol.108, pp. 99-104, ISSN 1389-1723

Barrajón-Simancas, N., Giese, E., Arévalo-Villena, M., Úbeda, J. & Briones, A. (2011). Amino acid uptake by wild and commercial yeasts in single fermentations and co-fermentations. *Food Chemistry*, Vol.127, pp. 441–446, ISSN 0308-8146

Bell, S.J. & Henschke, P.A. (2005). Implications of nitrogen nutrition for grapes, fermentation and wine. *Australian Journal of Grape and Wine Research*, Vol.11, pp. 242-295, ISSN 1322-7130

Bely, M., Sablayrolles, J.M. & Barre, P. (1990). Automatic detection of assimilable nitrogen deficiencies during alcoholic fermentation in enological conditions. *Journal of Fermentation and Bioengineering*, Vol.70, pp. 246-252, ISSN 1389-1723

Bisson, L.F. (1991). Influence of nitrogen on yeast and fermentation of grapes, *Proceedings of the International Symposium on Nitrogen in Grapes and Wine*, pp. 78-89, ISBN 0-9630711-0-6, Seattle, Washington, USA

Blouin, J. & Guimberteau, G. (2004). *Maduración y Madurez de la Uva*, Ediciones Mundi-Prensa, ISBN 8484764486, Madrid, Spain

Bouloumpasi, E., Souflerops, E.H., Tsarchopoulos, C. & Biliaderis, C.G. (2002). Primary amino acid composition and its use in discrimination of Greek red wines with regard to variety and cultivation region. *Vitis*, Vol.4, pp. 195-202, ISSN 0042-7500

Butzke, C.E. (1998). Survey of yeast assimilable nitrogen status in musts from California, Oregon, and Washington. *American Journal of Enology and Viticulture*, Vol.49, pp. 220-224, ISSN 0002-9254

Carrau, F.M., Medina, K., Fariña, L., Boido, E., Henschke, P.A. & Dellacassa, E. (2008). Production of fermentation aroma compounds by *Saccharomyces cerevisiae* wine yeasts: effects of yeast assimilable nitrogen on two model strains. *FEMS Yeast Research*, Vol.8, pp. 1196-1207, ISSN 1567-1356

Cooper, T.G. (1982). Nitrogen metabolism in *Saccharomyces cerevisiae*, In: *The Molecular Biology of the Yeast Saccharomyces. Metabolism and Gene Expression*, J.N. Strathern, E.W. Jones & J.B. Broach, (Eds.), pp. 399-462, Cold Spring Harbor Laboratory, ISBN 0879691492, New York, USA

ECC (1990). Commission Regulation VO 2676/90 concerning the establishment of common analytical methods in the sector of wine. *Official Journal of the European Community*, L272(3), pp. 1-192

Ferreira, V., Fernández, P., Peña, C., Escudero, A. & Cacho, J. F. (1995). Investigation on the role played by fermentation esters in the aroma of young Spanish wines by multivariate analysis. *Journal Science of Food Agriculture*, Vol.67, pp. 381- 392, ISSN 0022-5142

Franciolo, S., Torrens, J., Riu-Aumatell, M., López-Tamames, E. & Buxaderas, S. (2003). Volatile compounds by SPME-GC as age markers of sparkling wines. *American Journal of Enology and Viticulture*, Vol.53, pp. 158-162, ISSN 0002-9254

Franco, E. & Iñiguez, M. (1999). Estudio de la relación entre el color de la uva tinta y el color del vino. *Viticultura/Enolología Profesional*, Vol.63, pp. 23-34, ISSN: 1131-5679

Garde-Cerdán, T. & Ancín-Azpilicueta, C. (2008). Effect of the addition of different quantities of amino acids to nitrogen-deficient must of the formation of esters alcohols, and acids during wine alcoholic fermentation. *LWT-Food Science and Technology*, Vol.41, pp. 501-510, ISNN 0023-6438

Garde-Cerdán, T., Arias-Gil, M., Marsellés-Fontanet, A.R. Salinas, M.R., Ancín-Azpilicueta, C. & Martín-Belloso, O. (2008). Study of the alcoholic fermentation of must stabilized by pulsed electric fields. Effect of SO_2, In: *Progress in Food Chemistry,* E.N. Koeffer, (Ed.), pp. 73-103, Nova Science Publishers, Inc, ISBN 978-1-60456-303-0, New York, USA

Garde-Cerdán, T., Lorenzo, C., Lara, J.F., Pardo, F., Ancín-Azpilicueta, C. & Salinas, M.R. (2009a). Study of the evolution of nitrogen compounds during grape ripening. Aplication to differentiate grape varieties and cultivated systems. *Journal of Agricultural and Food Chemistry,* Vol.57, pp. 2410-2419, ISSN 0021-8561

Garde-Cerdán, T., Lorenzo, C., Carot, J.M., Esteve, M.D., Climent, M.D. & Salinas, M.R. (2009b). Differentiation of barrel-aged wines according to their origin, variety, storage time and enological parameters using fermentation products. *Food Control,* Vol.20, pp. 269-276, ISSN 0956-7135

Garde-Cerdán, T., Martínez-Gil, A.M., Lorenzo, C., Lara, J.F., Pardo, F. & Salinas, M.R. (2011). Implications of nitrogen compounds during alcoholic fermentation from some grape varieties at different maturation stages and cultivation systems. *Food Chemistry,* Vol.124, pp. 106-116, ISSN 0308-8146

Héberger, K., Csomós, E. & Simon-Sarkadi, L. (2003). Principal component and linear discriminant analyses of free amino acids and biogenic amines in Hungarian wines. *Journal of Agricultural and Food Chemistry,* Vol.51, pp. 8055-8060, ISSN 0021-8561

Henschke, P.A. & Jiranek, V. (1993). Metabolism of nitrogen compounds. In: *Wine Microbiology and Biotechnology,* G.H. Fleet, (Ed.), pp. 77-164. Harwood Academic Publishers, ISBN 10-0415278503, Victoria, Australia

Hernández-Orte, P., Guitart, A. & Cacho, J. (1999). Changes in the concentration of amino acids during the ripening of *Vitis vinifera* Tempranillo variety from the *Denomination d'Origine* Somontano (Spain). *American Journal of Enology and Viticulture,* Vol.50, pp. 144-154, ISSN 0002-9254

Huang, Z. & Ough, C.S. (1991). Amino acid profiles of commercial grape juices and wines. *American Journal of Enology and Viticulture,* Vol.42, pp. 261-267, ISSN 0002-9254

Lambrechts, M.G. & Pretorius, I.S. (2000). Yeast and its importance to wine aroma. A review. *South African Journal of Enology and Viticulture,* Vol.21, pp. 97–129, ISNN 0253-939X

Lorenzo, C., Pardo, F., Zalacain, A., Alonso, G.L. & Salinas, MR. (2008). Differentiation of co-winemaking wines by their aroma composition. *European Food Research and Technology,* Vol.227, pp. 777-87, ISNN 1438-2377

Mallouchos, A., Komaitis, M., Koutinas, A. & Kanellaki, M. (2002). Investigation of volatiles evolution during the alcoholic fermentation of grape must using free and immobilized cells with the help of solid phase microextraction (SPME) headspace sampling. *Journal of Agricultural and Food Chemistry,* Vol.50, pp. 3840-3848, ISSN 0021-8561

Marchetti, R. & Guerzoni, M.E. (1987). Effets de l'interaction souche de levure/composition du mout sur la production, au cours de la fermentation, de quelques métabolites volatils. *Connaissance de la Vigne et du Vin,* Vol.21, pp. 113-125, ISNN 0010-597X

Moreno-Arribas, M. V. & Polo, M. C. (2009). *Wine Chemistry and Biochemistry,* Springer, ISBN 9780387741161, New York, USA

Moyano, L., Zea, L., Villafuerte, L. & Medina, M. (2009). Comparison of odor-active compounds in Sherry wines processed from ecologically and conventionally grown Pedro Ximenez grapes. *Journal of Agricultural and Food Chemistry,* Vol.57, pp. 968-973, ISSN 0021-8561

Rapp A. & Versini G. (1991). Influence of nitrogen compounds in grapes on aroma compounds in wine, *Proceedings of the International Symposium on Nitrogen in Grapes and Wine*, pp. 156-164, ISBN 0-9630711-0-6, Seattle, Washington, USA

Ribéreau-Gayon, P., Glories, Y., Maujean, A. & Dubourdieu, D. (2006). *Handbook of Enology, Volume 2. The Chemistry of Wine Stabilization and Treatments,* Jonh Wiley & Sons, Ltd, ISBN 9780470010372, Chichester, England

Ruiz-Larrea, F., López, R., Santamaría, P., Sacristán, M., Ruiz, M.C., Zarazaga, M., Gutiérrez, A.R. & Torres, C. (1998). Soluble proteins and free amino nitrogen content in must and wine of cv. Viura in La Rioja. *Vitis,* Vol.37, pp. 139-142, ISSN 0042-7500

Shinohara, T. (1985). Gas chromatographic analysis of volatile fatty acids in wines. *Agricultural and Biological Chemistry*, Vol.49, pp. 2211-2212, ISSN 0002-1369

Shinohara, T. (1986). Factors affecting the formation of volatile fatty acids during grape must fermentation. *Agricultural and Biological Chemistry*, Vol.50, pp. 3197-3199, ISSN 0002-1369

Torrea, D., Fraile, P., Garde, T. & Ancín, C. (2003). Production of volatile compounds in the fermentation of chardonnay musts inoculated with two strains of *Saccharomyces cerevisiae* with different nitrogen demands. *Food Control*, Vol.14, pp. 565-571, ISSN 0956-7135

Ugliano, M. & Henschke, P.A. (2009). Yeasts and wine flavour, In: *Wine Chemistry and Biochemistry*, M.V. Moreno-Arribas & M. C. Polo (Eds.), Springer, pp. 313-392, ISBN 9780387741161, New York, USA

Usseglio-Tomasset, L. (1998). *Química Enológica,* Ediciones Mundi-Prensa, ISBN 9788471147011, Madrid, Spain

Uthurry, C.A., Suárez Lepe, J.A., Lombardero, J. & García del Hierro, J.R. (2007). Ethyl carbamate production by selected yeasts and lactic acid bacteria in red wine. *Food Chemistry*, Vol.94, pp. 262-270, ISSN 0308-8146

Valcarcel, M.J., Pérez, L., González, P. & Domecq, B. (1990). Efecto de las prácticas enológicas en vendimia sobre las levaduras responsables de la fermentación de mostos de Jerez, IV: Estudio industrial. *Alimentación, Equipos y Tecnología*, Vol.3, pp. 171-174, ISSN 0212-1689

Valero, E., Millán, C., Ortega, J.M. & Mauricio, J.C. (2003). Concentration of amino acids in wine after the end of fermentation by *Saccharomyces cerevisiae* strain. *Journal of the Science of Food and Agriculture*, Vol.83, pp. 830-835, ISSN 0022-5142

Versini, G., Orriols, I. & Dalla Serra, A. (1994). Aroma components of Galician Albariño, Loureira and Godello wines. *Vitis*, Vol.33, pp. 165-170, ISSN 0042-7500

Vilanova, M., Ugliano, M., Varela, C., Siebert, T., Pretorius, I.S. & Henschke, P.A. (2007). Assimilable nitrogen utilisation and production of volatile and non-volatile compounds in chemically defined medium by *Saccharomyces cerevisiae* wine yeasts. *Applied Microbiology and Biotechnology*, Vol.77, pp. 145–157, ISSN 0175-7598

9

Plant Extracts from Mexican Native Species: An Alternative for Control of Plant Pathogens

Francisco Daniel Hernández Castillo[1], Francisco Castillo Reyes[1], Gabriel Gallegos Morales[1], Raúl Rodríguez Herrera[2] and Cristobal N. Aguilar[2]
[1]Universidad Autónoma Agraria Antonio Narro &
[2]Universidad Autónoma de Coahuila
México

1. Introduction

Currently, control of plant pathogens requires employment of alternative techniques because traditional handling with synthetic chemicals has been caused various problems such as toxicity to users (Whalen *et al.*, 2003) and impairment of beneficial organisms (Anderson *et al.*, 2003). Another important aspect is that pathogenic organisms have generated resistance to the active ingredient of some synthetic fungicides in response to selection pressure due to high dose and continuous applications, causing great economic losses (Cooke *et al.*, 2003; Leroux, 2003). An economical and efficient alternative for disease control is the use of natural products derived from plants (secondary metabolites) (Wilson *et al.*, 1999), since it does not affect environment and their residues are easy to degrade. On the other hand, vegetal biodiversity in Mexico is available to be exploited, especially by their natural non-toxic, biodegradable compounds (Hernandez *et al.*, 2007). The potential use of plant extracts to control plant pathogens has been reported in different laboratory (Hernández *et al.*, 2010; Castillo *et al.*, 2010; Jasso de Rodríguez *et al.*, 2007; Lira *et al.*, 2003; Osorio *et al.*, 2010), greenhouse (Bergeron *et al.*, 1995) and field studies (Hernandez *et al.*, 2006, 2008). Based on the popular uses of plants in the Coahuila Southern region, botanical resources can be identifying by their antimicrobial potential against plant pathogens. However, still there is a lack of research in this field. As previously mentioned, there is a need for new plant disease management options with lower environmental and economic impact, which expresses a similar or greater effect in controlling pathogens. Mexico is one of the five countries with major biodiversity. It owns 10% of the world diversity with numerous endemic plant species. The arid and semi-arid areas cover 1,028,055 km^2, distributed in 19 states with less than 350 mm of rainfall per year, or 350-600 mm of annual rainfall, respectively. In Mexico, the Chihuahuan Desert is one of the most biologically rich deserts of the world. It covers an approximate area of 630,000 km^2, spanning the states of Chihuahua, Coahuila, Nuevo Leon, Durango, Zacatecas and San Luis Potosí, to until the Southwestern United States, corresponding to Arizona, New Mexico and Texas States (Fig. 1). In this desert are predominantly brushwood and grassland, among species highlighting the creosote bush (*Larrea tridentata*) (Jasso & Rodriguez, 2007).

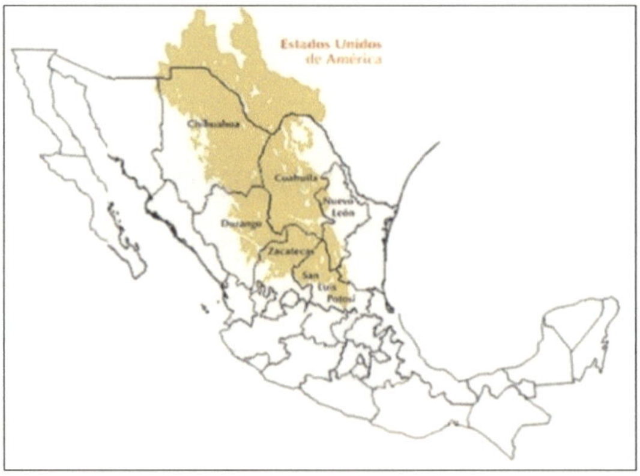

Fig. 1. Location of the Chihuahuan Desert.

2. Control of plant pathogens using plant extracts

2.1 Bio-fungicide potential of chemical groups present in plant extracts

The botanical bio pesticides represent an alternative for pest control with low environmental impact and high food safety. Several products derived from plants have shown an antimicrobial effect. Among the main compounds present in these extracts are: flavonoids, phenols, terpenes, essential oils, alkaloids, lectins and polypeptides. Some plant extracts containing these metabolites has been extracted in water or other solvents, depending on its polarity, and in powder form (Bautista *et al.*, 2003). The enormous diversity of secondary metabolites and biological properties present in plants, are still subject of study. The limited knowledge that currently exist about plant extracts, is an interesting point to begin studies with plants of almost any kind. However, there are some chemical derived from the knowledge base of the plants (Montes, 1996). Some families of plants may be more feasible for study, such as: *Solanaceae* for its high alkaloid content, or *Mimosaceae* that´s present species rich in tannins, or *Lamiaceae* and *Meliaceae* because their wide diversity of terpenoids. For production of active ingredients, there are factors that determine variability in quality and quantity of metabolites. A plant may have different concentrations of a chemical in different vegetal parts: roots, leaves, flowers and fruit and may even be absent in one or more parts, so it is convenient to collect integral samples (Montes, 1996) and also, knowing thee chemical content of plants used in a given region, either as an insecticide, fungicide, nematicide, among others.

2.2 Effectiveness of phytochemicals of native species against plant pathogens

In the context of this problem, one of our research projects has as objective to study the potential of phytochemicals from the Chihuahuan semidesert plant biodiversity as an alternative to control plant diseases caused by fungus and bacteria. The results have shown the added value of the Mexican botanical diversity because the wide range of potential applications of their resources that is geared mainly towards the collection of wild plants for the extraction and marketing of raw material; good examples are candelilla wax and hard fibers of yucca. In some cases, these raw materials are exported to countries where they are purified and transformed into finished products. A new use of these plants promises to change the structure and concept of these sources to become active materials for disease control. In the Table 1 is shown a listing of various plant species that we have studied against different species of plant pathogens with different habits of attack and producing different plant symptoms as root rots, leaf blights, anthracnose, fruit rot, rot grains and seeds, food molds, etc. as well as solvents used in the extraction of phytochemicals.

Source of plant extract	Plant pathogen	Solvents
Flourensia cernua	*Rhizoctonia solani*	Methanol
F. microphylla	*Phytophthora infestans*	Chloroform
F. retinophylla	*Alternaria sp*	Hexane
Origanum majorana	*Fusarium oxysporum*	Diethyl
Bouvardia ternifolia	*Colletotrichum coccodes*	Ethanol
Aloe vera	*Colletotrichum gloeosporoides*	Water
Larrea tridenta	*Pythium* sp.	Lanolin
Agave lechuguilla	*Botritys cinerea*	Cocoa butter
Yucca filifera	*Alternaria alternata*	
Opuntia ficus-indica	*Alternaria dauci*	
Lippia graveolens	*Penicillium digitatum*	
Carya illinoensis	*Phytophthora cinnamomi*	
	Colletotrichum truncatum	
	Fusarium verticillioides	
	Fusarium solani	
	Fusarium sambucinum	
	Clavibacter michiganensis subsp. *michiganensis*	
	Clavibacter michiganensis subsp. *nebraskensis*	

Table 1. Chihuahua semi-desert native plant species studied to determine their effect against various plant pathogens and solvents used for phytochemicals extraction.

The dose-response analysis of extracts from semi-desert plant species indicate that these phytochemicals have anti fungal and anti bacterial properties because most of the extracts inhibited mycelium or bacterial growth of various pathogens studied. This effect varies according to plant species and solvent used for phytochemicals extraction (Gamboa *et al.*, 2003b; Hernández *et al.*, 2006, 2008, 2010; Castillo *et al.*, 2010).

2.3 Factors involved in phytochemicals recovery from Chihuahuan semi-desert native plant species

The diversity of compounds in plant tissues is extensive from the chemical point of view, which has resulted in the identification of thousands of these compounds, with unknown biological functions, which represents a challenge in the search for compounds that are highly efficient for crop plant diseases control. The main groups of secondary metabolites present in plant tissues are polyphenols, terpenes and nitrogen compounds. Tannins (polyphenols) are phytochemicals widely distributed in the plant kingdom, found in roots, leaves, seeds and fruits. These compounds are secondary metabolites with a molecular weight range of 300-20 000 D (Gonzalez *et al.,* 2009). The tannins are non nitrogen compounds, flavor astringent, amorphous, mostly soluble in water and alcohol (Medina *et al* 2007). Its hydrophilic nature allows them associate with carbohydrates, alkaloids and proteins by hydrogen bonds, covalent bonds and hydrophobic interactions. The tannins are divided according to their sugar content, polymerization and esterification in hydrolysable tannins, condensed tannins and complex tannins (Fig. 2).

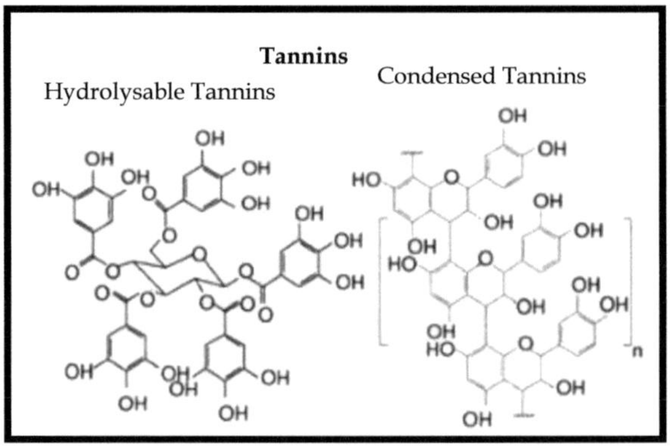

Fig. 2. Chemical structures of hydrolysable and condensed tannins

Hydrolysable tannins. These compounds are esters formed by a molecule of sugar (usually glucose) attached to a variable number of molecules of phenolic acids (gallic acid or its dimer, ellagic acid). By hydrolysis with acids, bases and hydrolytic enzymes may be broken the glycosidic bond to liberate the sugar and phenolic compounds. They have a central core consisting of a sugar or a shikimic acid analogue, which is esterified by gallic acid units or related compounds (C6-C1) (Mata *et al.,* 2008).

Condensed tannins. Proanthocyanidins are polymers or oligomers formed by covalent flavan-3ol (group of catechins) and flavanes4-ol (group of leucoantocianidinas). The term proanthocyanidins (PAS), is derived from the oxidation reaction that produces anthocyanidins (ACS) red in acid-alcohol solutions. Two abundant types of proanthocyanidins, which are formed by the condensation of catechin and epicatechin units that relate to cyanidin and are known as procyanidins and those whose monomeric units are gallocatechin and epigallocatechin, delphydinin resemble and are known as prodelphynidins. They have a structure similar to that of flavonoids. These substances are not hydrolysable by acids or enzymes. Strong acids, heat or oxidizing agents make them red or dark substances, insoluble in most solvents (Ramirez *et al.,* 2008).

Exploration of phytochemicals from native species has allowed recovery of them in form of resin using various solvents as indicated in Table 2. In most cases, methanol, chloroform and acetone are the most commonly used solvents for phytochemicals extraction. However, the use of non-conventional solvents allowed recovery of polyphenols (PT), equivalent to gallic acid and catechin with highly variable recovery rates. There are several factors involved in production and recovery of metabolites, such as the solvent used in the extraction process, for example in Table 2, is showed the amount of resin recovered from the same plant specie in relation to the solvent used. The solvent efficiency for most metabolites recovery is associated with its polarity, so it is important to perform studies about the specific implications of the solvent for high phytochemicals recovery.

Solvent	Fresh Leaf weight (g)	Dry weight of resin (g)	Recovery (%)
Methanol : Chloroform	460	87.8	19.1
Hexane	460	26.6	5.8
Diethyl	460	44.2	9.6
Ethanol	460	37.8	8.2

Table 2. Recovery of resin from *Flourensia cernua* leaves using four different solvents. Guerrero *et al.,* 2007.

In addition to solvents, there are other factors involved in the recovery efficiency of phytochemicals, such as environmental conditions during the plant growing season, in Fig. 3 it is showed that there is a differential in phytochemicals production as a consequence of locality or place of plant growth. These results refer that the ecological conditions where shrubs grown have an effect on the phytochemical compound characteristics and on their antifungal action, one last factor is the selection of plant species. In Table 3 are presented differences on phytochemicals production by different plant species, which could be correlated with the content of secondary compounds in their tissues.

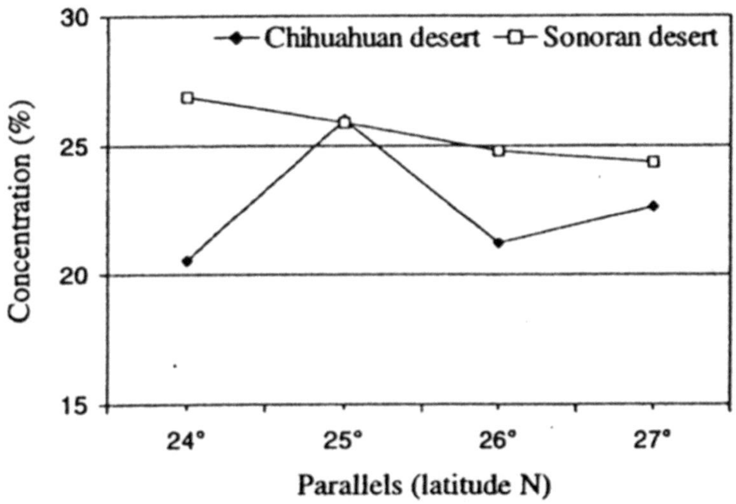

Fig. 3. Mean concentration of resin extracted from *Larrea tridentata* foliage with three different solvents. *Larrea tridentata* foliage was collected from four sampling locations in the Sonoran and Chihuahuan desert. Lira *et al.,* 2002.

Source of plant extract	Hydrolysable Tannins (mg/g)	Condensed Tannins (mg/g)	Total tannins
Larrea tridentata	17.3769 a	37.153 a	54.530 a
Carya illinoensis	1.0821 d	31.980 b	33.062 b
Opuntia ficus indica	1.1573 d	29.020 b	30.177 b
Agave lechuguilla	4.2952 c	22.629 c	26.924 c
Lippia graveolens	5.7996 b	19.090 d	24.889 c
Yucca filifera	0.7953 d	12.005 e	12.801 d
Flourensia cernua	4.7652 c	4.854 f	9.619 e

Table 3. Total tannins content in seven species from the Mexican plant semi-desert area. Means with the same letter are not statistically different according to the Tukey multiple range test ($P < 0.05$).

2.4 Plant extracts effect on microorganism's growth inhibition

Most plant pathogens have mycelia growth inhibition by effect of polyphenolic compounds and resins derived from Chihuahuan semi-desert plants. Inhibition ranging from 0 to 100% with a greater effect as concentration increase, i.e. as concentration of resin or polyphenols increases, the mycelia growth of plant pathogen is significantly reduced (Hernández et al., 2010; Castillo *et al.*, 2010). An example is shown in Fig. 4, where plant extracts obtained with three different solvents ffecting *R. solani* growth is showed, in general, phytopathogen growth is reduced as phytochemicals concentration increase, in some cases fungal radial growth was totally affected.

Inhibition of fungal mycelium growth by plant extract may be as effective that conferred by synthetic molecules. Table 4 shows the effect of synthetic molecules and phytochemicals on phytopathogens radial growth, both kinds of chemicals presented similar effects. This quality could be a plus for the use of plant extracts on disease control of crop fields, which could modifying the existing disease management systems while reducing the negative effect of some synthetic chemicals on the environment and develop a more friendly production system (Hernández *et al.*, 2006; Hernández *et al.*, 2008).

	Mycelia growth inhibition (%)		
Treatment	*B. cinerea*	*C. coccodes*	*F. oxysporum*
Control (Destilled H_2O)	0 d	0 f	0 d
Chemical control y	100 a	100 a	81.3 b
L. tridentata 1000	96 c	80.2 b	63.2 c
L. tridentata 2000	95.9 c	72.2 c	49.1 d
L. tridentata 4000	99.5 a	64.4 d	41.8 d

Table 4. Mycelia growth inhibition of *Botrytis cinerea, Fusarium oxysporum* and *Colletotrichum coccodes* after the incubation period containing different concentrations of *Larrea tridentata.* Lira *et al.*, 2006. y Chlorotalonil and prozycar were used at 2000 ul liter $^{-1}$, z Numbers Followed by the same letter do not differ significantly according to Tukey test ($P \leq 0.01$)

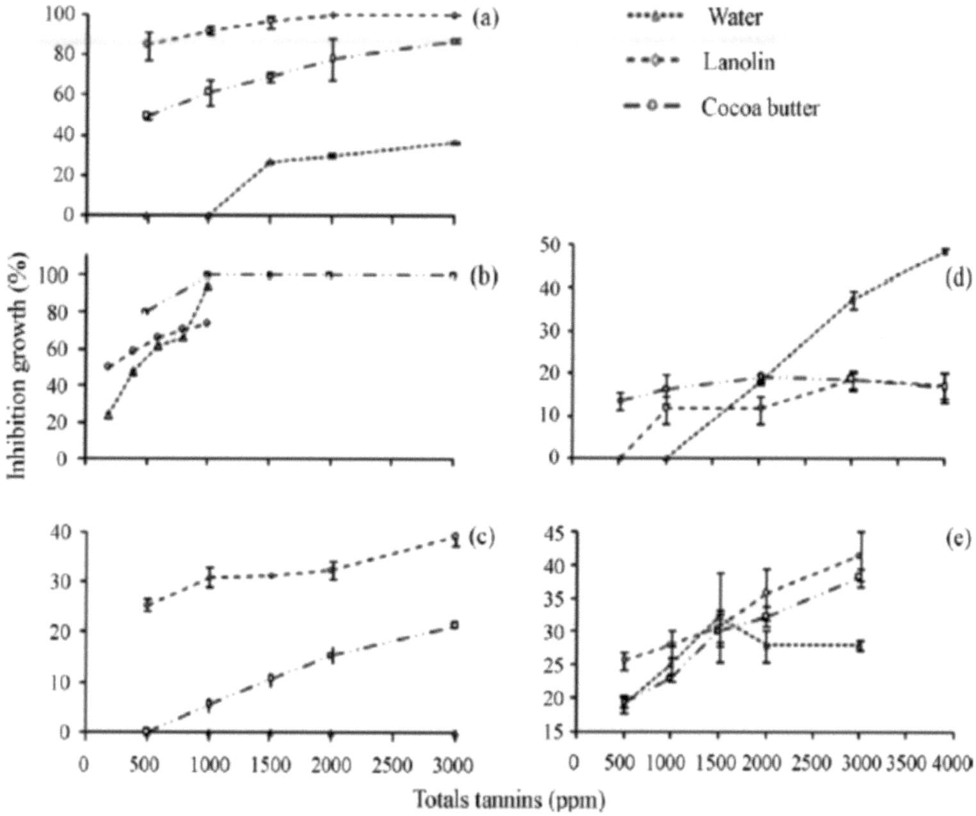

Fig. 4. Effect of plant extracts and total tannin concentration on inhibition of *R. solani* mycelia growth. (a) *Larrea tridentata* (b) *Flourensia cernua* (c) *Agave lechuguilla* (d) *Opuntia* sp. and (e) *Yucca* sp. Castillo, *et al.*, 2010.

In some extracts the overall effect on fungal mycelium growth inhibition can be maintained over time which gives fungicidal properties. Table 5 shows fungistatic and fungicidal action of some extracts on *P. infestans*, confirming the potential use of phytochemicals on plant disease control.

	Flourensia cernua		*Origanum mejorana*		*Bouvardia ternifolia*	
Dosis (ppm)	48 z	96	48	96	48	96
Metalaxil y	100.0 a	100.0 a	100.0 a	100.0 a	100.0 a	100.0 a
20000	88.44 ab	67.28 b	100.0 a	100.0 a	77.21 b	34.98 b
16000	81.63 b	48.56 c	100.0 a	100.0 a	57.14 c	1.23 c
12000	63.95 c	31.69 d	100.0 a	100.0 a	51.02 c	4.93 c
8000	49.66 c	9.15 e	100.0 a	100.0 a	22.45 d	0.0 c
4000	21.77 d	0.0 f	55.44 b	2.47 b	7.82 e	0.0 c
0	0.0 e	0.0 f	0.0 c	0.0 b	0.0 e	0.0 c

Table 5. Fungistatic and fungicidal effect of plant extracts obtained with methanol on *Phytophthora infestans* Mont (de Bary). z Hours, and y at 750 ppm. Gamboa *et al.*, 2003a.

This potential is effective also by low concentrations of some plant extracts which inhibited the fungal mycelium growth. Besides, availability of raw material for polyphenols extraction is high. Table 6 and Fig. 5 are presented the inhibitory concentrations IC_{50} of different plant extracts on *R. solani* growth.

Source of plant extract	Solvents	Fiducially Limits 95%		
		IC_{50} (ppm)	**Inferior**	**Superior**
Larrea trindetata	Water	$3.87X10^3$	$3.07X10^3$	$5.21X10^3$
Larrea trindetata	Lanolin	$1.85X10^2$	$6.86X10^1$	$2.93X10^2$
Larrea trindetata	Cocoa	$5.71X10^2$	$4.77X10^2$	$6.56X10^2$
Flourensia cernua	Water	$4.20X10^2$	$1.73X10^2$	$6.49X10^2$
Flourensia cernua	Lanolin	$2.12X10^2$	$7.96X10^1$	$3.11X10^2$
Flourensia cernua	Cocoa	$4.54X10^2$	---*	---*
Opuntia sp	Water	$3.83X10^3$	$3.24X10^3$	$5.19X10^3$
Opuntia sp	Lanolin	$2.08X10^4$	$1.06X10^4$	$9.44X10^4$
Opuntia sp	Cocoa	$4.9X10^8$	---*	---*
Agave lechuguilla	Water	NI	---	---
Agave lechuguilla	Lanolin	$1.70X10^4$	$7.08X10^3$	$2.21X10^5$
Agave lechuguilla	Cocoa	$6.72X10^3$	$4.14X10^3$	$2.79X10^4$
Yucca sp	Water	$5.74X10^4$	$1.42X10^4$	$1.00 X10^7$
Yucca sp	Lanolin	$8.96X10^3$	$5.14X10^3$	$2.99X10^4$
Yucca sp	Cocoa	$8.14X10^3$	$5.25X10^3$	$1.81X10^4$

Table 6. IC_{50} values for inhibition of mycelia growth *R. solani,* with different plant extracts. NI = Not inhibited to doses evaluated and * = Not permitted to identify fiducially limits.

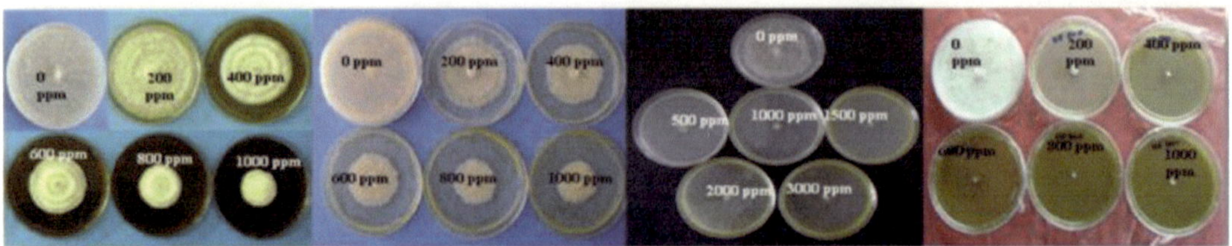

Water	Lanolin	Cocoa butter	Ethanol

Fig. 5. Inhibition of *R. solani* mycelia using different concentration of *F. cernua* extract.

The mechanism of action of these phytochemicals is variable, for example, toxicity of phenols for microorganisms is attributed to enzyme inhibition by oxidation of compounds. The mode of action of terpenes and essential oils has not been fully elucidated, but is postulated to cause cell membrane disruption by the lipophilic compounds. The postulated effect of alkaloids is that these compounds may alternate with DNA, while lectins and polypeptides are known that can form ion channels in the microbial membrane or cause competitive inhibition of adhesion of microbial proteins to host polysaccharide receptors (Cowan, 1999).

It has also been reported an excellent effect of plant extracts on growth inhibition of plant and food pathogenic bacteria. Table 7 shows the effect of plant extracts on growth of bacterial colonies, these plant extracts also reduce significantly the growth of food bacteria Figure 6.

		Bacteria Inhibition (%)		
		C. m. subsp. *michiganesis*	*C. m.* subsp. *nebraskensis*	
Source of plant extract	**Concentration (PPM)**	**8 Days**	**4 Days**	**6 Days**
Control (Distilled H_2O)	0	0	0	0
L. tridentata	500	100	100	100
L. tridentata	1000	100	100	100
L. tridentata	1500	100	100	100
L. tridentata	2000	100	100	100
F. cernua	50	100	100	100
F. cernua	150	100	100	100
F. cernua	300	100	100	100
F. cernua	450	100	100	100
A. lechuguilla	50	100	100	98.99
A. lechuguilla	150	100	100	100
A. lechuguilla	300	100	100	100
A. lechuguilla	450	100	100	100

Table 7. Effect of extracts from *Larrea tridentata, Flourensia cernua* and *Agave lechuguilla* on inhibition the growth of bacterial (*Clavibacter michiganensis* subsp. *Michiganensis* and *Clavibacter michiganensis* subsp. *nebraskensis*) colonies.

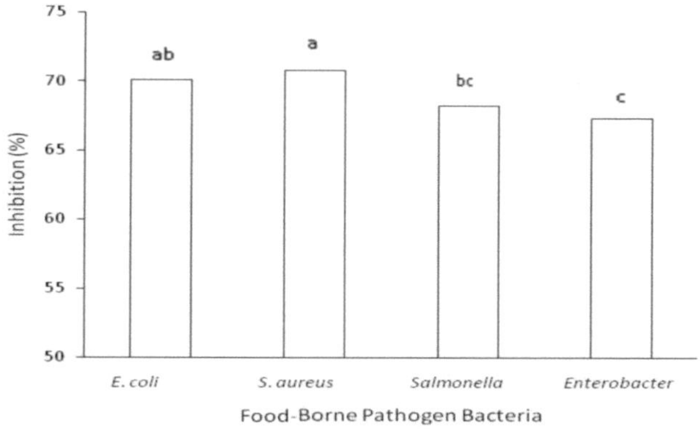

Fig. 6. Percentage of inhibition of food-borne bacterial growth because different plant extracts.

Most of the plant sources tested to date have demonstrated the antimicrobial potential of powders and extracts. Therefore, it is important to continue research for discover the active compounds responsible of the antifungal effect, and subsequently help to elucidate its biological effects and potential use. The available Mexican plant diversity should be used, especially because their biodegradable and nontoxic compounds.

2.5 Effect of solvent and extracts on spore production

Phytochemicals derived from semi-desert plants, shows not only action in arresting the growth of fungi and bacteria colony, but will also affect fungal sporulation, this action is presented in Table 8, showing the importance of the solvent used in phytochemical extraction and their effect on production of conidia for different fungal species.

Extracts	*Alternaria alternata*[x]	*Penicillium digitatum*[x]	*Colletotrichum gloeosporoides*[y]
Solvent			
Ethanol	0.93 b	0.24 a	5.50 c
Methanol: Chloroform	0.26 b	0.18 a	5.76 c
Hexane	4.40 a	0.19 a	7.77 b
Eter	3.33 a	0.24 a	9.29 a
Concentration			
0	3.13 a	0.61 a	8.07 a
500	2.78 ab	0.13 b	7.82 a
1000	2.66 ab	0.13 b	7.31 a
2000	1.64 ab	0.11 b	6.36 b
4000	0.94 b	0.08 b	5.80 b

Table 8. Comparison of four *Flourensia cernua* extracts and four concentrations on sporulation of three postharvest pathogens. [X] 1.0×10^5 conidia/ml, and [Y] 1.0×10^6 conidia/ml. Guerrero *et al.*, 2007

Likewise, one cans infer that the inhibition of sporulation is a function of the phytochemicals concentration used. Table 9, shows that conidia production is affected when phytochemicals concentration increase.

	Sporulation inhibition x 10^4 ml $^{-3}$		
Treatment	***B. cinerea***	***C. coccodes***	***F. oxysporum***
Control (Destilled H_2O)	8.3 a[z]	6.7 a	47.7 bcd
Chemical control	0.0 b	0.0 a	56.6 bc
L. tridentata 1000	2.2 b	4.2 abc	25.0 bcde
L. tridentata 2000	1.7 b	6.4 ab	20.3 cde
L. tridentata 4000	1.7 b	2.8 ab	15.8 de

Table 9. Effect of *Larrea tridentata* extracts on sporulation inhibition of *Botrytis cinerea, Colletotrichum coccodes* and *Fusarium oxysporum* after the incubation period (Lira *et al.*, 2006). Chemical controls used were chlorotalonil and prozycar at 2000 ul liter $^{-1}$. [z] Number followed by the same letter do not differ significantly according Tukey test ($p \leq 0.001$)

2.6 General description of Chihuahuan semi-desert plant species sources of phytochemical compounds with anti-fungal properties

Larrea tridentata is a xerophytes evergreen plant that can survive hundreds or thousands of years through vegetative reproduction (asexual), because the roots produce new sprouts or shoots which are then converted into new plants (Brinker, 1993). The plant shows variation in height from 0.5 to 4 m. This height is a function of ploidy level (diploid 86 cm, 112 cm hexaploid and tetraploid 138 cm). There is one main stem, but the thick branches grow vertically or obliquely from the crown and root side is dichotomous. Its leaves are small and bifoliate, dark green to yellowish green with thick cuticles and a resinous coating, have short petioles and grow opposite on the branches (Fig. 7). The flowers are yellow usually appear in late winter or early spring, but can bloom at any time after a rain, grow near the ends of young shoots and buds solitary with five petals. The fruit are small between 4 to 7 mm in diameter, have a fuzzy cover and contains 5 seeds (Jasso de Rodriguez *et al.*, 2006; Lira, 2003).

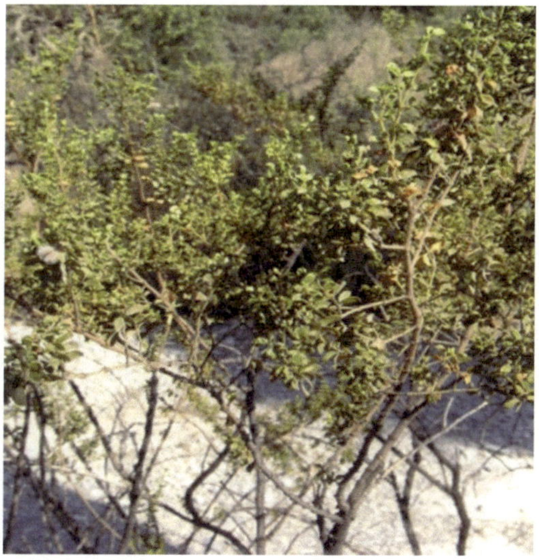

Fig. 7. *Larrea tridentata*

Secondary Metabolites: The main compounds reported in the literature are numerous. Distinguished by their higher content of dry weight basis of foliage phenolics, lignans, saponins, flavonoids, amino acids and minerals. The most important compound is nordihydroguaiaretic acid (NDGA) (Lira, 2003) found in the resin cell epidermal layers near the top and bottom of the leaves and stems.

Flourensia cernua D.C. Is a much-branched plant up to 2 m high, which exudes a resinous. It has slender branches, evergreen, light brown to gray with alternate leaves, composed of two leaflets, elliptic to oblong 17-25 mm long and 6.5-11.5 mm wide, acute at both ends, dark green, sometimes resinous paler underside and petiole of 1-2 mm (Hyder *et al.*, 2005). The flowers are in corymbs or panicles flower heads and has 12 to 20 flowers per capitulum. The fruit is a very hairy achene 6 mm long and 2 mm wide, laterally compressed, 2 to 4 edges uneven hair 2-3 mm long, nearly obscured by the long hairs of the achene (Jasso *et al.*, 2006).

Secondary Metabolites: The chemical composition of *F. cernua* resin is sesquiterpenoids and triterpenoids (Kingston *et al.*, 1975), polyacetylenes, p-acetophenones, benzofurans and benzopirans (Bohlmann and Grenz, 1977) and flavonoids (Dillon *et al.*, 1976; Rao *et al.*, 1970). Advanced Studies on phytochemistry of leaves reveal the presence of resins, flavonoids (deoxy flavonoids), phytoalexins, coumarins, phenolic compounds, benzofurans, p-coumaric acid. Some particular compounds include dehydroflourensic acid and flourensadiol (Kingston *et al.*, 1975) that enable the use of this species with biological activity against pathogens.

Opuntia ficus-indica (L.) Mill. This plant tree 3-5 m tall, crown wide, glabrous, stems of 60-150 cm wide, obovate cladodes of 30-60 cm long, 20-40 cm wide and 19-28 cm thick, dark green covered with a layer of wax. Spines usually absent or up to 2 per areola, short: only 0.5-1 cm, weak, whitish. Flowers (6-) 7-9 (-10) cm long are orange to yellow. The fruit is sweet, juicy, edible, 5-10 cm long and 4-8 cm wide, pyriform, slightly sunken in the navel, pulpy and thin shell (Fig. 8). The seeds are obovate to disc-shaped 3-4 mm in diameter (FAO, 1999).

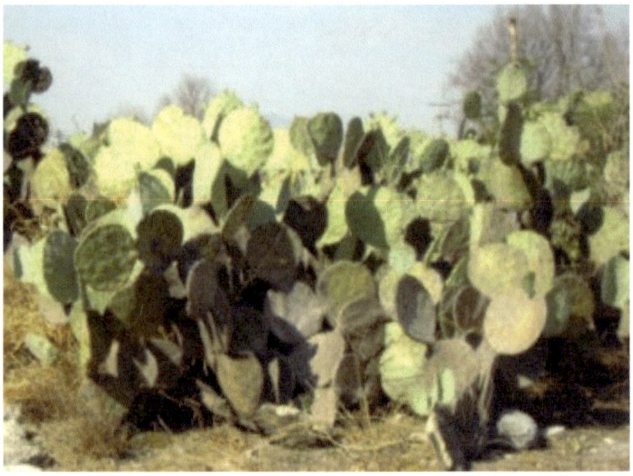

Fig. 8. *Opuntia ficus-indica*

Secondary Metabolites: According to the revised literature, has not been reported secondary metabolites present, although we did detect condensed polyphenols gallic acid equivalent, saponins and terpenes.

Lippia graveolens Kunth. Is an evergreen shrub, with life cycle of 3 to 10 years belonging to the family Verbenaceae, can reach up to 2.5 m tall with branched stems with many leaves 1-3 cm long and 0.5 to 1.5 cm wide, distributed in the opposite form, alternate and oval in shape with jagged edges, rough texture with light hairs. Presents individual inflorescences with small white flowers (Lahlou, 2004). The number of flowers per inflorescence is very variable most frequently found 10 flowers per inflorescence, its fruits are small capsules containing brown seeds, not more than 0.25 mm (Lahlou, 2004).

Secondary metabolites. The biological components with higher capacity are in the essential oil consisting mainly of thymol and carvacrol, as well as some phenolic acids and flavonoids with antimicrobial properties (Lambet *et al.*, 2001)

Yucca filifera Chabaud. Plant tree to over 10 m high, much branched with leaves up to 55 cm long and 3.6 cm wide, linear-oblanceolate, constricted near the base, rigid, usually rough on both surfaces with numerous coiled filaments white, easily breakable, so are most noticeable in young leaves (Fig 9). The escape of the foliage stands; panicle more or less cylindrical, pendulous, up to 1.5 m long, multiflora, extended flowers, pedicellate, pedicels up to 2.7 cm long, 3.8-5.2 perianth segments cm long, 0.7-2.5 cm wide, inner segments slightly shorter and wider, filaments 1-1.5 cm long; pistil 2.3-2.5 cm long, ovary 1.8-2 cm long and 0.4 to 0.5 cm in diameter. Hanging fruit, oblong, 5-8.8 cm long, 2.7-3.3 cm in diameter, ending in a peak of 0.2 to 0.7 cm long. Seed 8 x 2 mm, somewhat rough.

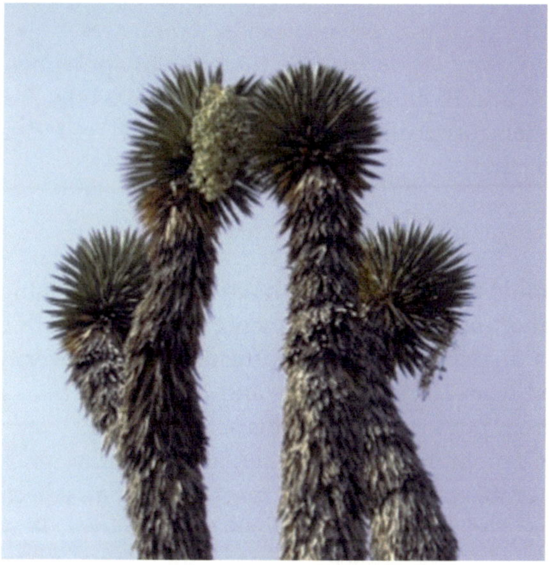

Fig. 9. Yucca filifera.

Secondary Metabolites: The leaves and roots of the *Yucca* genus contains saponins, steroidal sapogenins and a high content of ascorbic acid.

Carya illinoensis. Cultivated species belonging to the family Juglandaceae is a tree that can reach 50 meters in height with a trunk up to 2 m in diameter, its bark is cracked and rough, greyish. Its leaves are deciduous, compound, odd-pinnate, lanceolate, large, oval, toothed, petiole short 6 to 12 cm wide. The flowers are very small, apetalous, monoecious and are grouped in catkins (earrings) cylindrical pendants, light green. The fruit or drupe, consisting of pericarp, mesocarp and seeds (almonds). The pericarp, as the mesocarp is a segmented structure into four parts that opens dehydrated freeing the endocarp and seed. A portion of the mesocarp and endocarp is known as husk. The nuts consist of the endocarp and the seed typically measure 2 to 6 cm long and weigh 4 to 12 g each. The seed has two cotyledons separated by a center wall, which come from flowers carpels (Fig 10).

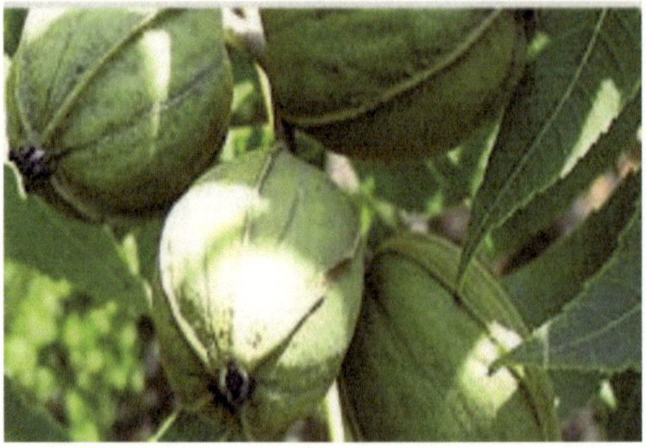

Fig. 10. Carya illinoensis fruits

Secondary metabolites. Depending on the analyzed part of the plant one cans find different active principles in leaves, naphthoquinones (juglone, plumbagin, beta-hydroplumbagin) in the pericarp, organic acids, tannins and naphthoquinones, in the cotyledons, unsaturated fatty acids, in the integument, polyphenols and tannins, and walnut, Vitamin A, B, C and E, minerals and iodine. Meanwhile, Sasaki (1964) reports that the walnut husk contains azaleatin (Quercetin 5-methyl ether) and caryatin flavonol (quercetin 3.5-dimethyl ether).

3. Conclusion

The from Mexican semi-desert plant species have the ability to inhibit the development of mycelium and sporulation of fungi and stramenopiles and growth of bacterial pathogens. Under field conditions a decrease in disease incidence and severity have been reported. Phytochemicals derived from *Larrea tridentata* and *Flourensia cernua* show a wide spectrum of action towards different phytopathogens, this activity occurs even with non-conventional solvents such as water, lanolin and cocoa butter. The use of natural extracts in controlling plant diseases has low or no environmental impact, so they may become a viable option for development of organic and sustainable agriculture. However, it is necessary to develop research on molecular and biochemical changes that these compounds may have on pathogen and plant.

4. Acknowledgment

The authors acknowledge the financial support for the development of research to the National Council of Science and Technology of Mexico (CONACYT) and Fitokimica Industrial, SA of CV. Francisco Castillo thanks CONACYT for the financial support for his Ph. D. studies.

5. References

Anderson, B.S., Hunt, J.W., Phillips, B.M., Nicely, P.A., Vlaming, V. de, Connor, V., Richard, N., & Tjeerdema, R. S. (2003). Integrated assessment of the impacts of agricultural drain water in the Salinas River. *Environmental Pollution*, Vol. 124, No. 3, (August 2003) pp. (523-532), ISSN 0269-7491

Arteaga, S., Andrade, C. A. & Cárdenas, R. (2005). *Larrea tridentata* (Creosote bush), an abundant plant of Mexican and US-American deserts and its metabolite nordihydroguaiaretic acid, *Journal of Ethnopharmacology*, Vol. 98, No. 3, (April 2005), pp. (231-239) ISSN 0378-8741

Bautista, B.S., García, E., Barrera, L., Reyes, N., & Wilson, C. (2003). Seasonal Evaluation of the postharvest fungicidal activity of powders and extracts of huamúchil (*Pithecellobium dulce*): action against *Botrytis cinerea, Penicillium digitatum* and *Rhizopus stolonifer* of strawberry fruit. *Postharvest Biology & Technology*, Vol. 29, No. 1, (July 2003), pp. (81-92), ISSN 0925-5214

Bergeron, C., Marston, A., Hakizamungu, E., & Hostettmann, K. (1995). Antifungal constituens of *Chenopodium procerum. International Journal of Pharmacognosy*, Vol. 33, No. 2, (); pp. (115-119).

Bohlmann, F., & Grenz, M. (1977). Über inhaltsstoffe der gattung *Flourensia, Chemische Berichte*,Vol. 110, No. 1, (Junuary 1977), pp. (295-300), ISSN 1099-0682

Castillo, F., Hernández, D., Gallegos, G., Méndez, M., Rodríguez, R., Reyes A. &. Aguilar, C.N. (2010). In vitro antifungal activity of plant extracts obtained with alternative organic solvents against *Rhizoctonia solani* Kühn. *Industrial Crops and Products*, Vol. 32, No. 3, (June 2010), pp. (324-328), ISSN 0926-6690

Cooke, D.E.L., Young, V., Birch, P.R.J., Toth, R., Gourlay, F., Day, J.P., Carnegie, S.F., & Duncan, J.M. (2003). Phenotypic and genotypic diversity of *Phytophthora infestans* populations in Scotland (1995-97). *Plant Pathology*, No.52 issue 2, pp (181-192), ISSN 0032-0862

Cowan, M. M. (1999). Plant products as antimicrobial agents. *Clinical Microbiology Review*, Vol. 12, No. 4, (October 1999), pp. (564-582), ISSN: 1098-6618

Dillon, M.O., Mabry, T.J., Besson, E., Bouillant, M.L., & Chopin, J. (1976). New flavonoids from *Flourensia cernua, Phytochemistry*, Vol. 15, No. 6, pp. (1085-1086), ISSN 0031-9422.

FAO. 1999. Agroecología, cultivo y usos del nopal. Roma, Italia. P 72.

Gamboa, A.R., Hernández, C.F.D., Guerrero, R.E. & Sánchez, A.A. (2003a). Inhibition of mycelial growth of *Rhizoctonia solani* Kühn and *Phytophthora infestans* Mont (de Bary) with methanolic plant extracts of Hojasén (*Flourensia cernua* DC), Marjoram (*Origanum majorana* L.) and trumpet [*Bouvardia ternifolia* (Ca.) Schlecht.]. *Mexican Journal of Phytopathology*, Vol. 21, No. 1, (Junio 2003), pp. (13-18), ISSN 0185-3309 (In Spanish)

Gamboa, A.R., Hernández, F.D., Guerrero, E., Sánchez, A., Villarreal, L.A., López, R.G., Jiménez, F., & Lira, S.R.H. (2003b). Antifungal effect of *Larrea tridentata* extracts on *Rhizoctonia solani* Kühn and *Phytophthora infestans* Mont. (De Bary). PHYTON-*International Journal of Experimental Botany*, Vol. 72, pp. (119-126), ISSN 1851 5657

González, G.E., Rodríguez, H.R.& Aguilar, G.C.N. (2009). Biodegradación de Taninos, CIENCIACIERTA No.17, http://www.postgradoeinvestigacion.uadec.mx/CienciaCierta/CC17/cc17taninos.html

Guerrero, R.E., Solís, G.S., Hernández, C.F.D., Flores, O.A. & Soval, L.V. (2007). *In vitro* biological activity of extracts from *Flourensia cernua* DC in post-harvest pathogens: *Alternaria alternata* (Fr.:Fr.) Keissl., *Colletrichum gloeosporoides* (Penz.) Penz y Sacc. y *Penicillium digitatum* (Pers.:Fr.) y Sacc. *Mexican Journal of Phytopathology*, Vol. 25, No.1, (Junio 2007), pp. (48-53), ISSN 0185-3309 (In Spanish)

Hernández, C. .F.D., Lira, S.R.H., Cruz, Ch.L., Gallegos, M.G., Galindo, C.M.E., Padrón, C.E. & Hernández, S.M. (2008). Antifungal potential of *Bacillus* spp. strains and *Larrea tridentata* extract against *Rhizoctonia solani* on potato (*Solanum tuberosum* L.) crop. *International Journal of Experimental Botany*, Vol. 77, pp. (241-252), ISSN 1851 5657

Hernández, C.F.D., Aguirre, A.A., Lira, S.R.H., Guerrero, R.E. & Gallegos, M.G. (2006). Biological efficiency of organic biological and chemical products against *Alternaria dauci* Kühn and its effects on carrot crop. *International Journal of Experimental Botany*, Vol. 75, pp. (91-101), ISSN 1851 5657

Hernández, L., A. Bautista, B., S. &Velázquez-del Valle, M. (2007). Prospective of plant extracts for controlling postharvest diseases of horticultural products. *Mexican Journal of Phytopathology*, Vol. 30, No. 2, (Junio 2007), pp. (119-123), ISSN 0187-7380 (in spanish)

Hernández,C.FD., Castillo, R.F., Gallegos, M.G., Rodríguez, H.R. & Aguilar, G.C.N. (2010). *Lippia graveolens* and *Carya illinoensis* organic extracts and there *in vitro* effect against *Rhizoctonia solani* Kuhn. *American Journal of Agricultural and Biological Sciences*, Vol. 5, No. 3, (Septiember 2010), pp. (380-384), ISSN 1557-4989.

Hyder, P.W., Fredrickson, E.L., Estell, R.E., Lucero, M.E. & Remmenga, M.D., (2005). Loss of phenolic compounds from leaf litter of creosote bush [*Larrea tridentata* (Sess. and Moc. ex DC.) Cov.] and tarbush (*Flourensia cernua* DC.). *Journal Arid Environments*, Vol. 61, No. 1, (April 2005), pp. (79–91), ISSN 0140-1963

Jasso C.D & Rodríguez, G. R. (2007). Mexican industrializable arid and semi-arid land species for sustainable agriculture, in: *agricultura sustentable y biofertilizantes*, Lira-Saldivar and Medina-Torres (eds.), pp 89-103, Mexico.

Jasso de Rodríguez, D., Angulo, S. J.L. & Hernández, C.F.D. (2006). An overview of the antimicrobial properties of Mexican medicinal plants, In: naturally occurring bioactive compounds, in: *Advances in phytomedicine*, Rai and Carpinella, (ed.), 325-377, IBSN 978-0-444-52241-2, Netherlands

Jasso de Rodríguez, D., Hernández, C.F.D., Angulo, S. J.L., Rodríguez, G.R., Villarreal, Q. J.A., & Lira, S.R.H. (2007). Antifungal Activity *in vitro* of *Flourensia cernua* and *Fusarium oxysporum. Industrial Crops and Products,* Vol. 25, No. 2, (Febrary 2007), pp. (111-116), ISSN 0926-6690

Kingston, D.G.L., Rao, M.M., Spittler, T.D., Pettersen, R.C., & Cullen, D.L. (1975). Sesquiterpenes from *Flourensia cernua*. *Phytochemistry*, Vol. 14, No. 9, (September, 1975), pp. (2033-2037), ISSN 0031-9422

Lahlou, M. (2004). Methods to study the phytochemistry and bioactivity of essential oils. *Phytotherapy Research*, Vol. 18, No. 6, (June 2004), pp. (435-448), ISSN 1099-1573

Lambert, R., Skandamis, P. , Coote, P. & Nychas, G.-J. (2001). A study of the minimum inhibitory concentration & mode of action of oregano essential oil, thymol and carvacrol, *Journal of Applied Microbiology*, Vol. 91, No. 3, (Septiember 2001), pp. (453–462), ISSN 1364-5072

Leroux, P. (2003). Mode of action of agrochemical towards plant pathogens. *Comptes Rendus Biologies*, Vol. 326, No. 1 (January 2003), pp. (9-21), ISSN 1631-0691

Lira, S.R.H. (2003). Estado actual del conocimiento sobre las propiedades biocidas de la gobernadora [*Larrea tridentata* (D.C.) Coville]. *Mexican Journal of Phytopathology*, Vol. 21, No. 2, (December 2003), pp. (214-222), ISSN 0185-3309

Lira, S.R.H., Balvantin, G.G.F., Hernández, C.F.D., Gamboa, A.R., Jasso de Rodríguez, D. & Jiménez, D.F. (2003). Evaluation of resin content and the antifungal effect of *Larrea tridentate* (Sesse and Moc. Ex D.C.) Coville extracts from two Mexican deserts against *Pythium* sp. Pringsh. *Mexican Journal of Phytopathology*, Vol. 21, No.2, (December 2003), pp. (97-101), ISSN 0185-3309 (In Spanish)

Lira, S.R.H., Gamboa, A.R., Villarreal, C.L.A., López, C.R.G. & Jiménez, D.F. (2002). Hydrosoluble extracts of *Larrea tridentata* from two desertic zones in the north of Mexico and their inhibitory effect on *Fusarium oxysporum*. *International Journal of Experimental Botany*, Vol. 71, pp. (167-172), ISSN 1851 5657

Lira, S.R.H., Hernández, S.M. & Hernández, C.F.D. (2006). Activity of *Larrea tridentata* (D.C.) Coville L. extracts and chitosan against fungi that affect horticultural crops. *Rev. Chapingo Serie Horticulture*, Vol. 12, No. 2, (December 2006), pp. (211-216), ISSN 0186-3231

Lira, S.R.H., Hernández, S.M., Chavéz, B.C., Hernández, C.F.D. & Cuellar, V.E. (2007). Biopesticides and biological control. CIQA, Monterrey, México. Pp 13-29. ISBN 968-844.054-X Mexico

Mata, G.M.A., Renovato, N.J. & Aguilar, C.N. (2008). Acido galico-fuentes, producción, usos potenciales y algunas propiedades, in : *Fitoquimicos sobresalientes del semidesierto mexicano*, Aguilar, C.N., Rodriguez R., and Jasso, D. (eds.), pp. 289- 302, IBSN 978-968-6628-760, Mexico.

Medina, M.M.A., Belmares, C.R.E., Rodriguez, H.R & Aguilar, C.N. (2007). Valorización comercial de los subproductos de la nuez para la producción de antioxidantes. Cienciacierta No. 9 *http://www2.uadec.mx/pub/pdf/cienciacierta9.pdf*

Montes, B. R. (1996). Natural plant products to combat pathogens. *Mexican Journal of Phytopathology*. Vol. 14, No. 1, (June 1996), pp. (9-14), (In Spanish)

Osorio, E., Flores, M., Hernández, D., Ventura, J., Rodríguez, R. and Aguilar, C. N. (2010). Biological efficiency of polyphenolic extracts from pecan nuts shell (*Carya illinoensis*), pomegranate husk (*Punica granatum*) & creosote bush leaves (*Larrea tridentata* Cov.) against plant pathogenic fungi. *Industrial Crops and Products*, Vol. 31, No. 1, (January 2010) pp. (153-157),

Ramirez, C.A., Favela,T.E, Saucedo,C.G., Roussos, S. & Augur, Ch. (2008). Catechina : estructura y biodegradacion, in : *Fitoquimicos sobresalientes del semidesierto mexicano*, Aguilar, C.N., Rodriguez, R., and Jasso, D. (eds.), pp.275-288, IBSN 978-968-6628-760, Mexico.

Rao, M.M., Kingston, D.G.I. & Splitter, T.D. (1970). Flavonoids from *Flourensia cernua*. *Phytochemistry*, Vol. 9, No. 1, (January 1970), pp. (227-228), ISSN 0031-9422

Sasaki, T. (1964). Components of pecan (*Carya pecan*). II. A new flavonol caryatin isolated from the bark of pecan and its structure. *Journal of the Pharmaceutical Society of Japan*, Vol. 84, No. pp. (47-51), ISSN 0031-6903

Seigler, D.S., Jakupcak, J., & Mabry, T.J. (1974). Wax esters from *Larrea divaricata*. Phytochemistry, Vol. 13, No. 6, (June 1974), pp. (983-986), ISSN 0031-9422

Whalen, M.M., Wilson, S., Gleghorn, C. & Loganathan, B.G. (2003). Brief exposure to triphenyltin produces irreversible inhibition of the cytotoxic function of human natural killer cells. *Environmental Research*, Vol. 92, No. 3, (July 2003), pp. (213-220), ISSN 0013-9351

Wilson, C.L., Ghaouth, A.E., & Wisniewski, M.E. (1999). Prospecting in nature´s storehouse for biopesticides. *Mexican Journal of phytopathology*, Vol. 17, No. 1, (June 1999), pp. (49-53), ISSN 0185-3309

10

Weed Biology and Weed Management in Organic Farming

Anneli Lundkvist and Theo Verwijst
Swedish University of Agricultural Sciences (SLU)
Sweden

1. Introduction

Weed biology, including the ecology, physiology and population dynamics of weed species, does not differ from plant biology apart from the notion that the plants under investigation are considered to be "unwanted". Weeds are unwanted and undesirable plants which interfere with the utilization of land and water resources and thus adversely affect human welfare (Rao, 1999). Weed biology research consequently aims to generate knowledge that is expected to be applied in the practical control of weeds, and should include integrated research, from basic to applied, with all elements contributing to real improvements in weed management (Moss, 2008). Management of weeds is performed for the benefit of different interests, ranging from clean and non slippery pavements, to minimizing yield losses in agriculture. The occurrence of weeds in agricultural crops leads to substantial yield reductions causing economic losses all over the world. Crop damage from weeds generally is larger than from other pests (Oerke, 2006). According to FAO (the Food and Agriculture Organization of the United Nations) and the environmental research organization, Land Care of New Zealand, weeds caused yield losses corresponding to $95 billion in 2009. This may be compared with yield losses caused by pathogens ($85 billion), and insects ($46 billion). The economic losses may even be larger if the costs for weed control measures are included (FAO, 2011).

The main reason for controlling weed abundance in agricultural crops is the risk for qualitative and quantitative reductions in crop yields. Black Nightshade (*Solanum nigrum* L.) is a problematic weed in crops such as peas (*Pisum sativum* L.), beans (*Vicia faba* L.) and soybean (*Glycine max* (L.) Merr.), where it not only causes a yield reduction in the crop, but also reduces crop quality by means of contamination with its poisonous seeds (Defelice, 2003). Common ragwort (*Senecio jacobaea* L.) is another poisonous species which does occur in temperate grasslands and pastures where it may lead to death of cattle and other livestock (Suter et al., 2007). Not only the fresh herbage is poisonous, but also its hay and silage remains toxic (Lüthy et al., 1981; Candrian et al., 1984).

A quantitative reduction in crop yield due to weeds foremost is ascribed to the ability of weeds to compete for resources such as light, water and nutrients, at the expense of the crop. The relative competitive ability of weed species is determined by two groups of interacting factors. The first one consists of species characteristics, such as propagation and dispersal features and other life cycle characteristics, and potential growth rate. The second

one is made up by the plant environment, which to a large extent is determined by the cropping system and its management. This implies that improvements in weed control in agriculture need to be based on both weed (and crop) ecology, and on the influence of the particular crop and management system on the population dynamics of weeds (Barberi, 2002). The influence of a particular management system may encompass both direct weed control methods such as different types of mechanical and chemical interference, and cultural weed control methods, such as crop choice and crop rotation (Bond & Grundy, 2001). The major difference with regard to weed control between conventional agriculture and organic farming is that the use of chemical weed control is prohibited in organic farming. Another difference is that artificial fertilizers cannot be employed, and thereby it is more difficult to adapt nitrogen levels to the immediate needs of a crop. This affects the relative competitive ability of crops and weeds, which interact with the immediate nutrient status of their environment. In conventional agriculture, chemical control may be employed with short notice and in a curative way, while in organic agriculture a longer time perspective should be taken to prevent yield losses due to weeds (Bastiaans et al., 2008). Direct and cultural methods need to be integrated in organic farming, with the long term goal to prevent the occurrence of weed-induced yield losses, while keeping down costs for weed control. This implies an integration of a complex biophysical system with an unpredictable market, thereby increasing risks for organic farmers.
What kinds of weed species do occur in agricultural crops and how can we control them in organic farming systems? Once we understand why particular weed species do grow abundantly in certain crop cultivation systems, we may alter the crops and crop management systems in such a way that long-term weed abundance decreases. In the following sections, a brief overview of important weed species and available weed control methods in organic farming will be described and some examples of progress in organic weed control are given from Sweden in the Northern part of Europe.

2. Classification of weed species

Given the fact that preventive rather than curative measures need to be used, weed control is one of the greatest challenges in organic farming. A first step for the organic farmer is to identify and recognize the weed species which actually are occurring on the fields, to be able to plan and perform effective short and long term weed control measurements. Weed species may be classified into groups for the purpose of planning and recording control measures against them in many different ways. Among those ways, a botanical classification (monocotyledons vs. dicotyledons) is useful in conventional farming, as selective, group specific herbicides are available. Weeds can also be grouped according to habitat requirements (preferred climate and soil types), invasiveness, economic importance or other criteria. Below, we use life cycle features and the mode of propagation to classify weeds for organic agriculture, as done for farmers in Sweden by Håkansson (2003) and by Lundkvist & Fogelfors (2004). An overview of the more commonly occurring weed species in Scandinavia and Finland, including classification criteria and cropping systems in which those species may occur as weeds, is given in Table 1. For more information about wild plant species that can occur as weeds in different environments, and means of controlling them, see the website 'Organic Weed Management' (Centre for Organic Horticulture, 2011), or for Nordic conditions the website 'Weed Advisor', developed at the Swedish University of Agricultural Sciences, Sweden, (Fogelfors, 2011) (under construction).

2.1 Annual species

Annual broad-leaved and grass weed species propagate by seeds. They grow and develop, flower, set seeds and die within a year after germination. Some annual species, such as *Erodium spp.* (Storksbill) may also display a biennial growth pattern, depending on the winter climate. The ability of short-lived plants to become successful weeds in different crops depends mainly on the germination biology of their seeds. An important seed characteristic is seed dormancy which gives weed species the ability to create a 'seed bank' in the ground. After seed shedding, the seeds may be dormant in the soil until the environmental conditions are favourable for germination. While being species specific and dependent on moisture and temperature, many weed species do have a seed bank with a half-life time of 5 years or more, which means that a fraction of seeds may be viable for many decades (Burnside et al., 1996). Annual weeds may also be classified according to the germination pattern of the seeds, which often varies through the growing season. Annual weed species may further be divided into winter and summer annuals, i.e. winter annuals have their main germination period in the autumn while summer annuals germinate mainly in spring.

In organic farming, both annual broad-leaved and grass weeds may cause yield losses since they are competing with the crop for resources like water, light and nutrients. Consequently, it is important to control them, early in the season before they start to compete with the crop or later in the season before they set seeds, to avoid an increase of the seed bank. For weed management methods, see section 3.

There are many important annual weed species which may lead to yield reductions in cropping systems. For example, the broad-leaved species Black bindweed (*Fallopia convolvulus* (L.) A. Löve), Cleavers (*Galium aparine* L.), Common chickweed (*Stellaria media* L.), Common ragweed (*Ambrosia artemisiifolia* L.), Fat-hen (*Chenopodium album* L.), Scentless mayweed (*Tripleurospermum inodorum* (L.) Sch. Bip), and grass weed species like Black-grass (*Alopecurus myosuroides* Huds.) and Wild oat (*Avena fatua* L) need to be controlled, foremost in annual crops.

2.2 Biennial species

Biennial species propagate through seeds and have a two year life cycle. They germinate and grow vegetatively during the first year, overwinter, and flower, set seeds and die during the second year. Soil cultivation effectively prevents biennial species to flower and set seed. Consequently, biennial species rarely are conceived as problematic weeds, except in perennial row crops and poorly established leys. An example of a biennial weed, occurring in more temperate regions, is Wild carrot (*Daucus carota* L.). Biennial species can be controlled in the same way as annual weeds, i.e. they should be removed early during the first season before they start to compete with the crop or later in the second season before the plants set seeds.

2.3 Perennial species

Perennial broad-leaved and grass weeds are more difficult to control compared to annual and biennial weed species since they propagate through both seeds and vegetative parts (roots and stems). A perennial plant may flower and set seed during several vegetation periods, by means of new shoots which are emerging yearly from the vegetative organs in the soil. These weeds may be divided in groups according to the way they propagate vegetatively, i.e. whether they have a stationary or a creeping root system.

2.3.1 Stationary perennials

This group overwinters by tap roots or by short below ground stem parts. Examples of important broad-leaved species are Curled Dock (*Rumex crispus L.*), Broad-leaved dock (*Rumex obtusifolius* L.), and Northern Dock (*Rumex longifolius* DC.). They often cause problems in leys and pastures, since they compete with the pasture species or arable crops and occupy area which could be utilized by more palatable crop species (Zaller, 2004). Although some vegetative regeneration takes place from underground parts, the vast majority of new plants develop from seeds (Cavers & Harpers, 1964). In leys and pasture, *R. crispus* is considered a very serious problem since it both decreases the quantity and the quality of the ley and pasture harvests (Cortney & Johnston, 1978; Oswald & Hagger, 1983). Dandelion (*Taraxacum* F.H. Wigg) is another example of a broad-leaved stationary perennial with stout tap roots, commonly found in pastures and lawns.

2.3.2 Creeping perennials

Creeping perennials spread vegetatively by means of roots, rhizomes or stolons, which elongate and produce new plants from reproductive buds on those organs. Rhizomes may produce roots and shoots from their internodes, while stolons do have their reproductive meristem at the apical end. Stolons often occur as areal runners, while roots and rhizomes spread below ground. Troublesome creeping perennial weed species in organic farming are Creeping thistle (*Cirsium arvense* (L.) Scop.), Field bindweed (*Convolvulus arvensis* L.), Perennial sow-thistle (*Sonchus arvensis* L.), and Common couch (*Elytrigia repens* (L.) Desv. ex Nevski).

Cirsium arvense is a deep-rooted, broad-leaved perennial that reproduces vegetatively and from seeds, but under most circumstances seed production contributes less to its weediness. The weediness of *C. arvense* can be attributed largely to its capacity for vegetative reproduction and regenerative growth from the numerous buds produced on the roots (Donald, 1994). *Cirsium arvense* is considered one of the world's worst weeds. This species causes problems in crop fields, grasslands and pastures as well as on fallow land and in nature conservation areas in temperate regions of both hemispheres (Holm et al., 1977; Donald, 1994).

Another broad-leaved species is *Convolvulus arvensis* which is a serious perennial weed found in many different crops (Weaver & Riley, 1982). After emergence of the seedling, a taproot is formed from which lateral roots are produced. They grow horizontally about 50-70 cm before turning down and forming secondary vertical roots. This growth pattern is then repeated. In this way, the species can spread rather rapidly over large areas (Centre for Organic Horticulture, 2011).

Sonchus arvensis is a competitive broad-leaved weed species with the main part of the root system 0-20 cm below soil surface (Lemna & Messersmith, 1990). The weed is usually found in spring sown crops (cereals, oilseed rape, potatoes and vegetables) where it can cause considerable yield losses. Compared with spring cereals, *S. arvensis* has shown to be very efficient in nitrogen uptake early in the growing season when nitrogen availability usually is quite low in organically managed fields (Eckersten et al., 2010). This is probably one reason for its increased abundance in organic farming in the northern parts of Europe.

A serious perennial grass weed is *Elytrigia repens*. Seedlings begin to develop rhizomes at the 4- to 6-leaf stage, around the time of first tillering (Palmer & Sagar, 1963). In most situations, vegetative reproduction is more important than propagation by seeds. The aerial shoots of the parent plant die back in the autumn and new primary shoots start to develop below-ground. These grow slowly until temperatures rise in spring, and shoots emerge above soil surface. New leaves are produced and previously dormant buds at the base of each shoot may grow out to form upright tillers or horizontal rhizomes. The rhizomes themselves form numerous lateral rhizomes, about two months after the first shoot emergence. *E. repens* usually occurs as a weed in open or disturbed habitats, rather than in closed plant communities. In compacted soil, the rhizomes grow more or less horizontally. Rhizome growth increases with nitrogen level. Rhizomes grow horizontally in summer before turning erect in autumn, ready to form new aerial shoots (Centre for Organic Horticulture, 2011).

2.4 Which weed species are favoured in which crops?

Sutherland (2004) distinguished weeds from non-weeds by means of life history traits of plant species, and concluded that life span was the most significant life history trait for weeds in general: Weeds were most likely to be annuals and biennials and less likely to be perennials than non-weeds. From Table 1, we see that annual plant species mainly occur as weeds in annual crops, implying that there is a strong interaction with the environment provided by an actual cropping system and the environment which is needed by certain plant species, to develop into large populations of weeds. Most of the annual species are able to develop during periods in which the crop is not present or not yet competitive. Some species, for example Common chickweed (*Stellaria media*), does tolerate a fair degree of shading, and may compete for water and nitrogen while situated below a crop canopy.

With regard to creeping perennials, they all have seedlings which hardly will establish in dense, competitive crops. But once established, they all are efficient users of nitrogen, and are conceived as strong competitors in most cropping systems. These weeds may escape effects of soil tillage, due to a deep position of their root system, and if they do not, their roots may be fragmented, each fragment being viable and able to sprout new shoots.

Instead of putting the question 'Which weed species are favoured in which crops?', one may ask the question 'Which crops have the best ability to compete and suppress weeds?'. In general, fast-growing crops, which close their canopy early, do have a good competitive ability and tend to suppress weeds much better then slow growing crops with more open canopies. Oats (*Avena sativa* L.), for instance, is considered to be a good competitor, while peas are on the other end of the scale (Lundkvist & Fogelfors 2004). Consequently, the core of weed control in organic farming is the use of suitable crop rotations in which crops with a weak competitive ability are alternated with strongly competing crops, or crops which allow for weed control at relative high frequencies throughout the growing season (see section 3).

Weed species	Monocotyledon, Dicotyledon	Annual (w/s), Biennial, Perennial	Crops in which the weed species mainly occur
Alopecurus myosuroides Huds.	Monocotyledon	Annual (w)	Autumn-sown annual crops
Apera spica-venti (L.) P. Beauv.	Monocotyledon	Annual (w)	Autumn-sown annual crops
Avena fatua L.	Monocotyledon	Annual (s)	Spring-sown annual crops
Capsella bursa-pastoris (L.) Medik.	Dicotyledon	Annual/biennial	Autumn-sown annual crops
Chenopodium album L.	Dicotyledon	Annual (s)	Spring-sown annual crops
Cirsium arvense (L.) Scop.	Dicotyledon	Perennial	Both annual and perennial crops
Convolvulus arvensis L.	Dicotyledon	Perennial	Both annual and perennial crops
Elytrigia repens (L.) Desv. ex Nevski	Monocotyledon	Perennial	Both annual and perennial crops
Erysimum cheiranthoides L.	Dicotyledon	Annual (w)	Annual crops
Fallopia convolvulus (L.) A. Löve	Dicotyledon	Annual (s)	Spring-sown annual crops
Fumaria officinalis L.	Dicotyledon	Annual (s)	Spring-sown annual crops
Galeopsis spp. L.	Dicotyledon	Annual (s)	Spring-sown annual crops
Galium aparine L.	Dicotyledon	Annual (w)	Autumn-sown annual crops
Lamium L.	Dicotyledon	Annual (w)	Annual crops
Lapsana communis L.	Dicotyledon	Annual (w)	Annual crops
Myosotis arvensis (L.) Hill	Dicotyledon	Annual (w)	Annual crops
Persicaria lapathifolia (L.) Gray	Dicotyledon	Annual (s)	Spring-sown annual crops
Poa annua L.	Monocotyledon	Annual/biennial	All crops
Polygonum aviculare L.	Dicotyledon	Annual (s)	Spring-sown annual crops
Ranunculus repens L.	Dicotyledon	Perennial	Perennial crops, First year leys
Rumex crispus L., *Rumex longifolius* DC., and *Rumex obtusifolius* L.	Dicotyledon	Perennial	Perennial crops
Sinapis arvensis L.	Dicotyledon	Annual (s)	Spring-sown annual crops
Sonchus arvensis L. – Dicotyledon – Perennial – Annual crops.	Dicotyledon	Annual (s)	Spring-sown annual crops

Spergula arvensis L. – Dicotyledon – Annual (s) – Spring-sown annual crops.	Dicotyledon	Perennial	Annual crops
Stellaria media L.	Dicotyledon	Annual (w)	Annual crops
Taraxacum F.H. Wigg	Dicotyledon	Perennial	Perennial crops, First year leys
Tripleurospermum inodorum (L.) Sch. Bip	Dicotyledon	Annual (w)	Autumn-sown annual crops, first year leys
Tussilago farfara L.	Dicotyledon	Perennial	Perennial crops
Veronica arvensis L. *Veronica persica* Poir.	Dicotyledon	Annual (w)	Annual crops
Viola arvensis Murr.	Dicotyledon	Annual (w)	Annual crops

Table 1. Commonly occurring weed species in Scandinavia and Finland. w = winter annual, s = summer annual. (Hallgren, 2000; Salonen et al., 2001; Riesinger & Hyvönen, 2005; Andreasen & Stryhn, 2008; Andreasen, & Streibig, 2011).

3. Strategies for weed management

Most weed control strategies aim at changing and/or reducing the relative competitiveness of the weed species, thereby favouring growth and development of the crop in comparison with the weed flora (Zimdahl, 2004).

Weed control strategies may be categorized in different ways. Often used terminology is biological, chemical, cultural, direct, indirect, mechanical, non-chemical, physical, and/or preventive weed control methods (Centre for Organic Horticulture, 2011; Larimer County Weed District, 2011). Biological control may be defined as the use of living agents to suppress vigor and spread of weeds. Such agents can be insects, bacteria, fungi, or grazing animals such as sheep, goats, cattle or horses, and consequently, biological control always implies an interaction of weed plants with organisms from another trophic level. Chemical control includes the use of herbicides to suppress and kill the weeds while cultural control may be defined as the establishment of competitive and desired vegetation, which prevents or slows down invasion by weedy species and is a key component of successful weed management. Direct weed control includes methods that aim to damage and kill weeds by direct physical force, compared to indirect methods which indirectly influence the weed floras, such as the choice of crop rotation or crops. Examples of mechanical methods are stubble cultivation, weed harrowing and hoeing while non-chemical methods include all control methods except herbicide use. Mechanical and thermal technologies are included in physical methods while the term 'preventive method' usually is employed when trying to stop weed infestation from the neighborhood to newly disturbed ground.

Bond & Grundy (2001) describe two types of methods: cultural methods (including pre-crop and post-harvest soil cultivation, crop rotation, crop cultivar choice, crop establishment, and limiting the introduction and spread of weeds) and direct control methods (mechanical control, thermal control, mulching, biological control).

Hatcher & Melander (2003) separate weed control methods into physical, cultural and biological weed control, where physical control includes mechanical methods (weed harrowing and hoeing) and thermal methods like flaming. Cultural control includes for example intercropping, weed cutting and mowing, and biological methods include the use of biocontrol agents like insects, fungi, and bacteria.

Below we have chosen to describe weed control methods in two major groups: cultural methods and physical weed control methods.

3.1 Cultural methods

Cultural methods aim at establishing a strong and competitive crop and thereby reducing the ability for the weed flora to grow and develop in the field.

3.1.1 Weed – crop competition

Competition is an interaction between plants which require the same limited resources like nutrients, water and light. Harper (1977) defines competition as 'An interaction between individuals brought about by a shared requirement for a resource in limited supply and leading to a reduction in the survivorship, growth and/or reproduction of the individuals concerned', and thereby points to the effects of competition. The aim of weed control is to ensure that as much resources as possible are accessible for the crop and not for the weeds and to reduce or delay growth and development of the weed flora. This is a valid short term goal, but also a long term goal, achieved by a reduction in replenishment of the weed seed bank, and avoidance of further seed dispersal and vegetative reproduction.

To illustrate the effects of removing competitive weeds on the growth of crop plants, a greenhouse experiment was performed in Sweden 2011 (Lundkvist & Verwijst, unpublished data). Spring barley and Charlock (*Sinapis arvensis*) were grown together in mixtures, where *Sinapis arvensis* was considered to be the weed species and barley the crop. In each box, six crop and weed plants i.e. a total of 12 plants were sown on 15 April. As control, boxes with six and 12 barley plants were used. At 6 May, weed plants were removed from some of the boxes. The results showed that barley displayed a nearly linear increase in biomass over time, when grown together with white mustard (solid line, Fig. 1). Total dry weight of the six barley plants at 12 May was about 3.8 g, which is much lower than the total dry weight of the six and 12 barley plants of the same age grown in monocultures, having dry weights of 9.5 and >12 g, respectively. The simulated weeding, performed at 6 May by means of removing the six white mustard plants per box, caused the growth rate of the remaining barley plants to accelerate (dotted line, Fig. 1) and led to significantly higher total dry weights of the unrestricted barley plants, compared to those which were restricted by the weed. On average, the solid line displays a slope of 0.23, with 95% confidence limits of 0.184 - 0.273, while the hatched line has a slope of 0.68, with 95% confidence limits of 0.500 - 0.854. Consequently, unrestricted growth is faster compared to restricted growth, which illustrates the importance of weed removal in the field.

Relative emergence time also strongly influences the competitive outfall between crops and weeds. When crop plants emerge before the weeds, they may be able to acquire more of the limited resources available than the weed plants, which will give the crop a competitive advantage. In two outdoor box experiments in Uppsala, Sweden, in 2006 and 2007, the effects of relative emergence time were studied on spring barley and perennial sow-thistle (*Sonchus arvensis*) (Fig. 2) (Eckersten et al., 2010, 2011a, 2011b). When the crop emerged 4 days before the weed, the stand was totally dominated by the crop 2 weeks after crop emergence (90% of the total aboveground biomass consisted of crop biomass). The opposite occurred when the crop emerged 8 or 26 days later than the weed (50% and 10% of the total aboveground biomass consisted of crop biomass, respectively).

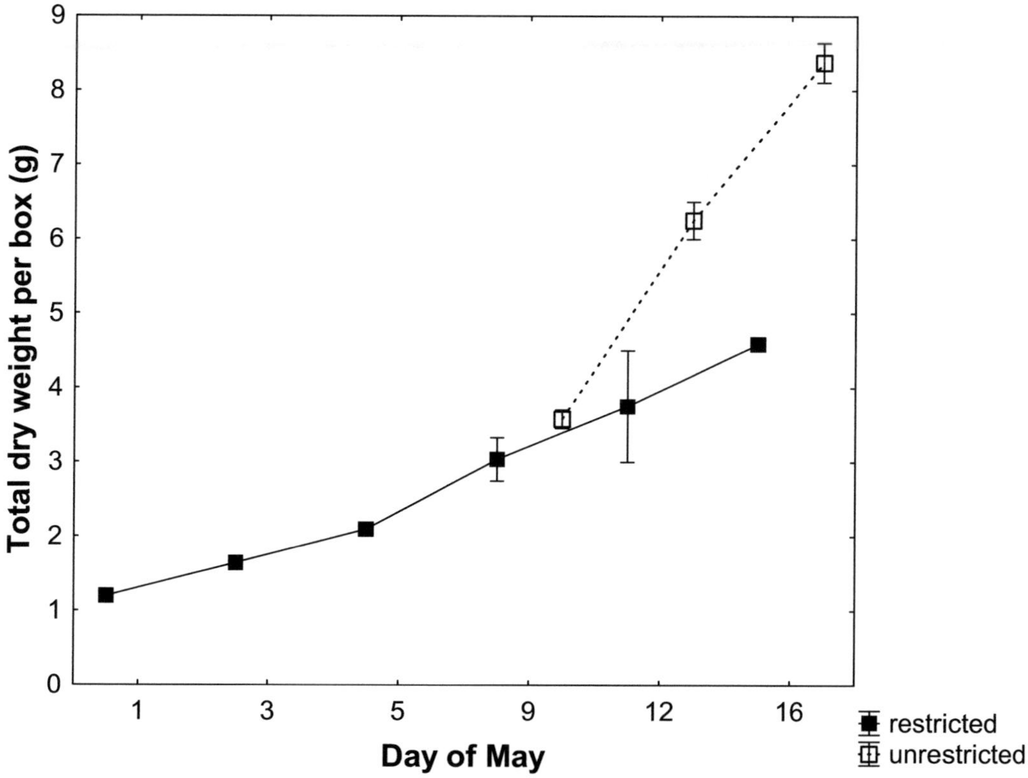

Fig. 1. Total dry weight of six barley plants per box over time. Growth was either restricted (six plants of white mustard were present over time) or unrestricted (the white mustard plants were removed on 6 May) (Lundkvist & Verwijst, unpublished data).

To assess the effects on *S. arvensis* competitive performance, its radiation and nitrogen (N) acquisition efficiencies and assimilate allocation were compared with spring barley at two N levels in the two outdoor box experiments mentioned above. First, shoot radiation use efficiency (RUE_{Shoot}) and nitrogen uptake efficiency (shoot uptake per soil mineral N per day; UPE) were estimated by calibrating a mechanistic model to above ground biomass and N observations (Eckersten et al., 2010). The RUE_{Shoot} was 44% lower whereas UPE was seven times higher in *S. arvensis,* than in barley. For *S. arvensis,* UPE was higher at the low N level than at high level, while the reverse was found for barley. Thereafter, it was tested whether the monoculture models could be applied to mixtures, assuming that intercepted radiation was partitioned between species proportional to their leaf area (Eckersten et al., 2011b). The mix-model was applicable to early stages, but underestimated shoot growth of both species grown in equal proportions, and overestimated *S. arvensis* shoot growth during late stages (415 -765 d°C after emergence). Conclusions were (i) that the growth of mixtures could be simulated as function of competition for radiation based on plant properties derived for monocultures, but needed additional modules for root/shoot biomass allocation, and (II) that the competitiveness of *S. arvensis* increased at low N supply due to a superior N acquisition efficiency compared to barley.

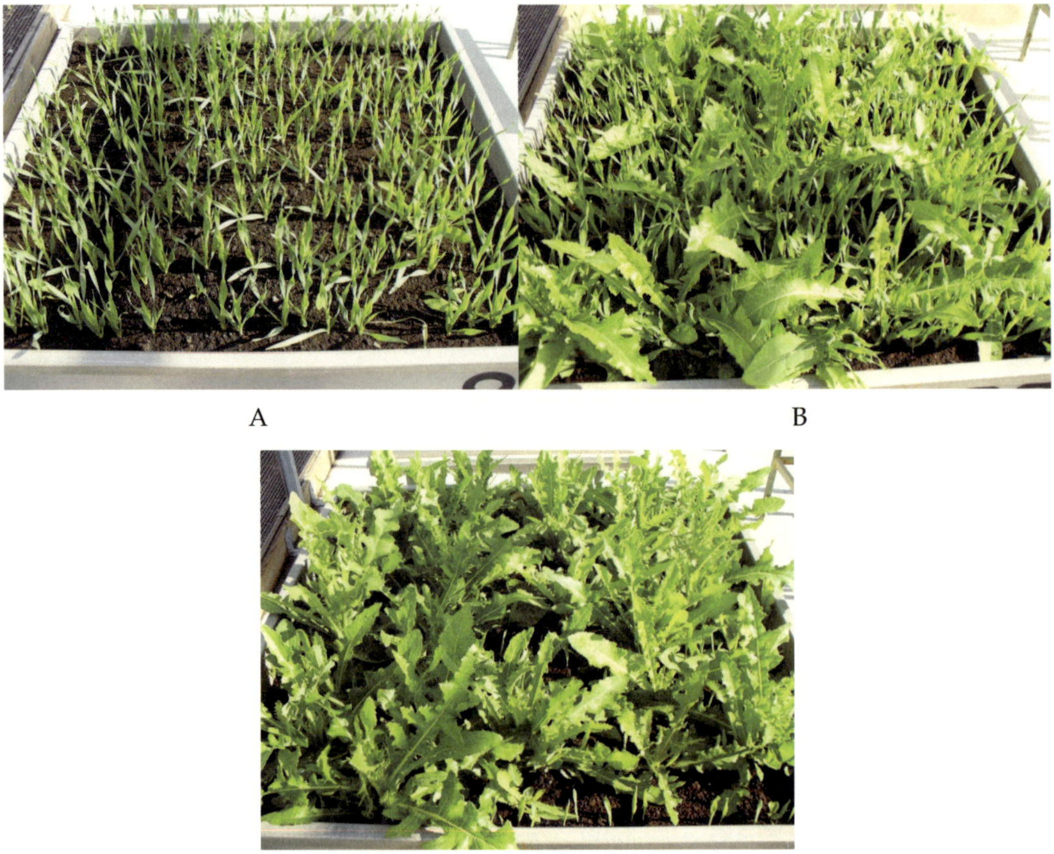

A B

C

Fig. 2. Effects of relative emergence time on growth and development of spring barley (*Hordeum distichon* L.) and perennial sow-thistle (*Sonchus arvensis*). A) Spring barley emerging 4 days before *S. arvensis*, B) Spring barley emerging 8 days after *S. arvensis*, and C) Spring barley emerging 26 days after *S. arvensis*. Photo: Anneli Lundkvist, 2007.

3.1.2 Crop and cultivar choice

The choice of crops and cultivars also is an important indirect weed control method. Different crops have different competitive abilities. In annual crops, cereals are considered to have the strongest competitive ability against weeds followed by oilseed rape, peas and potatoes/vegetables (Håkansson, 2003). Lundkvist et al. (2008) showed for example that peas, a weak competitor, had significantly higher weed biomass at harvest compared with oats and winter wheat. Autumn-sown cereals and oilseed rape also seem to have a stronger weed suppressing ability compared with corresponding spring-sown crops. Well established perennial leys or pastures are usually very competitive against weeds, while first year leys or pastures may be rather susceptible to weed competition. The relative competitive power is also affected by seed rate (relative plant density) and also time of sowing (relative emergence time) which affects the emergence of the crop in comparison with the weeds, see section 3.1.1.

Crop cultivars may differ in weed suppressing ability, and which cultivar the farmer chooses may also influence the biomass production of the crop. Important plant competition parameters seem to be early vigour and season growth, straw length, leaf area index, and rate of root system establishment (Drews et al., 2009; Olesen et al., 2004; Cousens et al., 2003; Gibson et al., 2003). Bertholdsson (2011) reported that the weed suppressing ability in wheat varieties depended mainly on early season crop growth and allelopathy, see section 3.1.4.

3.1.3 Crop rotations

The choice of crop rotation strongly affects the abundance and diversity of the weed flora (Bond & Grundy, 2001). Since different crops favour different types of weed species, it is important to change between annual and perennial crops in the crop rotation. Autumn- and spring-sown annual crops also favour different types of weed species, which makes it important to rotate between such crops within a crop rotation.

An example of organic crop rotations, well adapted to the farm situation, was reported by Lundkvist et al. (2008). To study the effects of organic farming on weed population development and crop yields, two different crop rotations were designed. One rotation was adapted for animals, containing perennial ley (six fields), and one without animals, including green manure (six fields) on an organic farm established in Central Sweden in 1987. Each field contained a fixed 1 m^2 reference plot in which all the weed observations were done each year. During the period 1988-2002, number of weed plants in spring and weed biomass at harvest were recorded in the reference plots. No differences in these two parameters were observed between the crop rotations. Number of weed plants in spring did not differ between annual crops and did not increase over the 15-year period. Neither did weed biomass at harvest nor weed species diversity change over the 15 years. The two crop rotations kept weed pressure at the same level as under the previous conventional farming practice. General observations in the field suggested that invasion of *Cirsium arvense* was occurring along the field borders. Competitive ability of the crops showed to be important in weed regulation. They concluded that to improve weed management in organic farming, advisors and farmers should recognize the importance of individual field and farm analyses to design location-specific, farm-adapted crop rotations.

To study the effects of different crop rotations on the performance of the perennial weeds *S. arvensis* and *C. arvense,* a field experimental study was performed in Central Sweden (Lundkvist et al., 2011b). The overall hypothesis was that biomass production of the two weed species would decrease with competition from a crop. The development of *S. arvensis* and *C. arvense* under crop competition was assessed during 2005-2009 by means of two field experiments, which each included five crop rotations (two rotations with annual crops only, and three with a sequence of both annual crops and perennial grass-clover ley), and two cultivation techniques. Statistical analyses showed that at the end of the crop rotations with perennial leys, the weeds were effectively suppressed (71-98%, P=0.001) and the cereal yields were higher (51-70%, P=0.001) compared with crop rotations with annual crops only (Fig. 3). The results showed that the weeds can be controlled effectively under Nordic conditions by using crop rotations including competitive perennial ley crops.

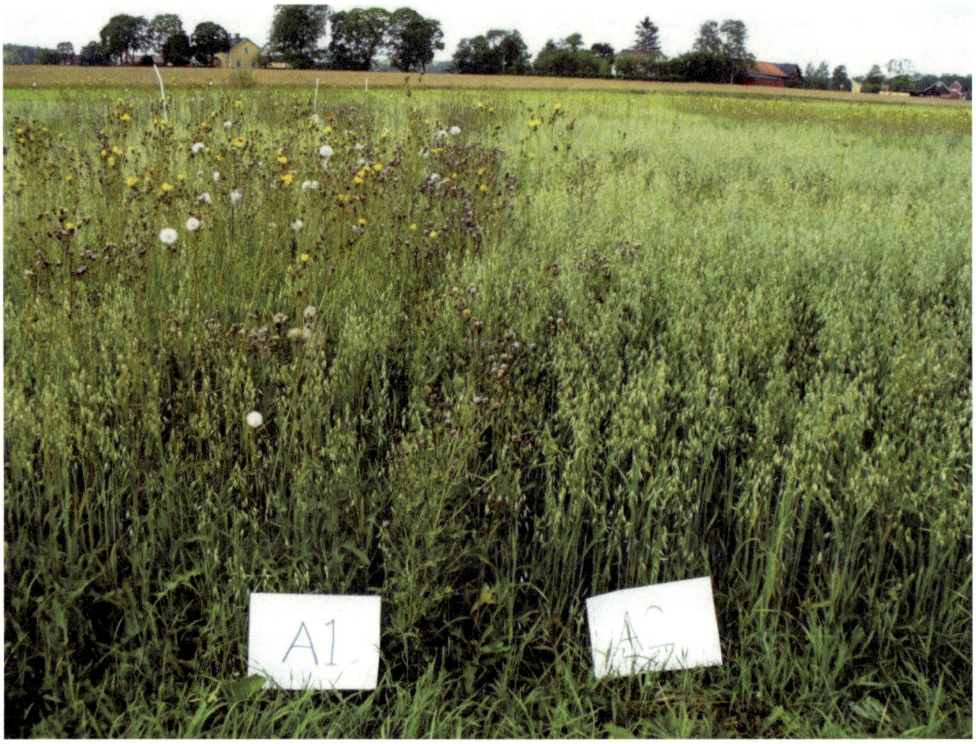

A B

Fig. 3. Occurrence of the perennial weed species *Sonchus arvensis* and *Cirsium arvense* in two different crop rotations in central Sweden 2005-2009. A) Crop rotation with annual crops only, showing a high abundance of the two weed species. B) Crop rotation including both annual crops and perennial leys, with low abundance of the two perennial weeds. Photo: Anneli Lundkvist, 2009.

3.1.4 Allelopathy

Rice (1984) defined allelopathy as the effect(s) of one plant on other plants through the release of chemical compounds in the environment, and this definition is largely accepted and includes both positive (growth promoting) and negative (growth inhibiting) effects. Muller (1969) and Olofsdotter et al. (2002) considered allelopathy as the effect of chemical interactions between plants and described competition as the removal of shared resources. Studies with the aim to find crop cultivars containing allelopathic compounds for improving weed suppressing ability have been performed and are ongoing (Olofsdotter et al., 2002; Bertholdsson, 2011) but thus far, the uptake of allelopathic traits in breeding programs has been slow and no typical allelopathic crop cultivars are available on the market at the moment (Kruse et al., 2000).

3.1.5 Biological control

Biological control methods aim at suppressing growth and development of weeds by using living agents like insects, bacteria, or fungi. Grazing animals like sheep, goats, cattle or horses may also be looked upon as 'tools' for biological weed control. Natural enemies may be used to reduce the abundance of certain weed species. Many studies have for example been performed with regard to the control of *C. arvense* with rust pathogens (Guske et al., 2004; Müller et al., 2011). To be successful in the long term, small numbers of the weed host must always be present to assure the survival of the natural enemy. One of the most successful examples of biological weed control is the control of St. Johnswort (*Hypericum perforatum* L.) on rangeland in the USA and Canada, by means of the leaf beetle *Chrysolina hyperici* Forster (Harris et al., 1969). Morrison et al. (1998) showed that part of this success may be attributed to the fungus *Colletotrichum gloeosporioides* Penz., which is transferred by the leaf beetle. Thus far, few weed species can be controlled effectively by weed species specific pathogens, but there are good opportunities for classical biological control of weeds to be developed for Europe as well (Sheppard et al., 2006).

3.2 Physical weed control methods

Physical weed control aims at directly suppressing/removing weed plants in the field to enhance the competitiveness of the crop. Physical control methods include both mechanical and thermal weed management. Regarding mechanical weed control, weeds are affected by tillage and soil cultivation in different ways: i) growing weeds and perennating organs are uprooted, dismembered, and buried, ii) the soil environment becomes changed in such a way that germination and establishment of weeds is promoted, and iii) weed seeds are moved vertically and horizontally which will affect the emergence, survival and competition of the weeds (Mohler, 2001). In Table 2, weed control effects of different physical control methods are summarized and below, the weed management methods are briefly discussed.

Implement	Positive weed control effect	Negative weed control effect
Plough	Disrupts growth and seed production. Buries seeds produced this year and buries perennial weeds and their below ground root/stem systems.	Weed seeds from the seed bank are moved up to the soil surface.
Cultivator/Disc cultivator	Disrupts weed growth and seed production. Buries seeds produced this year and buries /fragments perennial weeds and their underground root/stem systems.	May stimulate shoot development from below ground root/stem systems of perennial weeds.
Harrow	Destroys/kills small weed plants. Fragmenting root/stem parts of perennial weeds near the soil surface.	Stimulates weed seed germination. May spread viable root/stem parts of perennial weeds.
Roller	Improves germination conditions for the crop.	Improves germination conditions for the weed seeds.
Weed harrow	Covers small weed plants with soil and/or uproots them.	Stimulates weed seed germination. May more or less damage the crop.
Inter-row cultivator	Covers small weed plants with soil, uproots them or cuts them off.	May damage the crop.
Brush weeder	Covers small weed plants with soil or uproots them.	May damage the crop.
Weed mower	Cuts of weeds in growing crops.	If used after stem elongation, the crop will be damaged.

Table 2. Weed control effects of different types of tillage implements (after Lundkvist & Fogelfors, 2004).

3.2.1 Stubble cultivation

Stubble cultivation gives good control effects against perennial weeds by fragmenting their root systems (Håkansson, 2003) (Table 2). Development of new shoots is then triggered, which may deplete the carbohydrate stores of roots and rhizomes. Annual weeds also are controlled by stubble cultivation, causing disruption of their growth and seed setting. In Sweden, stubble cultivation is usually performed in the autumn after harvest, by using cultivators/disc cultivators, and the soil is often cultivated down to 10-15 cm (Lundkvist & Fogelfors, 2004).

To simulate different intensities of stubble cultivation and to assess the effects of different intensities of root fragmentation (5, 10 and 20 cm) on *Sonchus arvensis* on sprouting and shoot development, an outdoor box experiment was performed in Sweden in 2008 (Anbari et al., 2011). Shoot emergence time, shoot numbers, rosette size, and flower production were quantified as functions of root length and weight. Emergence of the first shoot per root and of later cohorts was delayed with decreasing root length and weight (Fig. 4). Number of shoots per root increased with root length and weight, but per unit root length and weight, short roots produced more shoots. The first emerging rosettes were, for rosettes of a given age, larger for longer roots, and total rosette area per root five weeks after planting increased with increasing root length and weight. The number of flowers and production of mature seeds were positively related to root length and weight, due to delayed sprouting of

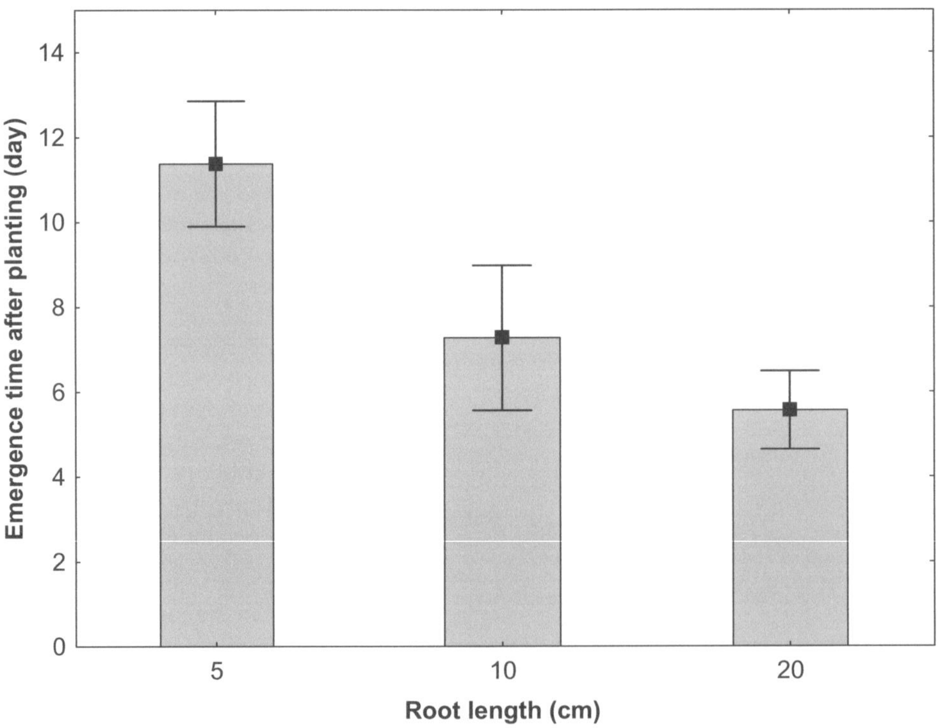

Fig. 4. Emergence time after planting (days) of the first shoot from *S. arvensis* roots of three length classes (5, 10, and 20 cm). Whiskers indicate 95% confidence interval (Anbari et al., 2011).

short and light roots. The proportion of flowers leading to mature seeds declined with shoot emergence time. By clarifying relationships between root size and growth parameters, this study showed that fractionating of *S. arvensis* roots delayed phenological development and hampered reproduction by seeds. The information may be used to refine mechanical weed control strategies for *S. arvensis*.

When farmers have large problems with perennial weeds in a field, fallow may be an interesting weed control method. During the fallow period, no crop is cultivated and soil cultivation is performed regularly. Fallow may be used during the whole growing season or parts of the season, combined with a crop grown before or after the fallow. Lundkvist et al. (2011b) studied the effects of short fallow on the performance of *S. arvensis* by means of field trials in Central Sweden. The overall hypothesis was that biomass production of *S. arvensis* would decrease with competition from a crop and with mechanical disturbance. To study the effects of short fallow in the spring, combined with competition of green manure crops, three field experiments were performed during 2005-2007, using short fallow techniques together with summer fallow and three green manure crops. Statistical analyses were done by ANOVA and comparisons were made by Student *t*-test. In the short fallow experiments the amount of *S. arvensis* was lower (75-93%; P=0.001) and the crop yields were higher (47-145%, P=0.001) in plots during the year after employment of short fallow together with green manure, compared with the control plots. Summer fallow was the most efficient method, followed by a combination of spring ploughing and disc harrowing. The results showed that *S. arvensis* can be controlled effectively under Nordic conditions by using short fallow.

3.2.2 Ploughing

Ploughing controls both annual and perennial weeds effectively (Table 2) (Lundkvist & Fogelfors, 2004). Perennial weed roots and/or belowground stem parts are cut off and buried in the soil. Since the plant parts are buried rather deep, shoots developing from those roots/stems usually have problems reaching the soil surface. Also annual weeds are efficiently controlled since the plants are buried in the soil, thereby interrupting their seed production. However, weed seeds from the seed bank will be moved up to the soil surface, and may eventually germinate and develop into new weed plants.

Early ploughing in the autumn is effective against annual weeds with late maturing seeds, and also against perennial weeds, since it stops their carbon assimilation and allocation of resources from shoots to storage organs. Late ploughing favours both perennial and annual weeds. Spring ploughing (which is often used on soils containing silt or fine sand) is also effective against perennial weeds like *C. arvense*.

3.2.3 Harrowing and seed bed preparation

In autumn, harrowing and seed bed preparation stimulate winter annual weed seeds to germinate while they stimulate both winter and summer annuals to germinate in spring (Table 2) (Håkansson, 2003). However, at the same time, weed plants that germinated early in the spring may be killed during sowing. During seed bed preparation, one aim is to avoid germination of weed seeds. Therefore, preparing a proper seed-bed implies killing of already emerged weeds, while applying as little soil cultivation as possible. Thereafter, sowing should take place as soon as possible to obtain an early crop establishment, thereby giving the crop and competitive advantage over the weeds.

3.2.4 Weed harrowing

The purpose of weed harrowing is to give crops a competitive advantage over weeds (Melander & Hartwig, 1995). Weed harrowing covers weeds and can kill weeds by uprooting them (Habel, 1954; Kees, 1962; Koch, 1964; Kurstjens & Kropff, 2001; Kurstjens et al., 2004). During harrowing, crop plants are sometimes covered with soil but often to a lesser extent than the weeds, and the crop usually recovers more quickly and out-grows the weeds before they have recovered from the harrowing (Bond & Grundy, 2001). Smaller weeds are easier to control via harrowing. Under favourable conditions, weed harrowing may provide similar efficacy as herbicides but usually the control effects from harrowing are lower than those which can be achieved with chemical control. Efficacy of harrowing depends on many factors including crop species and weeds present, the development stages of crop and weeds, weather, soil type and harrow type (Cirujeda et al., 2003; Hansen et al., 2007; Jensen et al., 2004; Rydberg, 1994). Weed harrowing may be divided into two categories; pre-emergence harrowing, and post-emergence harrowing. Pre-emergence harrowing (pre-wh) occurs after the crop is sown but before it emerges. This can be an effective control for early emerging weeds (Koch, 1959; Melander & Hartwig, 1995; Rasmussen, 1996) like *Sinapis arvensis*, *Galeopsis* spp., *Raphanus raphanistrum* L., and volunteers including *Brassica napus* L. Pre-wh may stimulate the germination of some weed species which can increase weed pressure (Kees, 1962). Post-emergence harrowing (post-wh) occurs after the crop has emerged and is challenging because both weeds and crop may be damaged by the harrow (Rasmussen et al., 2008) and the most sensitive development stage for mechanical disturbance often coincides for both the crop and the weeds.

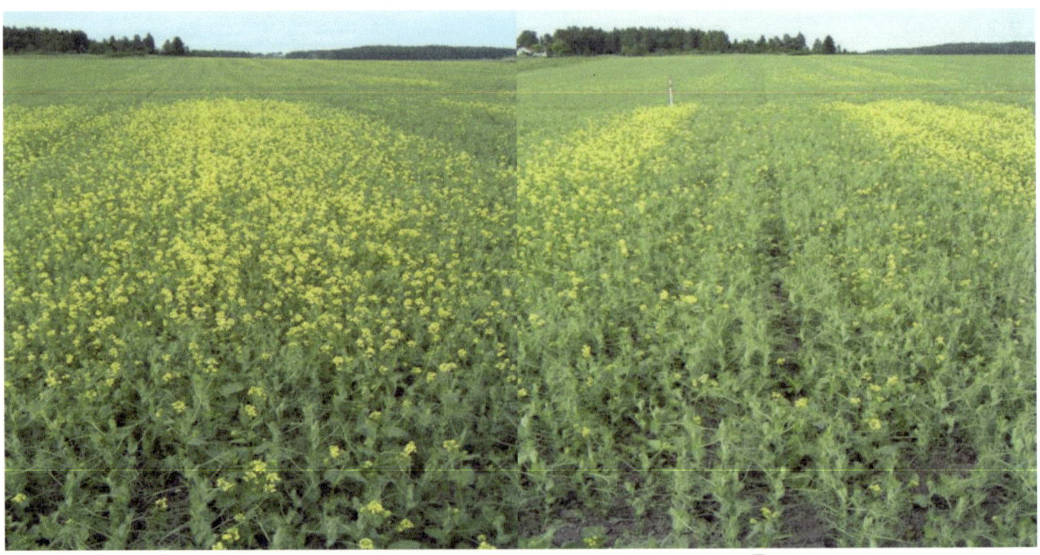

A B

Fig. 5. The weed control effect of pre-emergence weed harrowing four days after sowing against *Sinapis arvensis* (B) in peas in 2003 compared with the control plot (A) where no weed harrowing was performed (Lundkvist, 2009).

Given the increasing need for harrowing as a means of weed control and the lack of information on the effectiveness of the many combinations of pre-wh and post-wh treatments that are possible, particularly with respect to field sites in far northern Europe, a project was initiated to study the effects of different combinations of weed harrowing before and after crop emergence on weed control in field sites in Sweden (Lundkvist, 2009). The major hypotheses were (i) that combinations comprising both pre-wh and post-wh provide better weed control effect against annual weed infestations than treatments containing only pre-emergence harrowing, and (ii) that pre-emergence harrowing alone or in combination with post-emergence harrowing provides better control of early emerging weed species versus post-emergence harrowing alone. The results showed that a pre-emergence weed harrowing treatment alone or combined with weed harrowing shortly after crop emergence in peas and spring cereals is most effective against the early emerging weed species *S. arvensis* and *Galeopsis* spp. Post-emergence harrowing alone usually has low control effect on *S. arvensis* (Fig. 5, Table 3). The late emerging annual weed species *C. album* and *Polygonum lapathifolium* were most effectively controlled when pre-emergence weed harrowing was combined with one or two weed harrowing treatments after crop emergence. The best weed control was obtained by a combination of pre- and post-emergence harrowing, but these treatments also caused yield losses of 12-14% in spring cereals, while no yield losses were observed in peas (Lundkvist, 2009).

Treatment	En 2003 Peas	En 2004 Peas	Ua 2003 Peas	Ua 2004 Peas
Control (no weed harrowing)	120 (20)^{a}	747 (55)^{a}	133 (24)^{a}	158 (37)^{ab}
Early pre-wh (2-4 days after sowing)	21 (8)^{b}	656 (65)^{ab}	110 (35)^{a}	151 (18)^{abc}
Late pre-wh (6-8 days after sowing)	-	613 (257)^{b}	135 (24)^{a}	181 (22)^{ab}
Early + late pre-whs	-	571 (114)^{b}	137 (33)^{a}	184 (28)^{ab}
Early pre-wh + post-wh at crop growth stage DC 12-13	13 (1)^{bc}	607 (67)^{b}	59 (14)^{b}	115 (26)^{abc}
Late pre-wh + post-wh at crop growth stage DC 12-13	-	556 (60)^{b}	33 (6)^{bc}	93 (31)^{c}
Early pre-wh + post-whs, at crop growth stages DC 12-13 & DC 15-16	10 (1)^{c}	304 (101)^{c}	13 (3)^{cd}	-
Late pre-wh + post-whs, at crop growth stages DC 12-13 & DC 15-16	-	320 (141)^{c}	7 (3)^{d}	-
Post-wh at crop growth stage DC 12-13[1)]	100 (1)^{a}			
Post-wh at crop growth stage DC 15-16[1)]	120 (1)^{a}			
Post-whs at crop growth stages DC 12-13 & DC 15-16 [1)]	100 (1)^{a}			

Table 3. Total number of weed plants (m^{-2}) in the 4 field experiments with peas treated with different combinations of pre- (pre-wh) and post-weed harrowing (post-wh) at Enköping (En) and at Uppsala (Ua) in 2003-2004 (Lundkvist, 2009). Values indicate mean (SE) with n = 3. Mean in the same column with different superscript letters are significantly different ($P < 0.05$). [1)] Post-wh, without pre-wh, was performed in one experiment (En 2003, peas). (-) treatment not performed in the experiment.

3.2.5 Inter-row cultivators

Inter-row cultivators are designed to control weeds between the crop rows to a depth of 5-10 cm through soil coverage, uprooting or root cutting (see for example Mohler, 2001;

Melander et al., 2005). The method is most efficient against annual weeds but may also give some control effects on perennial weeds with a rather shallow underground root/stem system. Inter-row cultivation is usually carried out in row crops (i.e. crops like sugar beet, potatoes and maize grown with relatively large row spacing) but also used in small grain crops like cereals sown with a row spacing of 20-30 cm in organic farming.
To study the control effects of inter-row cultivation on *Sonchus arvensis*, three field experiments in oats were performed in central Sweden during 2006-2007 with an inter-row cultivator. The immediate control effect was rather good which is illustrated in Fig. 6. However, at the end of the season no significant effects were obtained on either weed biomass or crop yield probably due to a rather low soil nitrogen content which favoured the efficient nitrogen absorbing *S. arvensis* (Lundkvist et al., unpublished data).

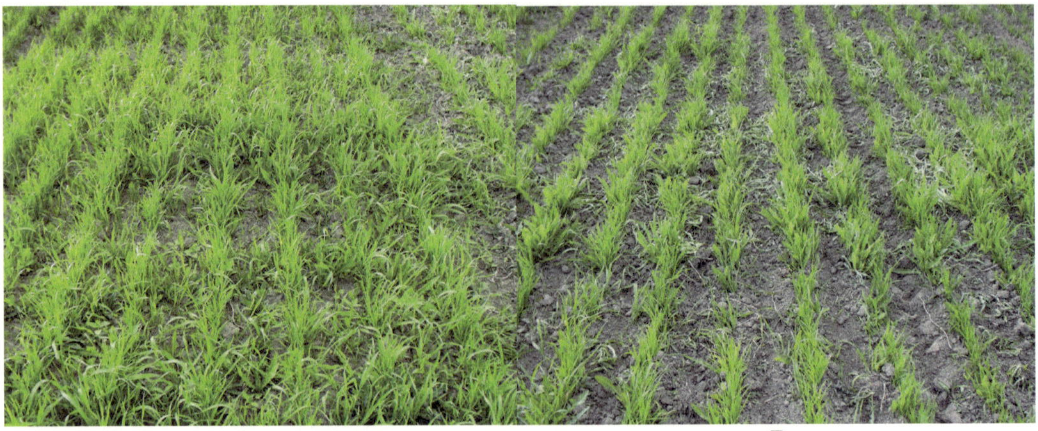

A B

Fig. 6. Effects of inter-row cultivation in oats with a large abundance of *Sonchus arvensis* in spring 2006. A) Control plot, B) Inter-row cultivation performed. Photo: Kurt Hansson.

3.2.6 Mowing

Mowing is a traditional weed control method by which growth and development of the weeds are disturbed by removing parts of their above ground biomass. Mowing is used in leys, near ditches and road verges and is often a rather efficient weed control method.
When mowing is combined with competition from a well established crop, proper weed control effects may be obtained (Graglia et al., 2006; Bicksler & Mausiunas, 2009). In Sweden, a selective weed mower 'CombCut' has been developed in such a way that it is possible to cut weed plants in a growing cereal crop without damaging the crop (http://www.jcs-innovation.se/enghem.html; Lundkvist et al., 2011a). CombCut combs through the field, down in the growing crop, cutting weeds which compete with the developing crop, while leaving the crop undamaged (Fig. 7). This is a novel weed control method since it is normally not possible to perform any type of mechanical weed control in cereals after crop emergence. Selective weed mowing is based on differences between the physical properties of crop and weed plants which - given a proper mowing timing, frequency and machine settings - can be used to control weeds in a growing crop without damaging the crop. Apart from counteracting vegetative weed biomass accumulation and competition with the crop, mowing may prevent weed seed formation, thereby preventing weed seed bank replenishment, and enhances the quality of seed crops.

The effects of the weed mower on weeds and crops are currently evaluated in an ongoing research project at SLU, Sweden (Lundkvist et al., 2011a). The hypotheses are that selective weed mowing (i) decreases the ability of the weeds to compete and reproduce in a crop, (ii) decreases the long term development of the weed populations, and (iii) increases the crop yields. To test these, we performed two field experiments and two outdoor pot experiments during 2008-2010 in Sweden. In the field experiments, the effects of selective mowing on *C. arvense* and spring wheat were determined by mowing at two different development stages of *C. arvense*. In pot experiment 1, effects of mowing two years in a sequence on *C. arvense* and spring barley were studied. In pot experiment 2, effects of different machine settings on spring barley were evaluated. Statistical analyses were done by ANOVA and comparisons were made by Student *t*-test. Preliminary results from the pot experiment 1 showed that growth of *C. arvense* was significantly reduced after mowing two years in a sequence (38-49%, P=0.001) compared with the control (Fig 8). When competition from spring barley was added, the reduction was even higher (66-79%, P=0.001). Also crop yields were significantly higher after mowing (76-94%, P=0.03) compared with the control (Fig 9). Machine settings had strong effects on the crop. A more aggressive setting caused stronger damage to the crop at later development stages. In the field experiments, no significant effects were obtained with regard to the crop yield due to large amounts of *C. arvense*. The results showed that selective mowing combined with crop competition seem to decrease the abundance of *C. arvense*.

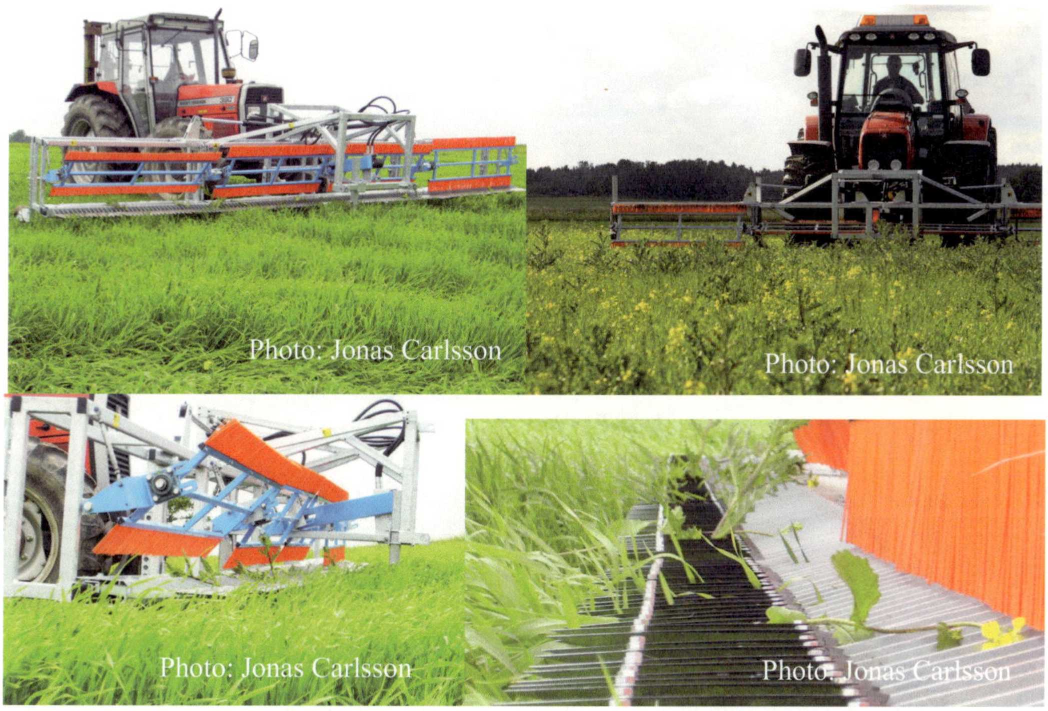

Fig. 7. Weed mower CombCut (upper left and right). Close up pictures of the brush reel (lower left) and the knives (lower right). Photo: Jonas Carlsson, JustCommonSence AB.

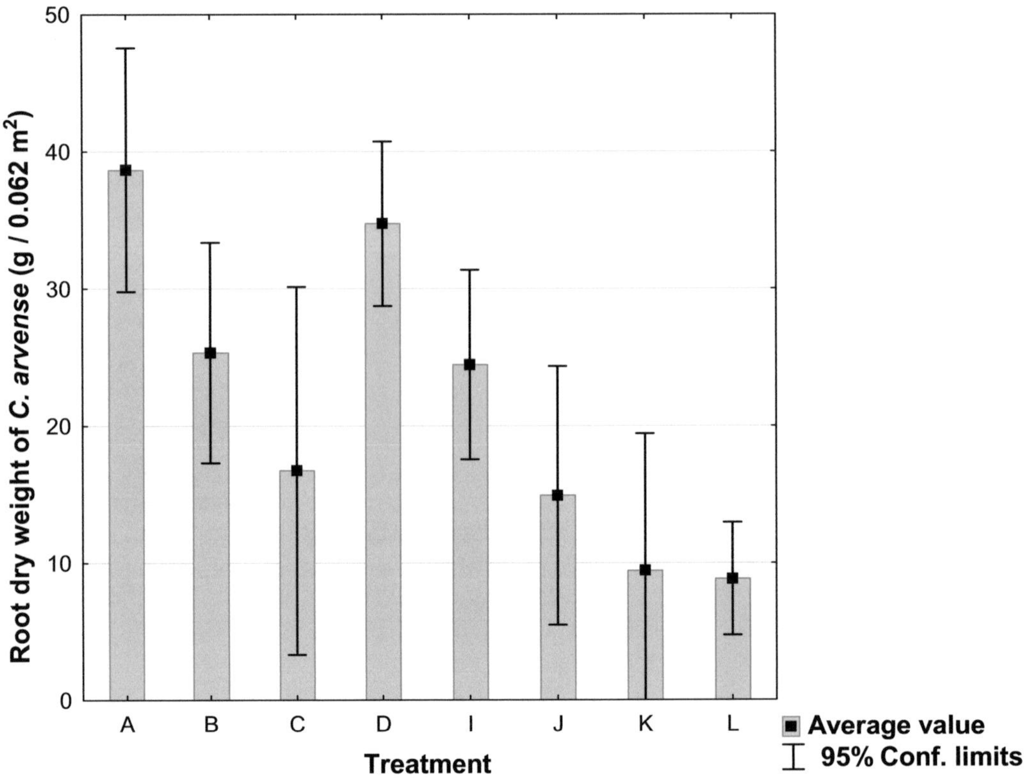

Fig. 8. Long term effects of selective mowing on *C. arvense* in pot experiment 1 in 2009

Root production of the weed (g/pot) in pots with *C. arvense* alone (A-D), and grown with spring barley (I-L). A, I = no mowing; B, J = early mowing; C, K = late mowing; D, L = early + late mowing; (Lundkvist et al. 2010).

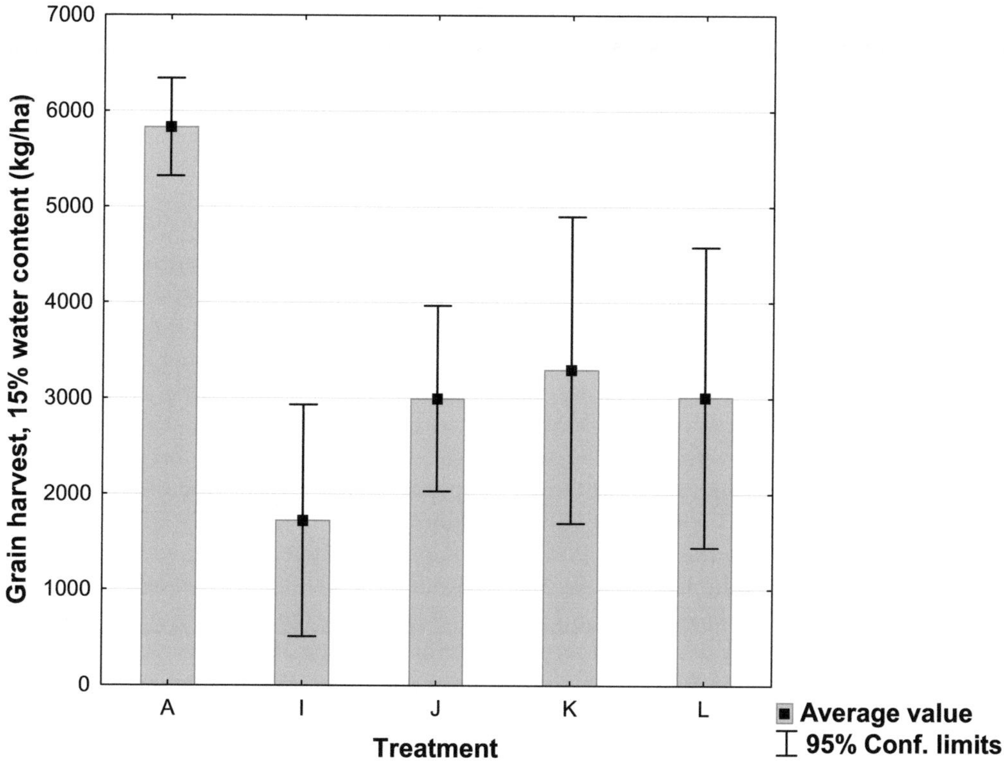

Fig. 9. Spring barley yield in pot experiment 1 in 2009.

A = spring barley, (without *C. arvense*), I = *C. arvense* + spring barley, no mowing, J = *C. arvense* + spring barley, early mowing, K = *C. arvense* + spring barley, late mowing, and L = *C. arvense* + spring barley, two mowings (Lundkvist et al., 2010).

3.2.7 Brush weeding

Brush weeding is used for controlling annual weeds through uprooting between and rather near the crop rows by using rotating brushes (see for example Mohler, 2001; Melander, 1997). This weed control method is mainly developed for post-emergence use in high-value vegetable crops, and further applications are restricted because of its low working capacity (Melander et al., 2005).

3.2.8 Ridging (potatoes and other row crops)

A ridger is a type of plough used to form ridges for covering the below ground parts of potatoes or other row crops, thereby protecting tubers from radiation and avoid greening. Ridging also works as a control method for annual weeds but also to some extent for perennial weed species by soil covering and/or up-rooting. The best control effect is obtained when the weeds are small, i.e. before they develop true leaves.

3.2.9 Flaming

When using flaming, weeds are briefly exposed to a propane or butane flame at 800-1000°C. The cell membranes are then disrupted and dehydration is rapidly occurring (Ascard 1995;

Ellwanger et al., 1973). This weed control method has a low working capacity and is mainly used against annual weeds before crop emergence in row crops such as onions, carrots, and sugar beets. Flaming may also be used after crop emergence (so-called selective flaming) when the crop plants have a protected terminal bud, like for example in cabbage (Holmøj & Netland, 1994).

4. Weed management strategies under climate change

A changing environment (either directional or with regard to parameter amplitudes) puts a selective pressure on plant species, and weeds are likely to be faster in adapting to changing environmental conditions represented by climate change than crops (e.g. Franks et al., 2007), due to their broader genetic variability. Altering crops to match changing environmental conditions is then one way to go, by means of devising appropriate crop breeding programmes which envisage climate change related to alterations of the environment. The geographic range of plant species is constrained by climatic limits, and changes in climate consequently will lead to alterations in the geographic distributions of weed species. For the temperate part of Europe, for example, a rise in temperature is favouring species from the Mediterranean region (Walther et al., 2002), and consequently, efforts have to be made to control invasive species (Sheppard et al., 2006). Ziska & Dukes (2011) recently published a book under the title "Weed biology and climate change" in which the major focus is on direct effects of elevated CO_2-levels on weed performance. Such effects have been proven to exist and have been quantified, including their interactions with plant water use and nitrogen uptake (e.g. Cotrufo et al., 1998; Poorter et al., 1996), However, from an agronomic point of view, not the direct effects of CO_2 on plant performance, but the globally changing precipitation and temperature patterns are the main causes of huge yield losses, and of changes in crop production systems and weed species distribution patterns.

While climate change already has been causing a number of catastrophic crop failures in many places of the world, the effects of a changing climate on crop production are expected to be less severe in the Northern parts of Europe. A significant climate warming is already occurring in Sweden (SMHI, 2006), and evaluation of existing climate scenarios (Eckersten et al., 2008) showed that a raise in air temperature by 4°C might be attained by the end of this century for the southern and middle parts of Sweden, and that an increase in growing season length is likely to occur due to an earlier temperature rise during spring. The actually monitored and for the future envisaged temperature rise will provide an enlarged time period to control annual and perennial weeds prior to sowing crops. A longer and warmer growing season also will lead to opportunities to grow other crops, including some that are commonly grown in rows. One such example is maize, of which the cultivation area in Sweden was increased with one order of magnitude only during the last decade. Due to shorter winters and longer vegetation periods, an increase of autumn sown crops also is envisaged in the Nordic countries. As outlined in section 2, specific cropping systems go along with a fairly specific weed flora, and consequently, choosing cropping systems in accordance with an increasing length of the vegetation period will bring about changes in the weed flora on the long run, favouring annual winter weeds in the Nordic situation. Frost-intolerant weed species may also be expected to shift their ranges further northwards with milder seasons, while milder seasons also provide opportunities for growing crops which under harsher conditions would be damaged.

In the context of climate change, the differences in photosynthetic pathways displayed by C_3 and C_4 plants may affect the competitive outcome between C_3 crops and C_4 weeds. An overall increase in atmospheric CO_2 would favour the C_3 crop over the C_4 weed, while an increasing temperature or reduced water availability would favour the C_4 weed. However, at Nordic latitudes, the growing season is characterised by long days, while most C_4 plants are short-day plants. This means that C_4 weeds will only flower if exposed to less than 12 hours of light per day, and consequently, are not likely to reproduce vigorously in a Nordic environment.

5. Conclusion

There are no simple standard solutions available for weed control in organic agriculture. While a conventional farmer may rely on herbicides, which can be applied with short notice to cure a field from an ongoing weed infestation, the organic farmer needs to take a long-term perspective while taking preventive measures to avoid yield losses. Direct and cultural methods need to be integrated in organic farming, with the long term goal to prevent the occurrence of weed-induced yield losses, while keeping down costs for weed control.
As certain crops do favour specific weed species, it is important to implement a crop rotation which suppresses the weed populations that have been expanding during a former cropping season. A proper crop rotation adapted to the actual farm situation is the core of organic farming. Early identification of an upcoming weed problem is necessary, and a wide range of control measures may be combined to keep weed populations at an acceptable level. Whatever crop is employed, soil bed preparation and management should be directed towards a rapid establishment and a maximum competitive ability of the particular crop under cultivation. Direct control measures need to be employed against weeds as early as possible, to prevent weeds from competing with a crop, but also in a later phase, to prevent weeds from replenishing the seed bank. Perennial weeds preferably should be prevented from establishment, but if they occur in fields, revising a planned crop rotation by, for example, employing a perennial ley, may contribute to a long-term solution.
Ongoing climate change in Nordic countries not only poses a threat to organic farming by means of favouring new and possibly invasive weeds. It also provides opportunities for prolonged weed control and use of new crops. Given the ongoing extension of the knowledge base for organic farming, the growing commitment of farmers devoted to organic farming, and national and European policies with clearly defined environmental goals, organic farming in the Nordic countries is well provided to meet its future challenges.

6. Acknowledgement

We kindly acknowledge the financial support from The Swedish Research Council for Environment, Agricultural Sciences and Spatial Planning, Stockholm, Sweden; Swedish University of Agricultural Sciences (SLU), and SLU EkoForsk, Uppsala, Sweden. We also want to thank Bengt Torssell, Henrik Eckersten, Johannes Forkman, Saghi Anbari, Håkan Fogelfors, Kurt Hansson, Jonas Carlsson, Tomas Svensson, Hugo Westlin, and Lars Ericson, for positive and constructive co-operations in many different ways during the years. Thanks also to Lennart Karlsson and Richard Childs for practical help and also to Martin Andersson, Astrid Adelsköld, Hanna Dahlén, Ingrid Persson, Ida Verwijst, Johanna Verwijst, Christine Kjällman, Lovisa Fogelfors, Stina Walde, Tove Landerstedt, Victoria

Stephien, and all the other skilled and hard working students that have helped us coping with all experiments through the years.

7. References

Anbari, S.; Lundkvist, A. & Verwijst, T. (2011). Sprouting and shoot development of *Sonchus arvensis* in relation to initial root size. *Weed Research*, Vol. 51, No. 2, (April 2011), pp. 142–150, ISSN 0043-1737.

Andreasen, C. & Streibig, C. (2011). Evaluation of changes in weed flora in arable fields of Nordic countries - based on Danish long-term surveys. *Weed Research*, Vol. 51, No. 3, (June 2011), 214-226, ISSN 0043-1737.

Andreasen, C. & Stryhn H. (2008). Increasing weed flora in Danish arable fields and its importance for biodiversity. *Weed Research*, Vol. 48, No. 1, (January 2008), pp. 1-9. ISSN 0043-1737.

Ascard, J. (1995). Effects of flame weeding on weed species at different developmental stages. *Weed Research*, Vol. 35, No. 5, (October 1995), pp. 397-411, ISSN 0043-1737.

Barberi, P. (2002). Weed management in organic farming: are we addressing the right issues? *Weed Research*, Vol.42, No. 3, (June 2002), pp. 177–193, ISSN 0043-1737.

Bastiaans, L.; Paolini, R. & Baumann, D. T. (2008). Focus on ecological weed management: what is hindering adoption? *Weed Research*, Vol. 48, No, 6, (December 2008), pp. 481-491, ISSN 0043-1737.

Bertholdsson, N-O. (2011). Use of multivariate statistics to separate allelopathic and competitive factors influencing weed suppression ability in winter wheat. *Weed Research*, Vol. 51, No. 3, (June 2011), pp. 273-283, ISSN 0043-1737.

Bicksler, A. J. & Masiunas, J. B. (2009). Canada thistle (*Cirsium arvense*) suppression with buckwheat or sudangrass and mowing. *Weed Technology*, Vol. 23, No. 4, (Oct. - Dec. 2009), pp. 556-563. ISSN 0890-037X.

Bond, W. & Grundy, A. C. (2001). Non-chemical weed management in organic systems. *Weed Research*, Vol. 41, No. 5, (October 2001), pp. 383-405, ISSN 0043-1737.

Burnside, O. C.; Wilson, R. G.; Weisber, S. & Hubbard, K. G. (1996). Seed Longevity of 41 Weed Species Buried 17 Years in Eastern and Western Nebraska. *Weed Science* 44, No. 1, (Jan. - Mar. 1996), pp. 74-86, ISSN 1550-2759.

Candrian, U.; Lüthy, J.; Schmid, P.; Schlatter, C. & Gallasz, E. (1984). Stability of pyrrolizidine alkaloids in hay and silage. *Journal of Agricultural and Food Chemistry*, Vol. 32, No. 4, (July 1984), pp. 935-937, ISSN 1520-5118.

Cavers, P. B. & Harper, J. L. (1964). Biological flora of the British Isles: *Rumex obtusifolius* L. and *Rumex crispus* L. *Journal of Ecology*, Vol. 52, No. 3, (Nov. 1964), pp. 737-766, ISSN 0022-0477.

Centre for Organic Horticulture, 2011. Organic Weed Management, In: *Centre for Organic Horticulture*. 20.07.2011. Available from <http://www.gardenorganic.org.uk/organicweeds/index.php>.

Cirujeda, A.; Melander, B.; Rasmussen, K. & Rasmussen, I. A. (2003). Relationship between speed, soil movement into the cereal row and intra-row weed control efficacy by weed harrowing. *Weed Research*, Vol. 43, No. 4, (August 2003), pp. 285-296, ISSN 0043-1737.

Cotrufo, M. F.; Ineson, P. & Scott, A. (1998). Elevated CO_2 reduces the nitrogen concentration of plant tissues. *Global Change Biology*, Vol. 4, No. 1, (January 1998), pp. 43-54, ISSN 1365-2486.

Cousens, R. D.; Barnett, A. G. & Barry G. C. (2003). Dynamics of competition between wheat and oat: 1. Effects of changing the timing of phenological events. *Agronomy Journal*, Vol. 95, No. 5, (September 2003), pp. 1293–1304, ISSN 1435-0645.

Defelice, M. S. (2003). The black nightshades, *Solanum nigrum* L. et al.—Poison, poultice, and pie. *Weed Technology*, Vol. 17, No. 2, (Apr 2003), pp. 421-427, ISSN 0890-037X.

Drews, S.; Neuhoff, D. & Köpke, U. (2009). Weed suppression ability of three winter wheat varieties at different row spacing under organic farming conditions. *Weed Research*, Vol. 49, No. 5, (October 2009), pp. 526-533, ISSN 0043-1737.

Eckersten. H.; Andersson, L.; Holstein, F.; Mannerstedt Fogelfors, B.;, Lewan, E.; Sigvald, R.; Torssell, B. & Karlsson, S. (2008). *An evaluation of climate change effects on crop production in Sweden*. Swedish University of Agricultural Sciences, Department of Crop Production Ecology, Report No 6, ISBN 978-91-576-7237-7, Uppsala, Sweden.

Eckersten, H.; Lundkvist, A. & Torssell, B. (2010). Comparison of monocultures of perennial sow-thistle and spring barley in estimated shoot radiation use and nitrogen uptake efficiencies. *Acta Agriculturae Scandinavica. Section B - Soil and Plant Science*, Vol. 60, No 2, (2010), pp.126-135, ISSN 0906-4710.

Eckersten, H.; Lundkvist, A.; Torssell, B. & Verwijst, T. (2011a). Effects of shoot radiation use and nitrogen uptake efficiencies on the competiveness of perennial sow-thistle (*Sonchus arvensis* L.), *Proceedings of 24th NJF Congress*, Food, Feed, Fuel and Fun - Nordic Light on Future Land Use and Rural Development, pp. 189, ISSN 1653-2015, Uppsala, Sweden. June 2011. 20.07.2011. Available from http://www.njf.nu/filebank/files/20110619$182028$fil$cyAOI5MQmtQWHa0Mh3Lh.pdf.

Eckersten, H.; Lundkvist, A.; Torssell, B. & Verwijst, T. (2011b). Modelling species competition in mixtures of perennial sow-thistle and spring barley based on shoot radiation use efficiency. *Acta Agriculturae Scandinavica. Section B - Soil and Plant Science*, DOI:10.1080/09064710.2011.555778, ISSN 1651-1913.

Ellwanger, T. C. Jr; Bingham, S. W. & Chapell, W. E. (1973). Physiological effects of ultra-high temperatures on corn. *Weed Science*, Vol. 21, No. 4, (Jul., 1973), pp. 296-299, ISSN 0043-1745.

FAO (Food and Agriculture Organization of the United Nations), (2011). The lurking menace of weeds. In: *Food and Agriculture Organization of the United Nations*. 20.07.2011. Available from: <http://www.fao.org/news/story/0/item/29402/icode/en/>.

Fogelfors, H. (2011). Weed Adviser for Farmers and Gardeners. In: *Swedish University of Agricultural Sciences*. 20.07.2011. Available from: <http://ograsradgivaren.slu.se/index.htm>.

Franks, S. J.; Sim, S. & Weis, A. E. (2007). Rapid evolution of flowering time by an anual plant in response to a climate fluctuation. *Proceedings of the National Academy of Sciences of the United States of America*, Vol. 104, No. 4, (January 2007), pp. 1278-1282, ISSN 1091-6490.

Gibson, K. D.; Fisher, A. J.; Foin, T. C. & Hill, J. E. (2003). Crop traits related to weed suppression in water-seeded rice (*Oryza sativa* L.). *Weed Science*, Vol. 51, No. 1, (Jan. - Feb. 2003), pp. 87-93, ISSN 0043-1745.

Graglia, E.; Melander, B. & Jensen, R. K. (2006). Mechanical and cultural strategies to control *Cirsium arvense* in organic arable cropping systems. *Weed Research*, No. 46, Vol. 4, (August 2006), pp. 304-312. ISSN 0043-1737.

Guske, S.; Schulz, B. & Boyle, C. (2004). Biocontrol options for *Cirsium arvense* with indigenous fungal pathogens. *Weed Research*, Vol. 44, No. 2 (April 2004), pp. 107-116. ISSN 0043-1737.

Habel, W. (1954). *Über die Wirkungsweise der Eggen gegen Samenunkräuter sowie die Empfindlichkeit der Unkrautarten und ihrer Alterstadien gegen den Eggvorgang*. Dissertation. Universität Hohenheim, Germany.

Hallgren, E. 2000. *Which weed species are most frequent and have the largest biomass proportions in different crops?* Rapporter från Fältforskningsenheten - Sveriges lantbruksuniversitet, Fältforskningsenheten, No 1, SLU, ISSN 1404-5974, Uppsala, Sweden.

Hansen, P. K.; Rasmussen, I. A.; Holst, N. & Andreasen, C. (2007). Tolerance of four spring barley (*Hordeum vulgare*) varieties to weed harrowing. *Weed Research*, Vol. 47, No.3, (June 2007), pp. 241-251, ISSN 0043-1737.

Harper, J. L. (1977). *Population Biology of Plants*. (1st edition), Academic Press Inc. Ltd, ISBN 0123258502, London, Great Britain.

Harris, P,; Peschken, D. & Milroy, J. (1969). The status of biological control of the weed *Hypericum perforatum* in British Columbia. *The Canadian Entomologist*, Vol. 101, No. 1, (January 1969), pp. 1-15, ISSN 0008-347X.

Hatcher, P. E. & Melander, B. (2003). Combining physical, cultural and biological methods: prospects for integrated non-chemical weed management strategies. *Weed Research*, Vol. 43, No. 5, (October 2003), pp. 303-322, ISSN 0043-1737.

Holm, L. G.; Plucknett, D. L.; Pancho, J. V. & Herberger, J. P. (1977). *The world's worst weeds: distribution and biology*. East-West Center/University Press of Hawaii, ISBN 0824802950, Hawaii, USA.

Holmøj, R. & Netland, J. (1994). Band spraying, selective flame weeding and hoeing in late white cabbage. In: *Acta Horticulturae 372 Symposium on Engineering as a Tool to reduce Pesticide Consumption and Operator Hazards in Horticulture*, Eds. R. Holmoy, N. Bjugstad, G. Redalen, K. Henriksen, H. Hagenvall, pp. 223-234. ISBN 978-90-66052-76-5, Ulvik, Norway.

Håkansson, S. (2003). *Weeds and Weed Management on Arable Land – An Ecological Approach* (first edition), CABI Publishing, ISBN 0-85199-651-5, Wallington, Oxon, UK.

Jensen, R. K.; Rasmussen, J. & Melander, B. (2004). Selectivity of weed harrowing in lupin. *Weed Research* , Vol. 44, No. 4, (August 2004), pp. 245-253, ISSN 0043-1737.

Kees, H. (1962). *Untersuchungen zur Unkrautbekämpfung durch Netzegge und Stoppelbearbeitungsmassnahmen*. Dissertation. Universität Stuttgart-Hohenheim, Germany.

Koch, W. (1959). *Untersuchungen zur Unkrautbekämpfung durch Saatpflege und Stoppelbearbetungsmassnahmen*. Dissertation. Universität Stuttgart-Hohenheim, Germany.

Kruse, M.; Strandberg, M. & Strandberg, B. (2000). *Ecological Effects of Allelopathic Plants – a Review*. National Environmental Research Institute, NERI Technical Report No. 315, ISBN 87-7772-540-9, Silkeborg, Denmark.

Kurstjens, D. A. G. & Kropff, M. J. (2001). The impact of uprooting and soil-covering on the effectiveness of weed harrowing. *Weed Research*, Vol. 41, No. 3, (June 2001), pp. 211-228, ISSN 0043-1737.

Kurstjens, D. A. G.; Kropff, M. J. & Perdok, U. D. (2004). Method for predicting selective uprooting by mechanical weeders from plant anchorage forces. *Weed Science*, Vol. 52, No. 1 (Jan. - Feb., 2004), pp. 123-132, ISSN 1550-2759.

Larimer County Weed District, (2011). Methods of weed control. In: *Larimer County Weed District*, 20.07.2011, Available from: < http://www.larimer.org/weeds/>.

Lemna, W. K. & Messersmith, C. G. (1990). The biology of Canadian weeds 94. *Sonchus arvensis* L. *Canadian Journal of Plant Science*, Vol. 70, No. 2, (April 1990), pp. 509-532, ISSN 0008-4220.

Lundkvist, A. (2009). Effects of pre- and post-emergence weed harrowing on annual weeds in peas and spring cereals. *Weed Research*, Vol. 49, No. 4, (August 2009), pp. 409-416, ISSN 0043-1737.

Lundkvist, A. & Fogelfors, H. (2004). *Ogräsreglering på åkermark (Weed Control on Arable Land)*. Department of Ecology and Crop Production Science, Swedish University of Agricultural Sciences, ISBN 1404-2339, Uppsala, Sweden.

Lundkvist, A.; Salomonsson, L.; Karlsson, L. & Dock-Gustavsson, A-M. (2008). Effects of organic farming on weed flora composition in a long term perspective. *European Journal of Agronomy*, Vol. 28, No. 4, (May 2008), pp. 570-578, ISSN 1161-0301.

Lundkvist, A.; Verwijst, T.; Westlin, H. & Carlsson, J. (2010). Utvärdering av tistelskärare 2008-2010. Slutredovisning. In: *Välkommen till SLU EkoForsk*, 20.07.2011. Available from: *<http://www.slu.se/sv/centrumbildningar-och-projekt/ekoforsk/projekt-2008-/tistel-2008/>*.

Lundkvist, A.; Verwijst, T. & Westlin, H. (2011a). Control effects on creeping thistle (*Cirsium arvense* (L.) Scop.) by selective mowing in spring cereals. *Proceedings of 24th NJF Congress, Food, Feed, Fuel and Fun – Nordic Light on Future Land Use and Rural Development*, p. 190, ISSN 1653-2015, Uppsala, Sweden. June 2011. 20.07.2011. Available from: http://www.njf.nu/filebank/files/20110619$182028$fil$cyAOI5MQmtQWHa0Mh3Lh.pdf.

Lundkvist, A.; Fogelfors, H.; Ericson, L. & Verwijst, T. (2011b). The effects of crop rotation and short fallow on the abundance of perennial sow-thistle (*Sonchus arvensis* L.). *Proceedings of 24th NJF Congress, Food, Feed, Fuel and Fun – Nordic Light on Future Land Use and Rural Development*, p. 76, ISSN 1653-2015, Uppsala, Sweden. June 2011. 20.07.2011. Available from: http://www.njf.nu/filebank/files/20110619$182028$fil$cyAOI5MQmtQWHa0Mh3Lh.pdf.

Lundkvist, A.; Verwijst, T.; Westlin, H. & Carlsson, J. (2011c). Weed cutter CombCut®, In: *Landtechnische Lösungen zur Unkrautregulierung im Ökolandbau*, Eds. B. Wilhelm & O.

Hensel, pp. 271-276, Universität Kassel, Fachgebiet Agrartechnik, Witzenhausen. In press.

Lüthy, J.; Zweifel, U.; Karlhuber, B. & Schlatter, C. (1981). Pyrrolizidine alkaloids of *Senecio alpinus* L. and their detection in feeding stuffs. *Journal of Agricultural and Food Chemistry*, Vol. 29, No. 2, (March 1981), pp. 302–305, ISSN 1520-5118.

Melander, B. (1997). Optimization of the adjustment of a vertical axis rotary brush weeder for intra-row weed control in row crops. *Journal of Agricultural Engineering Research*, Vol. 68, No 1, (September 1997), pp. 39–50. ISSN 0021-8634.

Melander, B.; Rasmussen, I. A. & Barberi, P. (2005). Integrating physical and cultural methods of weed control - examples from European research. *Weed Science*, Vol. 53, No. 3, (May - Jun. 2005), pp. 369-381, ISSN 1550-2759.

Mohler, C. L. (2001). Mechanical management of weeds, In: *Ecological Management of Agricultural Weeds*, Editors: Liebman, M; Mohler, C. L. & Staver, C.P, pp. 139-209, Cambridge University Press, ISBN 0-521-56068-3, Cambridge, UK.

Morrison, K. D.; Reekie, E. G. & Jensen, K. I. N. (1998). Biocontrol of common St. John'swort (*Hypericum perforatum*) with *Chrysolina hyperici* and a Host-Specific *Colletotrichum gloeosporioides. Weed Technology*, Vol. 12, No. 3, (Jul. - Sep. 1998), pp. 426-435, ISSN 0890-037X.

Moss, S. R. (2008). Weed research: is it delivering what it should? *Weed Research*, Vol. 48, No. 5, (October 2008), pp. 389-393, ISSN 0043-1737.

Muller, C. H. (1969). Allelopathy as a factor in ecological process. *Vegetatio*, Vol. 18, No 1/6 (1969), pp. 348-357, ISSN 0042-3106.

Müller, E.; Jud, P. & Nentwig, W. (2011). Artificial infection of *Cirsium arvense* with the rust pathogen *Puccinia punctiformis* by imitation of natural spore transfer by the weevil *Ceratapion onopordi. Weed Research*, Vol. 51, No. 3 (June 2011), pp. 209-213. ISSN 0043-1737.

Oerke, E-C. (2006). Crop losses to pests. *The Journal of Agricultural Science*, Vol. 144, No. 1, (Feb 2006), pp. 3-43, ISSN 0021-8596.

Olesen, J. E.; Hansen, P. K.; Berntsen, J. & Chirensen, S. (2004). Simulation of above-ground suppression of competing species and competition tolerance in winter wheat varieties. *Field Crops Research*, Vol. 89, No. 2-3, (Oct 2004), pp. 263-280, ISSN 0378-4290.

Olofsdotter, M.; Jensen, L. B. & Courtois, B. (2002). Review. Improving crop competitive ability using allelopathy - an example from rice. *Plant Breeding*, Vol. 121, No. 1, (February 2002), pp. 1-9, ISSN 0179-9541.

Oswald, A. K. & Hagger, R. J. (1983). The effects of *Rumex obtusifolius* on the seasonal yield of two mainly perennial ryegrass swards. *Grass and Forage Science*, Vol. 38, No. 3, (September 1983), 187-191, ISSN 1365-2494.

Palmer, J. H. & Sagar, G. R. (1963). *Agropyron Repens* (L.) Beauv. (*Triticum repens* L.; *Elytrigia repens* (L.) Nevski). *Journal of Ecology*, Vol. 51, No. 3 (Nov. 1963), pp. 783-794. ISSN 0022-0477.

Poorter, H.; Roumet, C. & Campbell, B. D. (1996). Interspecific variation in the growth response of plant to elevated CO_2: a research for functional types. In: *Carbon*

Dioxide, Populations, and Communities, Körner, C. & Bazzaz, F. A. (Eds.), pp. 375-412, Academic Press INC., ISBN 0-12-420870-3, San Diego, CA, USA.

Rao, V. S. (1999). *Principles of Weed Science*, (2nd edition), Science Publishers, ISBN 9781578080694, Enfield, New Hampshire, USA.

Rasmussen, J. (1996). Mechanical weed management. *Proceedings of Second International Weed Control Congress*, pp. 943-948, ISBN 87-984996-1-0, Copenhagen, Denmark, June 1996.

Rasmussen, J.; Bibby, B. M. & Schou, A. P. (2008). Investigating the selectivity of weed harrowing with new methods. *Weed Research*, Vol. 48, No. 6, (December 2008), pp. 523-532, ISSN 0043-1737.

Rice, E. L. (1984). *Allelopathy*, (2nd edition), Academic Press, ISBN 0125870558, Orlando, USA.

Riesinger, P. & Hyvönen, T. (2006). Weed occurrence in Finnish coastal regions: a survey of organically cropped spring cereals. *Agricultural and Food Science*, Vol. 15, No. 2, (2006), pp. 166-182, ISSN 1795-1895.

Rydberg, T. (1994). Weed harrowing – the influence of driving speed and driving direction on degree of soil covering and the growth of weed and crop plants. *Biological Agriculture and Horticulture*, Vol 10, No. 3, (1994), pp. 197–205. ISSN 0144-8765.

Salonen, J.; Hyvönen, T. & Jalli, H. (2001). Weeds in spring cereal fields in Finland – a third survey. *Agricultural and Food Science in Finland*, Vol. 10, No. 4, (2001), pp. 347-364, ISSN 1795-1895.

Sheppard, A. W.; Shaw, R. H. & Sforza, R. (2006). Top 20 environmental weeds for classical biological control in Europe: a review of opportunities, regulations and other barriers to adoption. *Weed Research*, Vol. 46, No. 2, (April 2006), pp. 93-117, ISSN 0043-1737.

SMHI (Swedish Meteorological and Hydrological Institute), (October 2006). Klimat i förändring – En jämförelse av temperatur och nederbörd 1991-2005 med 1961-90. In: *SMHI (Swedish Meteorological and Hydrological Institute)*, 20.07.2011, Available from: http://www.smhi.se/publikationer/klimat-i-forandring-1.6397.

Suter, M.; Siegrist-Maag, S.; Connely, J. & Lüscher, A. (2007). Can the occurrence of *Senecio jacobaea* be influenced by management practice? *Weed Research*, Vol. 47, No. 3, (June 2007), pp. 262-269, ISSN 0043-1737.

Sutherland, S. (2004). What makes a weed a weed: life history traits of native and exotic plants in the USA. *Oecologia*, Vol. 141, No. 1, (Sep. 2004), pp. 24-39, ISSN 0029-8549.

Walther, G-R.;, Post, E.; Convey, P.; Menzel, A.; Parmesan, C.; Beebee, T. J. C.; Fromentin, J-M.; Hoegh-Guldberg, O. & Bairlein, F. (2002). Ecological responses to recent climate change. *Nature*, Vol. 416, (March 2002), pp. 389-395, ISSN 0028-0836.

Weaver, S. E. & Riley, W. R. (1982). The Biology of Canadian Weeds. 53. *Convolvulus arvensis* L. *Canadian Journal of Plant Science*, Vol. 62, No. 2, (April 1982), pp. 461-472. ISSN 0008-4220.

Zaller J. G. (2004). Ecology and non-chemical control of *Rumex crispus* and *Rumex obtusifolius* (*Polygonaceae*): A review. *Weed Reseach*, Vol. 44, No. 6, (December 2004), pp. 414-432, ISSN 0043-1737.

Zimdahl, R. L. (2004). *Weed – Crop Competition. A review.* (2nd edition), Blackwell Publishing Ltd., ISBN 0813802792, Iowa, USA.

Ziska, L. H. & Dukes, J. S. (2011). *Weed Biology and Climate Change.* Blackwell Publishing Ltd., ISBN 978-0-8138-1417-9, Iowa, USA.